THE BRAIN AND BEHAVIOR
Assessing Cortical Dysfunction
Through Activities of Daily Living (ADL)

Guðrún Árnadóttir, MA, BMROT

Reykjavík City Hospital
Reykjavík, Iceland

with 108 illustrations

THE C. V. MOSBY COMPANY

St. Louis • Baltimore • Philadelphia • Toronto 1990

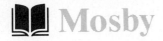

Editor Richard A. Weimer
Assistant Editor Adrianne Cochran
Production/editing CRACOM Corp.
Design Candace Conner

Printed in the United States of America

The C.V. Mosby Company
11830 Westline Industrial Drive, St. Louis, Missouri 63146

Library of Congress Cataloging-in-Publication Data

Árnadóttir, Guðrún, 1955-
    The brain and behavior: assessing cortical dysfunction through
activities of daily living (ADL)/Guðrún Árnadóttir.
      p.   cm.
    Includes bibliographical references.
    ISBN 0-8016-0334-X
    1. Brain damage—Diagnosis.   2. Clinical neuropsychology.
  3. Cerebral cortex—Diseases.   I. Title.
    [DNLM: 1. Activities of Daily Living.   2. Brain—physiopathology.
  3. Central Nervous System Diseases.   WL 300 A742b]
    RC387.5.A76   1990
    616.8′0475—dc20
    DNLM/DLC
    for Library of Congress   89-14581
                                            CIP

GW/D/D 9 8 7 6 5

To my mother

Foreword

In the emerging science of occupation, the importance of an interdisciplinary knowledge base cannot be overstated. At the same time, however, the key focus upon daily occupations, those familiar units of activity that define and give meaning to our life, must be maintained. The maintenance of an appropriate balance between knowledge from other fields and from within occupational science is most critical in the practice of occupational therapy. With increasing pressures to document our science base, we may easily shortcut the process of scientific development by accepting more familiar sciences as a practice base without using the core of occupation to choose the elements that we can uniquely provide as health professionals. It is this shortcut that we must avoid, for the full development of our science and our practice and for the greatest benefit to our patients.

The development of occupational science has been the vision of the University of Southern California Occupational Therapy Department for many years. Out of its rich traditions has come the constant effort to strengthen the professional practice of occupational therapy upon a science base. From the department's founder, Margaret Rood, through the conceptual leadership of Mary Reilly, the professional leadership of Florence Cromwell, and the research contributions of A. Jean Ayres, that goal was acknowledged. The process of academic recognition of occupational science as a field of doctoral study began under the guidance of Elizabeth Yerxa and has become a reality with the work of Florence Clark. Each of these and other leaders have contributed to a new stage of the development. In addition, these occupational therapists, theorists, and scientists have inspired others to participate in this monumental process. Colleagues and students, in particular, have been motivated to contribute to the growing understanding of occupation.

As a faculty member in the University of Southern California Department of Occupational Therapy, I have guided the work of many students in the research thesis process. For them and for me, it has been a professional growth process and an exciting intellectual process. When Guðrún Árnadóttir received the Fulbright Scholarship to study with us at USC, a very special process began. Guðrún brought her rehabilitation experience and knowledge base and began to combine it with the new ideas with which her course work involved her. Her guidance committee, of which I was the chair, included Dr. Yerxa, Dr. Clark, and Dr. Shirley Vulpe. Dr. Ayres acted as an expert reviewer of content during the instrument development process. Each contributed to the further development of a strong researcher, scientist, and clinician. The synthesis that resulted, however, belonged to Guðrún Árnadóttir alone.

The blend of neuro-psycho-occupational information in this book represents an ongoing development of concepts, methods, and attitudes that speak to the core of occupational science. The preliminary stages of development of the instrument, which measures performance of routine occupations such as dressing, yet reflects on the meaning of such performance in terms of the integrity of the neurological processes underlying such occupations is an exciting clinical and research challenge. Árnadóttir's OT-ADL Neurobehavioral Evaluation (A-ONE), in addition to its clinical usefulness, should provide a stimulus for continued study and further understanding of the complex phenomenon of human occupation. I am excited by this potential and feel sure that others will be too.

Ruth Zemke, PhD, OTR, FAOTA
Associate Professor, USC OT
May 1989

Preface

Lately, within the field of occupational therapy there has been a growing awareness of the importance of having occupational therapists evaluate patients with cognitive perceptual deficits in a way unique to this discipline, that is, with a functional emphasis. Traditionally, occupational therapists have used standardized procedures that evaluate independence in primary activities of daily living (ADL) separately from cognitive perceptual function. This is unfortunate, since the "traditional" cognitive perceptual evaluation includes items not oriented to the discipline of occupational therapy; that is, they do not focus on how or why such dysfunction interferes with daily activities. With this in mind, I combined theories of neurobehavior with principles of occupational therapy to develop an assessment tool that directly links functional performance in daily activities to neurobehavioral deficits: the Árnadóttir OT-ADL Neurobehavioral Evaluation (A-ONE). This book presents the A-ONE, indicating with examples how it can be used most effectively, and delineates the concepts on which it is based.

This book is intended for the practicing therapist as well as for students of occupational therapy. It provides guidance in evaluating cognitive perceptual dysfunction from a functional viewpoint, so that the effects of neurobehavioral deficits on task performance can be studied. The level of discussion is complex at times, based on the assumption that therapists and students who use this book have a knowledge of neuroanatomy, neuro-

physiology, neurology, occupational performance, activity analysis, and ADL. Throughout the text are tables that condense and simplify complex information. Illustrations are based on clinical situations encountered in actual cases.

Part I presents the background necessary for the development of a system for performing a neurobehavioral ADL evaluation. It reviews the literature on functional neuroanatomy, neurophysiology, and neurobehavior and relates it to observations of patients' neurobehavioral performance during ADL. The material presented is not intended to replace classic texts in neuroanatomy or neuropsychology or to serve as a historical overview of neurobehavioral deficits. Rather, it is intended to provide structured observation procedures that can aid occupational therapists in evaluating the functional level of patients with neurobehavioral dysfunction of cortical origin. The material has been simplified to provide a holistic picture of brain function, and specificity has therefore been sacrificed to a degree.

Chapter 1 outlines the main components of the occupational performance frame of reference, which include performance skills, including self-care activities, and performance components, including neurobehavioral concepts. Chapters 2 and 3, which review the gross anatomy and function of the cerebral hemispheres, define the terminology used in the remainder of the book in establishing the theoretical basis for the design of the A-ONE. Chapter 4 reviews a few of the studies used in tracing neuronal processing of the central nervous system during functional activities and touches on some proposed processing models. Chapter 5 discusses the causes of cortical CNS dysfunction, and Chapter 6 reviews a selection of other evaluation methods used with CNS-damaged patients. Chapter 7 provides examples of occupational performances in self-care, or primary ADL activities, from a neurobehavioral viewpoint. Thus it attempts to interpret neurobehavioral dysfunction in terms of functional performance observed during the self-care activities of patients suffering from CNS dysfunction. Chapter 8 discusses neurobehavioral impairment by focusing on processing deficits. Some considerations related to treatment of patients are also mentioned.

Part II presents the A-ONE and its manual. The A-ONE is an ADL tool that implements concepts from the discipline of occupational therapy and from current theory on neurobehavior to aid therapists in clinical reasoning and decision making. These concepts are defined in the glossary. Used properly, the A-ONE yields direct information regarding neurobehavioral deficits, how they interfere with function, and possibly how they relate to the localization of lesions and processing mechanisms that underlie dysfunction. This part of the book is intended for experienced therapists with a theoretical background in occupational therapy and research methods as well as practical experience in patient evaluation. The A-ONE is intended to generate questions that facilitate clinical decision making regarding, for example, treatment methods, prognosis, and independence levels. Its aim is not to specify treatment methods but to provide practical information that can be immediately implemented in treatment. It is also meant for monitoring progress. The A-ONE puts the occupational therapist in a unique position to evaluate the daily functional performance of patients with neurobehavioral dysfunctions and the manner in which their task performance is affected by neurobehavioral impairments.

The A-ONE instrument evaluates skill in performance of ADL and examines the effect of neurobehavioral dysfunction on task performance. It can also identify problem areas, which can then be tested in a more specific way if necessary. The A-ONE is not intended to replace other forms of evaluation procedures, such as neuropsychological tests, neurological examination, tests of speech and language pathology, and neuroimaging, but rather to complement these methods. Viewing the individual from all possible aspects by using a combination of evaluative methods to explore behavior, as well as CNS structure and processing patterns, can provide a more complete evaluation of patients than any one method alone. Comparative studies that examine the combined findings of behavioral and technological evaluations can provide more effective evaluation and thus can lead to the development of more effective treatment strategies, thereby benefiting patients.

The inspiration for the A-ONE grew from indications of the link between brain and behavior noted while observing neurologically impaired patients performing self-care tasks. These observations were accompanied by analysis of patients' task performance using the well-known activity analysis, which I was introduced to by Dr. A. Cooper and her colleagues at the University of Manitoba in Canada during undergraduate studies in occupational therapy. While I was doing graduate work at the University of Southern California in the United States, these ideas evolved into a master's thesis titled "Development of the Árnadóttir OT-ADL Neurobehavioral Evaluation (A-ONE) and Comparison to Neuroimaging." The thesis committee members included the chairperson, Dr. R. Zemke, who recommended this work for publication, Dr. F. Clark, Dr. E. J. Yerxa, and Dr. S. Vulpe, who also provided personal support during the writing of this book. Dr. Yerxa greatly influenced me during this project through her courses in the USC master's program. Similarly the influence of Dr. A. J. Ayres' unique work in occupational therapy is evident, and her personal support regarding the publication was invaluable. Extensive editorial comments from Dr. L. Llorens helped shape this book into its present form.

The following individuals also are gratefully acknowledged for their contributions and assistance at various stages of the book's development: Sigrún Garðarsdóttir, Peggy Helgason, Dr. V. Henderson, Dr. þorlákur Karlsson, Hope Knútsson, Dr. M. Nuwer, Sigrún Ólafsdóttir, L. D. Parham, Jóhannes Pálmason, T. Sasao, Lillý Sverrisdóttir, and Dr. M. Vulpe. In addition, my thanks to the staff and editors at The C.V. Mosby Company and CRACOM for their assistance.

The development of the A-ONE would have been impossible without the contribution of many therapists, other staff members, and patients at various facilities: in Iceland, the Reykjavík City Hospital, Reykjalundur Rehabilitation Center, and the National Hospital of Iceland; in the United States, the UCLA Medical Center, Reed Neurological Institute, Daniel Freeman Memorial Hospital, and the University of Southern California.

The following foundations provided financial support for different parts of the work: the Science Fund of the Reykjavík City Hospital in Iceland, the Icelandic Council of Science, the Alpha Association of the Phi Beta Kappa Alumni in Southern California, and the California Foundation of Occupational Therapy.

A review of the development of this book would not be complete without mentioning the contribution of Dr. R. Bergland. Through his writings and conversations conveying the beauty that radiates from some people with neurobehavioral problems, he has helped me appreciate some of the mysteries of the brain. My interest in working with those who have neurobehavioral dysfunctions has guided me through this project. I hope that I have succeeded in communicating this interest to other therapists so that they may seek the most appropriate treatment for those with neurobehavioral dysfunctions and thereby help the "hidden star" described by Dr. Bergland to shine as brightly as possible. The search for illumination should lead therapists in the same way that the search for perfection without limits led Jonathan Livingstone Seagull (Bach, 1973) toward his goal, where the hunger for perfect speed was fed by practice.

Guðrún Árnadóttir

Contents

Introduction

Current neurobehavioral theory is concerned with how environmental stimuli are processed within the central nervous system (CNS) to effect behavioral and emotional responses. Llorens defines processing of stimuli as "the recognition, interpretation, storage, and retrieval of information to which meaning is attributed from the past and present experience" (1986, p. 104). Task performance in daily activities is a result of behavioral responses. The mechanism of nervous-system processing and neurobehavior is thus a complex interaction of processing and response.

The performance of daily activities requires adequate functioning of specific parts of the nervous system. Consequently, dysfunction of certain components of the CNS may result in impairment of specific aspects of activities of daily living (ADL). For example, a massive posterior inferior parietal lesion in the left hemisphere may cause bilateral motor apraxia. Ideomotor apraxia is defined by Ayres (1985) as a breakdown in planning and programming of action. This neurobehavioral impairment can make object manipulation difficult for such functional activities as combing the hair and brushing the teeth or holding a spoon when eating. A small precentral lesion in the primary motor area may, on the other hand, cause muscle paralysis of the contralateral side, but not apraxia. The paralysis would require that the patient perform some daily activities with one-handed techniques, and performance of others might be impossible. Thus, neurological dysfunctions that can

be observed through the patient's engagement in daily activities point to localization and indicate the extent of neurological damage. By analyzing the performance of ADL components, the integrity of CNS activity can be evaluated. Such analysis would provide additional information for the traditional judgments made about independence in functional performance through an ADL evaluation.

Because neurobehavioral deficits often interfere with independence, it would be beneficial for therapists to be able to detect these while observing ADL, thereby gaining understanding of the factors that underlie functional dependence. Such information would aid therapists in understanding the reasons for the functional impairments. Subsequently, therapists could speculate regarding the most pertinent treatment for the neurobehavioral deficits that are causing functional dependence.

Tools used by occupational therapists to assess cognitive and perceptual function do not usually include structured observations of ADL performance, although ADL assessment tools are among those most often used by occupational therapists to assess occupational role performance. ADL assessments traditionally provide information on functional dependence. However, assessment instruments for ADL are usually not administered simultaneously with tests of cognitive and perceptual function to make a systematic determination of neurobehavioral dysfunction. Such dysfunction is, however, a common factor in failure to achieve

1

independence in self-care skills. Thus neurobehavioral dysfunction may not be measured in terms of the identification of deficits or addressed in the devleopment of treatment aims. In addition, few studies have been conducted to investigate the connection between the results of cognitive evaluation and actual functional performance.

I believe that a systematic evaluation of ADL can be used as a structure for clinical reasoning to aid in detecting neurobehavioral dysfunction and also in assessing functional independence in self-care activities. Self-care activities are non-role-specific, cross-cultural occupational performance skills that reflect the core concept of occupational therapy, which is *purposeful activity*. By *activity analysis,* performance in self-care skills can be analyzed so that different neurobehavioral performance components necessary for task completion can be examined as well as the effects of their dysfunction on self-care performance. For therapists to use this type of clinical reasoning to speculate regarding the location of a lesion and the resulting processing disturbance, guidelines for the interpretation of results are needed. Such guidelines could be included in an evaluative instrument to make it usable for most therapists, not simply for neurobehavioral specialists. Such an instrument could thus further enable inferences to be made about CNS structures and functions on the basis of behavior, in addition to aiding in the identification of impairments of performance. However, if an instrument is to be practical for clinical purposes and accessible to most therapists, it cannot be too complicated. Still, a certain degree of complexity is necessary for the instrument to meet its purpose of gathering information regarding the specification of neurobehavioral deficits that interfere with function and the CNS processes responsible for dysfunction.

Scientific revolutions have been described by Kuhn (1970) as involving five repeatable steps: (1) preparadigm, (2) paradigm, (3) anomalies, (4) crisis, and (5) the evolution of new paradigms. According to him, a paradigm is an accepted model or pattern of practice. Further, "The paradigms in-clude law, theory, application and instrumentation" (Kuhn, 1970, p. 10). The literature on neurological function and dysfunction has indicated a paradigm shift in terms of the methods used for information gathering and the way CNS function is viewed. The emphasis on localization of certain functions within specific cortical areas emerged about 100 years ago. Clinical observations were matched with postmortem studies to gain information (Geschwind, 1979a and b; Lassen et al., 1978; Springer and Deutsch, 1981). Then animal studies (Heilman, 1983) and direct electrical stimulation of the brain during surgery (Lassen et al., 1978), as well as development of different neuropsychological paradigms for assessment of specific behavior (Heilman, 1983), added to the localization maps. These additions fit the ideas of processing mechanisms.

More recently, computerized methods using chemical factors and electrophysiological techniques have been developed to study CNS (Duffy, 1985; Lassen et al, 1978; Restak, 1984). In my view, these newer methods have evolved from the previous paradigms because of the external influences of the scientific revolution, which provided the necessary technology. These new studies build on the knowledge from previous studies and add to them. Still more complete information could be gathered by combining these studies with clinical neurobehavioral observations, such as those performed in occupational therapy. This might increase understanding of the CNS, which would further enhance knowledge of its functions, the effects of its dysfunctions, and the mechanisms of its recovery.

In other words, during the past few years there has been a paradigm shift in the evaluation methods used to examine the nervous system. A combination of behavioral, processing, and structural evaluations promises to enhance knowledge of the CNS, thus introducing a potential for an investigation of treatment effectiveness or even the establishment of new treatment strategies. It is therefore desirable for therapists to be able to associate a patients' neurobehavioral deficits in self-care dysfunction with the probable lesion site as identified by technological methods or neuropsychological testing.

On the basis of this identified need, I have constructed an instrument that directly links functional performance in daily activities and neurobehavior: *The Árnadóttir OT-ADL Neurobehavioral Evaluation (A-ONE)*. This evaluation, which is based on occupational therapy principles, tests ADL and neurobehavioral components simultaneously. It thus combines neurobehavioral theory with core principles from the practice of occupational therapy. The occupational therapy background includes the method of activity analysis, ADL evaluation tools, and principles from the occupational performance frame of reference. The A-ONE is intended to reveal more direct information than previously available functional evaluations have provided regarding neurobehavioral deficits and how they relate to localization of lesions and of processing sites that underlie dysfunctions. Further, with future improvement and research, it is hoped that the A-ONE will contribute to knowledge development within the field of occupational therapy.

Neurobehavioral theory provides a part of the theoretical base for the development of the A-ONE. Neurobehavioral theory is, in turn, based on functional neuroanatomy and neurophysiology. Addressing such areas as stimulation of the sensory systems, the processing of such stimulation within the CNS, and the generation of behavioral responses, this theory links brain processes to behavior and emotional responses (Llorens, 1986). Occupational therapists assess and treat behavior as it is manifested through function in the performance of various tasks. All tasks provide sensory stimuli, and the ADL comprise a group of such tasks. ADL components can thus be utilized as multiple sensory stimuli that work in a combined fashion to elicit neurobehavior. These ADL can be analyzed according to their specific nature, be it visual, auditory, tactile, proprioceptive, or vestibular.

ADL can also be divided into primary components, which include the self-care activities of feeding, hygiene and grooming, dressing, and transfer behavior, as well as communication; and secondary components, which include employment and household and leisure activities. Primary ADL skills are associated with the most basic environmental tasks that individuals have to perform, and they precede the secondary skills in the developmental sequence. The evaluation and treatment of primary ADL skills are routine procedures in most settings where occupational therapy is practiced; they can be performed in any setting where occupational therapists work, and they require a minimum of equipment. For these reasons, the primary ADL components were chosen to assess neurobehavioral deficits. Such deficits can also be detected through evaluation of secondary ADL skills, sometimes termed *instrumental ADL,* by use of the same strategies. I believe that a combination of primary and secondary ADL evaluations would eventually provide the most complete neurobehavioral assessment. Further, I believe that the A-ONE could prompt reconsideration of treatment strategies because it identifies neurobehavioral deficits, as well as the extent of their interference with functional independence, and furthermore relates the neurobehavioral impairment to CNS dysfunction. Thus, the A-ONE puts the occupational therapist in a unique position to evaluate the daily functional performance of patients with neurobehavioral dysfunctions and how their task performance is affected by neurobehavioral impairments and then to develop and evaluate suitable treatment for use in therapy.

PART
I

Review of the Literature

This section provides a theoretical base for the Árnadóttir OT-ADL Neurobehavioral Evaluation (A-ONE). The gross anatomy of the cerebral cortex, its function, and neuronal processing are reviewed as a basis for the illustration of how neurobehavioral dysfunction can be detected by a functional evaluation, and how the results can be related to organic central nervous system (CNS) dysfunction. Causes of neurobehavioral deficits are outlined and related to different patterns of dysfunction. Different methods for assessing the CNS and neurobehavior are discussed, as well as impairments related to dysfunction of the cerebral cortex and processing disturbances. Although subcortical structures also play an important role in behavior, this review is limited to the function and dysfunction of the cerebral cortex.

CHAPTER
1

Theoretical Base

A théory, according to Yerxa (1983), is a guiding set of ideas and concepts that allows knowledge to be developed and tested. Theoretical ideas enable us to have a sense of understanding about the world: they help to explain and to predict. Further, they may aid in creating a change or even in controlling a phenomenon.

When science is used as a process to describe phenomena, the formation of a theory before research is done is the strategy of choice (Reynolds, 1971). This method involves the development of a theory by process description, an evolutionary process that starts with an idea. Then it moves on to conceptualization, a classification system in which typology, or a guiding set of concepts must be developed; these are the building blocks for the theory and must be mutually exclusive and exhaustive. Concepts are evaluated by agreement and intersubjectivity of the scientific community involved (Reynolds, 1971). This requires operational definitions of the theoretical concepts, in addition to conceptual definitions. Finally, the conceptualization evolves into relational statements. According to Yerxa (1983), theory is composed of a collection of such statements. A statement generated from a theory, based on its typology, is selected for comparison with the results of empirical research designed to test the statement's correspondence with the theory (Reynolds, 1971). According to Reynolds, the reason for the strategy of creating a theory and then designing research is to develop theory through the continuous interaction of theory

and research. This continuity is also reflected in the writings of Ayres (1972), who states, "Theoretical models, like children, follow a developmental sequence. The sequence, unlike that of children, may never be completed" (p. 3).

Yerxa (1983) describes the process of theory development as a cycle that generates knowledge: ideas are generated from practice; theoretical statements are formulated from these ideas and are tested by research, providing further knowledge, which is then implemented in practice, and so on.

Dickoff et al. (1968) describe theory for a practice discipline as a conceptual framework that is aimed at a specific purpose. According to these authors, there are four levels of theories that could be viewed on a developmental continuum. The first, most primitive theory level includes the "factor-isolating" theories, which provide names for things; in other words, they develop terminology. The second level is composed of "factor-relating" theories, which develop interrelations among factors. The third level includes "situation-relating" theories, which have the property of making predictions regarding situations. Subsequently, as these theories predict that one situation will cause another, they may promote or inhibit consequent situations. The fourth and most mature theory level, according to Dickoff et al., is that of "situation-producing" theories, or prescriptive theories. These theories specify goals as aims of activities and prescribe activities to reach the goals. They also provide a "survey list" to supplement the prescription of such goal-oriented activities. As will become evident later on, the theory presented here provides statements relating factors that are based on different classes of concepts.

RELATIONAL STATEMENTS

The Introduction proposed a relation between the behaviors of the individual with CNS damage and the structural and processing abnormalities caused by the damage. In terms of theory, this would be considered a relation between two statements. Additionally, it was proposed that dysfunction of certain definite CNS components may result in impairment of specific ADL aspects: ADL components could be used as sensory stimuli to elicit behavioral responses in order to assess the neurobehavior of an individual with CNS damage. Such evaluations can be obtained through skillfully administered occupational therapy (OT) ADL assessments, which can predict the structural damage or information-processing dysfunction within the brain. Thus ADL observation is a method that can be used to evaluate the integrity of CNS activity. Further, it was reasoned that the results of the occupational therapy ADL assessment could be compared with results of other evaluation techniques, such as brain imaging, which reflect cerebral dysfunction directly. These statements were developed from the idea that occupational therapy evaluations have an analytic value when organized in a systematic way.

CONCEPTS

The concepts used as the basis of the relational statements are drawn from different sources, which can be divided into two categories: (1) neurobehavior and (2) occupational therapy assessment based on activity analysis. Each of these can be subdivided. Previously, neurobehavioral theory was based on knowledge of neuroanatomy and neurophysiology obtained from postmortem studies and clinical observations. In recent decades knowledge of brain function has increased tremendously because of experimental analyses of animal behavior, as well as advances in electrophysiology and neurochemistry. These advances have led to the development of new evaluation methods for study of the nervous system, including, for example, several brain-imaging methods. Current neurobehavioral theory refers to information processing within the central nervous system, which occurs as a result of sensory information from the individual and the surrounding environment. This processing leads to functional behavioral and emotional responses.

Occupational therapists assist neurologically impaired patients to function at their optimal levels in the environment. To do so, they assess the patients' behavior and their environment, as well as the interaction between the two. The most powerful tool used by occupational therapists for such assessment is activity analysis.

Activity analysis is defined as the process of examining activities in detail by breaking them down into their components (Trombly, 1983), in order to understand and evaluate tasks (Llorens, 1986). Activity analysis is used in the theory developed here to identify different behavioral components and possible manifestations of CNS dysfunction, during primary activities of daily living. The behavioral components are classified as *performance components,* whereas ADL skills are classified as *performance skills* under the occupational performance frame of reference reviewed later in this chapter. Instruments assessing ADL were chosen because they are the traditional tools of occupational therapy, they are commonly used by these therapists, and they are of significance to the patients.

Guidelines for interpreting the results of an occupational therapy ADL evaluation relating to specific neurobehavioral deficits were developed. The impairments identified can then be used to generate a hypothesis about the localization of cerebral dysfunctions. This process is in agreement with the assumption made by Llorens (1986) that "skillfully administered [activities] can elicit behavioral responses," from which inferences about the "level or quality of sensory perception, sensory integration, emotion, cognition, and motor output" (p. 105) can be made. According to Llorens, activities provide stimulation through the senses. These stimuli are processed through the action of the nervous system and result in thought, motor, and glandular responses. The theory introduced in this book is concerned with a description of phenomena and attempts to provide a guiding set of ideas, presented in the form of an OT-ADL assessment, which follows Reynolds' (1971) suggestion for theory development with the purpose of furthering science.

TYPOLOGIES

The typologies used to develop the Árnadóttir Occupational Therapy Activities of Daily Living Neurobehavioral Evaluation (A-ONE) are also varied. One category was concerned with traditional occupational therapy components of primary activities of daily living (see, for example, the A-ONE in Chapter 10). This typology has been accepted by the community of occupational therapists. Another category was drawn from the neurological literature, including the different abnormalities that have been related to neurobehavior. Because of functional overlap and processing complexity within the brain, the deficits cannot be considered completely mutually exclusive. However, they are exhaustive, for their purpose, and they have been accepted, although not necessarily exclusively agreed upon by the scientific community by which they are used. The typology incorporated in the A-ONE Neurobehavioral Impairment Subscales, which were used to combine the OT-ADL assessments with the symptomatology of the neurological literature, is presented here for the first time and has not yet been approved by any scientific community. However, experts in the field of neurology and occupational therapy were asked to evaluate it before it was used.

DEFINITION OF TERMS

For a theory to be developed, it is necessary to define the underlying concepts. These definitions have to be conceptual as well as operational if the relation between concepts is to be explored. The glossary provides conceptual definitions of the concepts used in the A-ONE instrument. The test manual in Part II of this book provides operational definitions for the concepts to be measured by the instrument. Fig. 1-1 outlines the theoretical base for the A-ONE instrument: Activity analysis was used for analyzing occupational performance skills, occupational performance components, neurobehavioral function and dysfunction, and cortical function and dysfunction. Components were then synthesized into the present form of the A-ONE.

OCCUPATIONAL PERFORMANCE FRAME OF REFERENCE FOR OCCUPATIONAL THERAPY

Occupational performance is one of the frames of reference for occupational therapy. According to Pedretti and Pasquinelli-Estrada (1985), this frame serves as a unifying conceptual system in agreement with the definition of occupational therapy, as well as the philosophical base of the occupational therapy profession and "the position of the American Occupational Therapy Association on purposeful activities" (p. 1). As such it is a suitable guide for occupational therapy practice.

Occupational performance refers to the ability of an individual to accomplish the tasks required by the role of that individual. Roles take into account the developmental stage of the individual. Examples of roles are homemaker, student, and employee. The roles of a preschooler and a retired employee reflect the relation of developmental stages and roles. The occupational performance skills of individuals in the various roles include: self-care, work, and play or leisure. These skill-concepts reflect the core concept of occupational therapy, namely, purposeful activity. These skills are influenced by what is called the *life space* of individuals, which refers to their cultural background as well as their human and non-human environment (Pedretti and Pasquinelli-Estrada, 1985).

The foundation for occupational performance comprises functional elements termed *performance components,* which are behavioral patterns based on learning and developmental stages. The perfor-

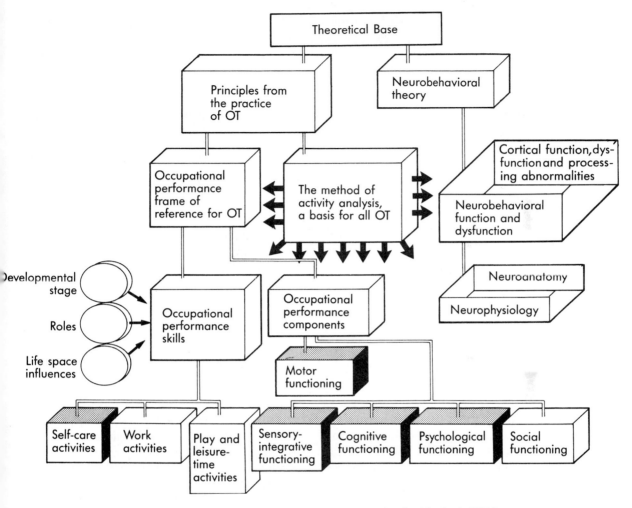

FIG. 1-1 Theoretical base for the factor-relating theory that is operationalized by the A-ONE instrument. Shading on the boxes for occupational performance skills and components indicate that these areas are addressed by the A-ONE instrument.

mance components include (1) sensory-integrative functioning, (2) motor functioning, (3) social functioning, (4) psychological functioning, and (5) cognitive functioning. Each of the performance components can be further subdivided (Fig. 1-2). Body scheme, posture, and visual perception are thus, for example, classified as some of the subunits of the sensory-integrative component, whereas communication, concentration, problem solving, conceptualization, time management, and integration

of learning are considered to be cognitive components. The motor components include, among other subunits, muscle strength, tone, and functional use of the body and its extremities. The psychological components include emotional states, defense mechanisms, self-identity, and self-concept (Pedretti and Pasquinelli-Estrada, 1985).

Some of the main concepts of this frame of reference are role performance, development, purposeful activity, adaptation, and the factors influ-

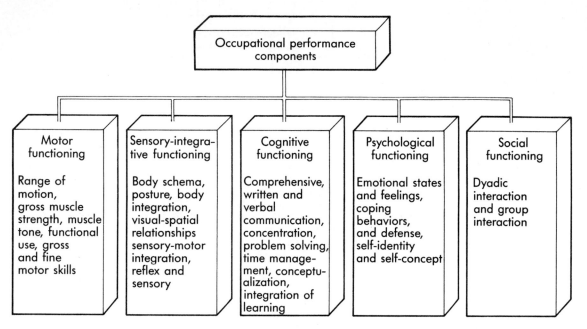

FIG. 1-2 Occupational performance components and their subcomponents. (Reprinted with permission of the American Occupational Therapy Association, Inc., © 1974, A curriculum guide for occupational therapy educators, p. 12.)

encing it. Participation in meaningful selected tasks should be in accord with the individual's role. Such tasks aim toward maximal occupational performance allowing for functional independence. These occupational therapy concepts and principles guide the actions of the therapists who prescribe occupational therapy treatment within this frame of reference (Pedretti and Pasquinelli-Estrada, 1985).

According to Pedretti and Pasquinelli-Estrada, purposeful activity, the key concept in the philosophical base of occupational therapy, refers to an activity that is meaningful to the client. It requires and elicits functional coordination of the physical, emotional, and cognitive systems. These authors state, "Activity is not only viewed as the core of occupational therapy but also as the unique feature of the profession" (p. 7). Additionally, purposeful activities characterize the tools used by the occupational therapy profession. The message from the occupational performance frame of ref-

erence is that occupational therapists should evaluate role dysfunction and use purposeful activities in the remediation of dysfunction. Evaluation should address the ability to plan and perform purposeful activities as well as the person's ability to meet the functional demands made by the environment. It should also consider the performance components and how they affect performance skills. The dysfunction addressed under this frame of reference is dysfunction in occupational performance, be it dysfunction of the performance skills or of the performance components that result in impaired performance skills. The A-ONE is an instrument designed to detect dysfunction of self-care skills, which is reflected by the Functional Independence Scale, and of specifically defined performance components, reflected by the Neurobehavioral Scale.

The occupational therapy concepts in the factor-relating theory proposed by this book are activities of daily living (ADL). ADL assessment

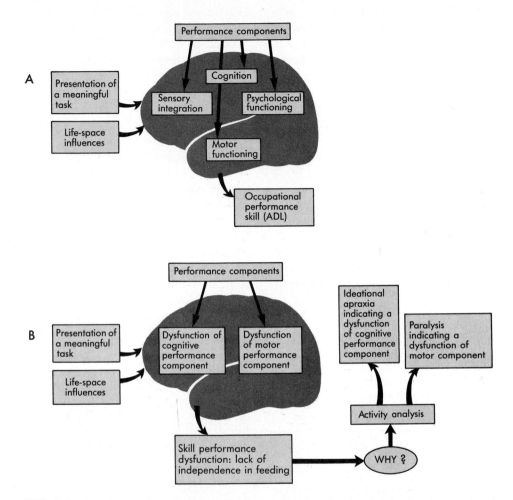

FIG. 1-3 Occupational performance. **A,** Occupational performance function. Presentation of a meaningful task that takes into account the developmental stage and the role of the individual results in successful task performance of an ADL skill. **B,** Occupational performance dysfunction. Presentation of a meaningful task reveals dysfunction of skill performance. Activity analysis reveals information regarding dysfunction in occupational performance components that contributes to the skill performance dysfunction.

tools are used to evaluate functional independence in the performance of self-care skills, which are classified as purposeful activities. By activity analysis, the self-care skill performance is analyzed, so that the different performance components can be examined as well as the effects of their dysfunction on self-care performance. Thus the pre-

sentation of a meaningful task, such as feeding, provides information that calls for a goal-directed, purposeful response. It calls for a combination of external environmental factors, such as food and cutlery, as well as internal performance components, such as visual-spatial relationships, muscle tone, and emotional state. Thus to carry out the behavior required to participate in or perform this task, which is a part of the individual's role and essential to productive living, different performance components must be brought into play. The quality of the response, when analyzed with the required performance components in mind, reveals information not only about independence in the self-care performance skill but also regarding performance-component dysfunctions or neurobehavioral dysfunctions—the problems that interfere with independence. These would be problems such as misjudging distances when reaching out for a cup, or the lack of an idea regarding how to use cutlery. Thus, the occupational performance frame of reference, which delineates a particular aspect of the occupational therapy in agreement with its philosophy and definition, is a central theme that supports the appropriateness of the A-ONE and its concepts for use in the discipline of occupational therapy (Fig. 1-3).

RESEARCH

According to Yerxa (1983), theoretical statements are tested through research, in order to explore whether the statements can be confirmed or not. The studies reported in Part 2 of this book are concerned mainly with the development of the A-ONE, an ADL evaluation intended to be sensitive to neurobehavioral deficits. This instrument was developed to provide behavioral information that could be used to identify CNS dysfunction and the reasons for the lack of functional independence of patients with such disorders. Because the idea behind the studies generated typology and relational statements, the studies were designed to test the validity of the relational statements and to obtain preliminary data that would shed further light on the meaning of test performance, as a first step contributing to theory development. According to Yerxa (1983), an instrument can be used to operationalize concepts from a theory. It is hoped that this instrument, which is basically an organization of ideas, will serve to combine the science of neurobehavior and principles from occupational therapy, and that by doing so, it will add to the knowledge of the central nervous system and neurobehaviors and thereby lead to increased benefits to patients.

CHAPTER

2

Gross Anatomy of the Cerebral Hemispheres

The human nervous system is composed of two divisions: the central and peripheral nervous systems. The central nervous system (CNS) can be subdivided into six areas: the spinal cord, brain stem, cerebellum, thalamus, basal ganglia, and the cerebral hemispheres (Barr and Kiernan, 1983; Felten and Felten, 1982). The cerebral hemispheres are paired structures composed of gray matter, which consists of a collection of nerve cells termed the *cerebral cortex,* and white myelinated axons of nerve cells that connect different areas in the hemispheres (Daube and Sandok, 1978). This chapter reviews the literature on the gross anatomy of the cerebral hemispheres to acquaint the reader with the terminology used in subsequent chapters in establishing the theoretical base for the design of the Árnadóttir OT-ADL Neurobehavioral Evaluation (A-ONE). The discussion of the anatomy of the brain is derived from the excellent reviews of Barr and Kiernan (1983) and Daube and Sandok (1978), as well as from *Gray's Anatomy* (Williams and Warwick, 1980) and Netter's illustrations (1983). Investigation methods used to examine the cerebral cortex and pertinent electrical and chemical components related to functional anatomy are also reviewed.

THE CEREBRAL CORTEX

The cerebral cortex is a layer of nerve cells approximately 5 mm thick that forms the outer surface of the cerebral hemispheres. It forms the *gyri,* or the cerebral convolutions, of the brain and the intervening grooves, called *sulci*. Fissures, which are deeper than the gyri, separate larger components of the brain (Barr and Kiernan, 1983). A longitudinal fissure divides the cerebrum into left and right hemispheres. Each hemisphere has three surfaces: superolateral, medial, and inferior (Barr and Kiernan, 1983; Netter, 1983). The transverse cerebral fissure separates the cerebral hemispheres above from the cerebellum, midbrain, and diencephalon below (Barr and Kiernan, 1983). Because of the similarity in the gross anatomy of the two hemispheres, the text in the following discussion will refer to only one hemisphere. The lateral fissure, or fissure of Sylvius, extends from the inferior surface of the hemisphere, laterally between the frontal and temporal lobes. The central sulcus of Rolando runs from the superior border of the hemisphere downward and forward on the lateral surface toward the lateral fissure (Barr and Kiernan, 1983; Netter, 1983). The calcarine sulcus on the medial surface of the hemisphere extends from the posterior end of the corpus callosum to the occipital pole (Barr and Kiernan, 1983). The parieto-occipital sulcus is also mainly situated on the medial surface of the cerebrum. It extends from the calcarine sulcus and runs toward the superior margin. It cuts the superior margin and runs for a short distance on the superolateral surface (Barr and

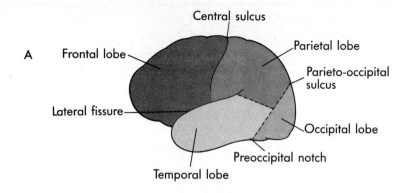

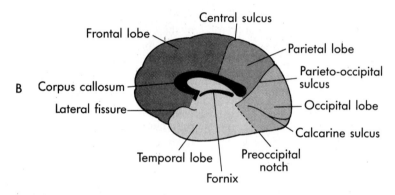

FIG. 2-1 Lobe division of the cerebral hemispheres. **A,** Lateral surface. **B,** Medial surface.

Kiernan, 1983; Netter, 1983). The inferior margin of the hemisphere has a shallow indentation, the preoccipital notch, about 5 cm from the occipital pole (Netter, 1983). The features just described divide the cerebral cortex into four sections: the frontal, parietal, occipital, and temporal lobes (Fig. 2-1) (Netter, 1983).

The frontal lobes

Laterally, the frontal lobe is composed of the area in front of the central sulcus, above the lateral fissure. The medial boundary of the frontal lobe includes the anterior part of the corpus callosum. The lobe is bounded posteriorly on the medial side by an imaginary line drawn between the central sulcus at the superior surface and the corpus callosum, as illustrated in Fig. 2-1 (Barr and Kiernan, 1983). There are three main sulci (precentral sulcus, superior sulcus, and inferior sulcus) on the superolateral surface of the frontal lobe, which divide it into four gyri (precentral gyrus, superior, middle, and inferior frontal gyri) as illustrated in Fig. 2-2. On the inferior surface of the frontal lobe there are two sulci (olfactory sulcus and orbital sulcus) and two main gyri (gyrus rectus and the orbital gyri). Medially, the cingulate sulcus separates the cingulate gyrus from the medial frontal gyrus.

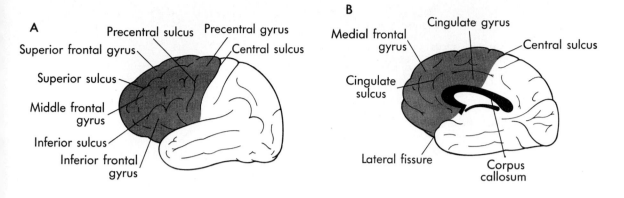

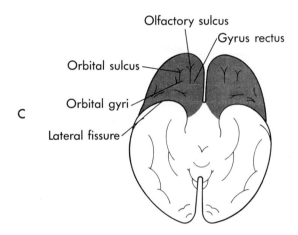

FIG. 2-2. Gyri and sulci of the frontal lobe. **A,** Lateral surface. **B,** Medial surface. **C,** Inferior surface.

The parietal lobes

The parietal lobe has two boundaries based on anatomical landmarks on the lateral surface: the central and the lateral sulci. It also has boundaries consisting of two hypothetical lines. One of these is drawn between the parieto-occipital sulcus and the preoccipital notch; the other is drawn from the middle of the previously established line to the lateral sulcus, as illustrated in Fig. 2-1. Medially, the parietal lobe is distinguished from the frontal lobe by the earlier mentioned imaginary line between the central sulcus above, the corpus callosum and calcarine sulcus below, and the parieto-occipital sulcus posteriorly (Barr and Kiernan, 1983). The parietal lobe has two main sulci on the lateral surface (postcentral sulcus and intraparietal sulcus), which divide it into three main gyri (postcentral gyrus, superior parietal lobule, and inferior parietal lobule), as shown in Fig. 2-3. The inferior parietal lobule is further composed of two gyri: the supramarginal gyrus, which surrounds the upper ends of the lateral fissure, and the angular gyrus,

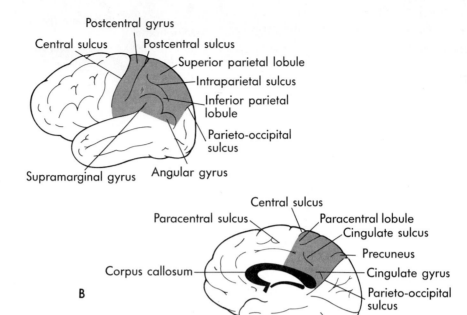

FIG. 2-3 Gyri and sulci of the parietal lobe. **A,** Lateral surface. **B,** Medial surface.

which surrounds the superior temporal sulcus. Medially, the cingulate sulcus extends from the frontal lobe over to the parietal lobe, where it gives off the paracentral sulcus before it terminates in the marginal and subparietal sulci. These sulci form the paracentral lobule, which is composed of extensions from the pre- and postcentral gyri on the lateral surface. The area above the subparietal sulcus is continuous with the superior parietal lobule on the lateral suface, it is called the *precuneus* area.

The occipital lobes

The occipital lobe occupies mainly the medial surface of the hemisphere. On this surface it is separated from the parietal lobe by the parieto-occip-ital sulcus and the calcarine sulcus, as already described, and from the temporal lobe by the imaginary line between the tip of the calcarine sulcus and the preoccipital notch. On the lateral surface it is separated from the temporal and parietal lobes by an imaginary line from the parieto-occipital sulcus to the preoccipital notch (see Fig. 2-1) (Barr and Kiernan, 1983; Netter, 1983). The cuneus on the medial surface of the hemisphere is the area between the parieto-occipital sulcus and the calcarine sulcus. Laterally, there are two sulci (transverse occipital sulcus and calcarine sulcus). Inferiorly, there are two sulci (occipito-temporal sulcus and collateral sulcus), which run across the temporal and occipital lobes, and two gyri (medial

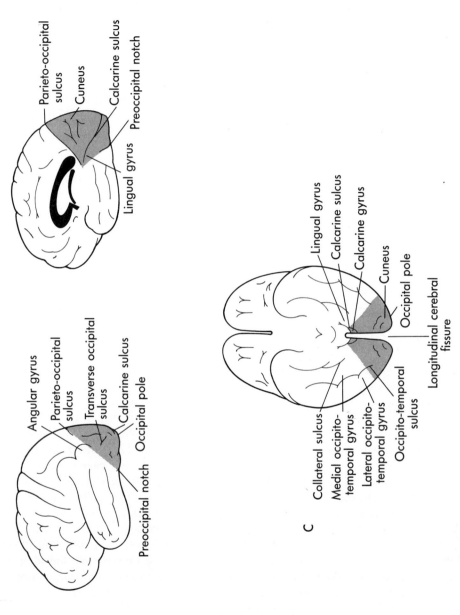

FIG. 2-4 Gyri and sulci of the occipital lobe. **A**, Lateral surface. **B**, Medial surface. **C**, Inferior surface.

occipito-temporal gyrus and lateral occipito-temporal gyrus). See Fig. 2-4 for sulci and gyri of the occipital lobe.

The temporal lobes

The landmarks of the temporal lobe are, laterally, the lateral fissure and the imaginary lines previously mentioned (see Fig. 2-1). Inferiorly, an imaginary line drawn between the anterior end of the calcarine sulcus and the preoccipital notch separates the temporal lobe from the occipital lobe (Barr and Kiernan, 1983). The temporal lobe is divided laterally by two sulci (superior and inferior temporal sulci) into three gyri (superior, middle, and inferior temporal gyri [Fig. 2-5]). The superior temporal gyrus runs into the supramarginal gyrus at the level of the parietal lobe, and the middle temporal gyrus meets with the angular gyrus of the inferior parietal lobule (Barr and Kiernan, 1983; Netter, 1983). The surface of the superior temporal gyrus, which forms the "floor" of the lateral fissure, forms small gyri, the transverse temporal gyri, which are also called *Heschl's convolutions*. On the inferior and medial surfaces of the temporal lobe are three sulci (collateral sulcus, rhinal sulcus, and occipito-temporal sulcus) and four gyri (lingual gyrus, parahippocampal gyrus, and medial and lateral occipito-temporal gyri). The lateral occipito-temporal gyrus is continuous with the inferior temporal gyrus on the lateral surface of the hemisphere. The most anterior part of the parahippocampal gyrus becomes the uncus. The parahippocampal gyrus and the lingual gyrus are continuous. The dentate gyrus lies between the parahippocampal gyrus and the hippocampus (Barr and Kiernan, 1983; Netter, 1983).

The insula

The insula, or island of Reil, is usually considered separately from the four main lobes of the cerebral cortex. It lies at the bottom of the lateral fissure, overlapped by the other lobes. It has two main sulci (central and circular sulci). It has two long and several short gyri, as well as the limen, which is the inferior part of the insula (Barr and Kiernan, 1983; Netter, 1983).

The limbic lobes

The cingulate and the parahippocampal gyri on the medial aspect of the temporal and frontal lobes are connected by the isthmus. Together with the hippocampus, they form what is sometimes called the *limbic lobe* of the cerebral hemisphere, shown in Fig. 2-6 (Barr and Kiernan, 1983). According to Daube and Sandok (1978), the limbic lobe includes structures on the medial surface of the cerebrum, which have been found to be functionally and anatomically related. These include the uncus, the hippocampus, the parahippocampal gyrus, the fornix, the orbitofrontal cortex, and the cingulate gyrus (Barr and Kiernan, 1983; Daube and Sandok, 1978). Damasio and Van Hoesen (1983) include the cortical areas connecting the cingular and parahippocampal gyri in the definition of the limbic cortex. Thus they include the subcallosal gyrus beneath the anterior corpus callosum in the frontal lobe, the posterior orbitofrontal area, the anterior insular area, the temporal pole and perirhinal cortices as an anterior connection between the two previously mentioned gyri, as well as the cortical area around the anterior part of the calcarine fissure and the area posterior to the splenium of corpus callosum. The term *limbic system,* on the other hand, refers to a much more extensive collection of structures, including the limbic cortex, subcortical structures (amygdala, anterior thalamus, dentate gyrus, habenula, interpeduncular nucleus, mammillary bodies of the hypothalamus, and the septum), and interconnecting pathways (the cingulum, fimbria, fornix, habenulointerpeduncular pathway, mammillotegmental tract, mammilothalamic tract, medial forebrain bundle, stria medullaris thalamus, stria terminalis, uncinate fasciculus, and the ventral amygdalofugal pathway). The limbic structures are thus linked by a circular pathway, called the *Papez circuit,* named after its discoverer (Barr and Kiernan, 1983; Daube and Sandok, 1978; Walsh, 1987).

CORTICAL CONNECTIONS

As indicated earlier, the white matter of the hemispheres is made up of the myelinated axons of nerve cells that connect different areas of the hemi-

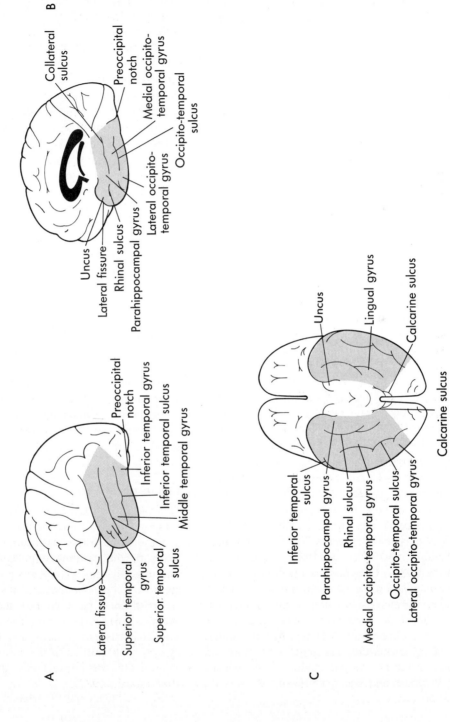

FIG. 2-5 Gyri and sulci of the temporal lobe. **A,** Lateral surface. **B,** Medial surface. **C,** Inferior surface.

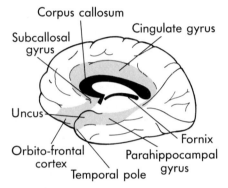

Corpus callosum

Cingulate gyrus

Subcallosal
gyrus

Uncus

Orbito-frontal
cortex

Temporal pole

Fornix

Parahippocampal
gyrus

FIG. 2-6 The limbic lobe.

spheres. There are three types of fiber connections associated with the cerebral cortex that influence its function. Association fibers connect different areas within the same hemisphere. There are two types of association fibers: long and short. Long association fibers lie rather deep. They are gathered into bundles that connect different lobes. Short association, or arcuate, fibers connect adjacent gyri. They lie beneath the cortex, arching around the bottom of the sulci (Barr and Kiernan, 1983; Daube and Sandok, 1978; Walsh, 1987; Williams and Warwick, 1980). Commissural fibers connect homologous areas in the two hemispheres. Most of these pass through the corpus callosum. Projection fibers connect the cortex with subcortical nuclear structures, including the thalamus, hypothalamus, brain stem, cerebellum, and spinal cord (Barr and Kiernan, 1983; Daube and Sandok, 1978; Walsh, 1987; Williams and Warwick, 1980).

Association fibers

Fig. 2-7 illustrates examples of long association-fiber bundles. The fibers of these bundles are of different lengths, and they enter and leave the bundles at different points. The cingulum, on the medial surface, contains fibers that connect the cingulate gyrus in the frontal and parietal lobes, the parahippocampal gyrus of the temporal lobe, and the septal area below the anterior part of the corpus callosum. The superior longitudinal fasciculus, or arcuate fasciculus, connects the frontal, parietal, and occipital lobes on the lateral surface. It also sends fibers to the posterior temporal lobe. This fiber bundle provides an important connection between the sensory and motor language areas (Barr and Kiernan, 1983; Walsh, 1987). The inferior longitudinal fasciculus connects the occipital and temporal poles. This fiber bundle is, however, not as clear-cut as many others. The inferior occipito-frontal fasciculus extends inferiorly from the frontal lobe to the occipital lobe. It shares a common association fiber bundle with the uncinate fasciculus, which connects the orbitofrontal area with the temporal pole (Barr and Kiernan, 1983; Walsh, 1987). Fig. 2-7 also includes an example of short association fibers, or arcuate fibers. The illustration demonstrates fibers in the association cortex of the parietal lobe, which receive fibers from the adjacent gyri, or the somesthetic area of the same lobe.

Commissural fibers

There are three fiber systems of commissural fibers, which connect the two hemispheres. The largest of these is the corpus callosum (Fig. 2-8). It has four parts: the rostrum, genu, trunk, and splenium. This fiber system is very extensive and connects most cortical parts of the hemispheres. The anterior and posterior forceps connect the frontal and the occipital poles respectively. The anterior commissure connects the inferior and middle temporal gyri. A small portion of this system also connects adjacent olfactory cortical areas (Barr and Kiernan, 1983; Walsh, 1987).

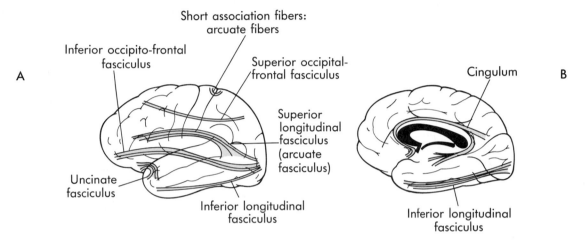

FIG. 2-7 Association fibers. **A,** Lateral view, including both long and short association fibers. **B,** Medial view.

Projection fibers

Projection fibers connecting cortical areas to subcortical nuclei can bring information both to and from the cortex. Afferent information to the cortex comes mainly from the thalamus. It projects to all areas of cortex. Efferent information from various cortical areas is provided to the thalamus and other subcortical nuclei (basal ganglia, hypothalamus, red nucleus, reticular formation, corticobulbar and corticospinal nuclei). Information is carried to and from the cortex via the corona radiata and the internal capsule, which projects to the thalamus and other subcortical nuclei. Anteriorly, the internal capsule contains fibers connecting the dorsomedial

thalamic nucleus and prefrontal cortex. The genu, which is the middle of the internal capsule viewed in a transverse plane and its adjacent region of the posterior limb, projects between the ventral anterior and ventral lateral nuclei of the thalamus to motor and premotor areas of the frontal lobe. Posteriorly, the internal capsule projects between the somesthetic areas and the association cortex in the parietal lobe to the ventral posteriolateral and ventral posteriomedial thalamic nuclei. The posterior thalamic radiation establishes a connection between the thalamus (lateral geniculate) and the cortex of the occipital lobe. In addition, the inferior thalamic radiation connects thalamic nuclei (medial

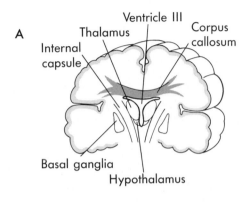

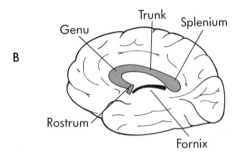

FIG. 2-8 Commisural fibers. **A,** Coronal section of corpus callosum connecting the two hemispheres. **B,** Sagittal section of corpus callosum, including its subcomponents.

geniculate) with the cortex of the temporal lobe, as shown in Fig. 2-9 (Barr and Kiernan, 1983; Daube and Sandok, 1978; Walsh, 1987).

THE THALAMUS

The thalamus is one of four components of the diencephalon. It is a paired structure composed of a group of nuclei: the dorsolateral nuclei, dorsomedial nuclei, lateral posterior nuclei, pulvinar, medial geniculate body, lateral geniculate body, ventral anterior nuclei, ventral posterior nuclei, ventral lateral nuclei, midline nuclei, medial tha-

lamic nuclei, lateral thalamic nuclei, intralaminar nuclei, and ventricular nuclei (Daube and Sandok, 1978). These nuclei relay information to and from the cortex (Fig. 2-10).

The hypothalamus is also one of the four components of the diencephalon. It is connected to the pituitary gland by the infundibulum, which is a unidirectional tract containing axons terminating in the posterior pituitary gland. The periventricular region of the thalamus surrounds the third ventricle. The mamillary bodies are located in the anterior hypothalamus. The medial forebrain bun-

A

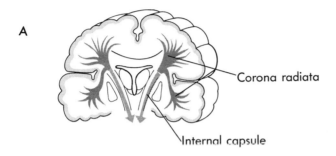

Corona radiata

Internal capsule

B

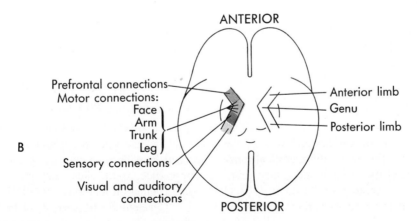

ANTERIOR

Prefrontal connections
Motor connections:
   Face
   Arm
   Trunk
   Leg
Sensory connections
Visual and auditory
   connections

Anterior limb
Genu
Posterior limb

POSTERIOR

FIG. 2-9 Projection fibers. **A,** Coronal view of the internal capsule and corona radiata. **B,** Transverse section of the internal capsule connecting cortex and subcortical structures.

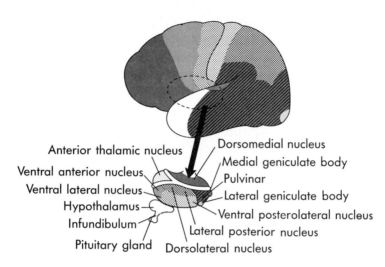

Anterior thalamic nucleus
Ventral anterior nucleus
Ventral lateral nucleus
Hypothalamus
Infundibulum
Pituitary gland

Dorsomedial nucleus
Medial geniculate body
Pulvinar
Lateral geniculate body
Ventral posterolateral nucleus
Lateral posterior nucleus
Dorsolateral nucleus

FIG. 2-10 Thalamus. The dotted area indicates the structural relation of thalamus to cortex. The thalamus and some of its nuclei are illustrated in the drawing indicated by the arrow. Different shades indicate different thalamic nuclei. The shades further indicate which cortical areas connect with which thalamic nuclei. The structural relation of the hypothalamus and the pituitary gland to the thalamus are also shown.

dle connects the hypothalamus with the limbic cortex. There are extensive interconnections between the hypothalamus and the limbic system. The hypothalamus also receives fibers from the dorsomedial thalamic nucleus, and has reciprocal connections with the anterior nuclei of the thalamus. It has further connections with the reticular activating system of the midbrain.

Bear in mind that although this book is limited to the functions of the cerebral cortex, the cortex does not function in isolation; cortical functions are influenced by and influence other structures in the CNS. The reader is referred to classical texts in neuroanatomy for a more thorough review of the CNS.

Anatomical landmarks of the four lobes of the cerebral cortex, as well as subdivisions of these lobes into gyri by fissures, have been outlined in this section. Cortical fiber connections, important

to functions and neuronal processing, have also been mentioned. The functions and signs of dysfunction of the different lobes will be reviewed later to further establish the basis for the evaluation method proposed by this book.

ANATOMICAL ASYMMETRY OF THE CEREBRAL CORTEX

Some reports of anatomical asymmetries were found in reviewing the literature. These are discussed here because of their potential functional importance, and because they may be detected by some evaluation methods, such as CT scans.

Geschwind and Levitsky (1968) reported the existence of anatomical asymmetries in the right and left superior temporal lobes of humans. According to them, the planum temporale was larger in the left hemisphere in 65% of the 100 brains they studied postmortem. On the right side, however, only 11% were larger. The left planum was reported to be considerably longer than the right planum on the average. The planum is important in auditory comprehension, as will be evident in Chapters 3 and 4.

Galaburda, LeMay, Kemper, and Geschwind (1978) also reported that structural asymmetries between the hemispheres were found upon post-mortem studies of human brains, as well as in radiological examination, and that these asymmetries between the hemispheres may relate to left-right differences in cortical function. They suggested, for example, that language lateralization could be based on auditory asymmetries. They reported two major differences in the two hemispheres. The first is in the temporo-parietal cortex on the left side, which can exceed its counterpart on the right by approximately seven times. They also reported that the left planum temporale is larger in the majority of right-handed persons. The left occipital lobe and the right frontal lobe were also reported to be more extensive than their counterparts on CT scans, according to these authors. These differences are reported to be much less striking in left-handed individuals.

According to Galaburda et al., pneumoencephalography studies have revealed ventricular asymmetry. They also pointed out that frontal and occipital asymmetries of the lateral ventricles are correlated with hand preference. According to them, the left posterior horn of the lateral ventricles is longer in right-handed subjects than its counterparts in 60% of cases, whereas the right posterior horn is reported to be longer in only 10% of cases. In left-handed and ambidextrous individuals, a longer left occipital horn was found in only 38% of cases, while 31% had a longer right posterior horn. Further, angiographic studies are reported to have revealed that the left Sylvian fissure was longer, and placed more horizontally, than its counterpart in the right hemisphere in humans.

From the preceding reports of structural hemispheric differences, it is evident that, when looking at evaluation techniques such as CT scans and CMEEG's that reveal images of brain structure

or are based on accurate electrode placement on the scalp, awareness of the reported anatomical differences and information regarding the handedness of the individuals is important. Some slight anatomical discrepancies between the hemispheres that are observed on x-ray films or neuroimaging computer printouts may be explained in this way and may turn out to be normal, when handedness of the person is considered.

BLOOD FLOW OF THE CORTEX

Cerebral blood flow is necessary for cerebral function. Dysfunction of specific parts of the arterial system can lead to localized specific neurological signs and thus to neurobehavioral dysfunction, as will be evident in Chapter 5. Therefore, the anatomy and the function of this system is discussed in this section. Some of the assessment methods described in Chapter 6 also relate to the arterial system.

The internal carotid system

The internal carotid system is one of two arterial systems involved with blood supply to the cerebral cortex; the other is the vertebral system. The internal carotid artery arises from the common carotid artery (Barr and Kiernan, 1983; Daube and Sandok, 1978; Netter, 1983; Williams and Warwick, 1980). The internal carotid arteries on each side terminate in the smaller anterior cerebral arteries and the middle cerebral arteries (Fig. 2-11). On its way to the cerebral cortex, the internal carotid arteries supply parts of the limbic system, anterior inferior thalamus, and anterior part of the internal capsule. The two anterior cerebral arteries are connected by the anterior communicating artery. The anterior cerebral artery travels in the longitudinal fissure, and arches around the genu of the corpus callosum. Its branches extend over the anterior medial border of the hemispheres over to the parietal lobes, and also supply a strip of the lateral surface (Barr and Kiernan, 1983; Netter, 1983).

The middle cerebral arteries run laterally and then posteriorly in the lateral fissure. They divide into branches distributed to the lateral surfaces of

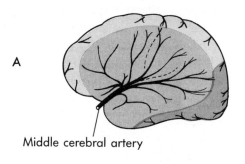

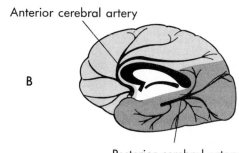

FIG. 2-11 The cerebral arteries. **A,** Lateral surface of the cerebral cortex. This surface is mainly supplied by the middle cerebral artery. **B,** Medial surface of the cerebral cortex. This surface is supplied by the anterior cerebral artery from the internal carotid arterial system, as well as the posterior cerebral artery from the vertebral arterial system. Shading indicates areas of arterial distribution.

the cerebral hemispheres and the insula (Netter, 1983; Williams and Warwick, 1980). Orbital branches supply the inferior frontal gyri and the lateral orbital surfaces of the frontal lobes. The frontal branches supply the precentral, middle, and inferior frontal gyri. The parietal branches supply the postcentral gyri and the inferior parietal lobes. The temporal branches supply the lateral surface of the temporal lobe (Netter, 1983; Williams and Warwick, 1980).

The vertebral system

The vertebral system initiates with the two vertebral arteries, which arise from the subclavian ar-

teries on each side. The two vertebral arteries join at the level of the pons, to form the basilar artery. The basilar artery, ascending on the middle anterior surface of the pons, divides to form the posterior cerebral arteries. These ascend posteriorly around the midbrain and reach the medial surfaces of the cerebral hemispheres. The arteries give off temporal branches, which run over the inferior surface of the temporal lobes, as well as calcarine and parieto-occipital branches, which run to the posterior part of cortex. These arteries, located inferiorly and posteriorly on the medial sides of the hemispheres, send branches to supply a peripheral strip on the lateral cortical surfaces, as shown in

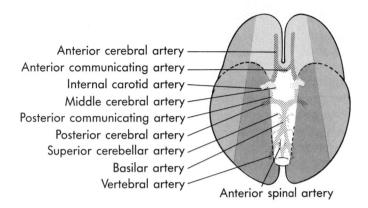

Anterior cerebral artery
Anterior communicating artery
Internal carotid artery
Middle cerebral artery
Posterior communicating artery
Posterior cerebral artery
Superior cerebellar artery
Basilar artery
Vertebral artery

Anterior spinal artery

FIG. 2-12 The vertebral arterial system and circle of Willis. Shading indicates areas of arterial distribution.

Figs. 2-11 and 2-12 (Barr and Kiernan, 1983; Netter, 1983).

Major anastomotic channels provide communication between the arterial systems supplying the brain. The circle of Willis, situated in the cisterna interpeduncularis at the base of the brain, connects the basilar and internal carotid arterial systems (Fig. 2-12). It consists of (1) the anterior communicating artery, which unites the two anterior cerebral arteries, which are branches of the internal carotid arteries, and (2) two posterior communicating arteries, which arise from the internal carotid arteries and join the corresponding posterior cerebral arteries, which are branches of the basilar artery (Liebman, 1979; Netter, 1983; Werner, 1980; Williams and Warwick, 1980). There are also corticomeningeal anastomoses between the three major cerebral vessels (Daube and Sandok, 1978; Matthews and Miller, 1975; Werner, 1980) and anastomoses between extra- and intracranial arteries where a branch from each of the external carotid arteries communicates with a branch from the internal carotid arteries (Daube and Sandok, 1978).

If the collateral cerebral circulation is adequate, occlusion of the internal carotid artery, for example, will cause no neurological deficit. However, if it is not adequate, occlusion causes infarc-

tion in the cortical area nourished by the anterior or middle cerebral arteries, or both (Gowers, 1974). The severity of the dysfunction also depends on how rapidly occlusion develops. When occlusion occurs slowly, the collateral circulation may have time to take over, resulting in only moderate impairment; such compensation does not occur with a rapidly developing occlusion (Daube and Sandok, 1978; Liebman, 1979; Matthews and Miller, 1975; Gowers, 1974). See Chapter 5 for a discussion of cerebral vascular disorders resulting in neurobehavioral dysfunction.

THE VENTRICULAR SYSTEM

The brain and the surrounding nervous structures house four cavities, called *ventricles* (Fig. 2-13). There are two lateral ventricles, one in each hemisphere. These have three horns, an anterior horn reaching forward to the frontal lobe, a posterior horn reaching back toward the occipital lobe, and an inferior horn stretching over to the temporal lobe. The two lateral ventricles connect with the third ventricle, located at the level of the thalamus and separating its two parts. The third ventricle is connected with the fourth ventricle, located at the level of the pons and medulla, by a canal, the *cerebral aqueduct*. The fourth ventricle communicates with the subarachnoid space surrounding

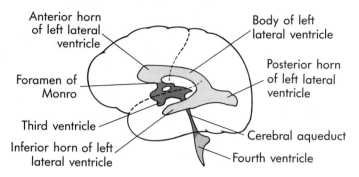

FIG. 2-13 The ventricular system.

the brain and other CNS structures. The subarachnoid space is formed by the meninges surrounding the brain. It in turn connects with the venous sinuses (Barr and Kiernan, 1983; Daube and Sandok, 1978; Netter, 1983).

The ventricular cavities are filled with cerebral spinal fluid (CSF). This fluid enters the ventricular system via vascular organs, termed the *choroid plexus,* located in the different ventricles. There are different theories about the origin of the CSF. It is either considered to be produced by the choroid plexus or more likely to be filtered into the ventricles via the choroid plexus. The CSF is thought to serve different functions. It has been related to a buffer system serving the purpose of absorbing forces that might be harmful for the CNS. It is also thought to remove leftover products from cerebral metabolism and to contribute to the blood-brain barrier system, mentioned later in this chapter, in communication between the extra- and intracellular environments of the brain (Barr and Kiernan, 1983; Daube and Sandok, 1978; Netter, 1983). However, others believe that the ventricles have a more important role in nervous function, perhaps one of the most important roles there is. According to Bergland (1985), "More and more evidence suggests that the brain was given its hollow form to fulfill endocrine functions" (p. 136). He points out the close proximity of the third ventricle to the pituitary gland. Bergland considers the brain to be a "hormonally driven gland" (p. 93),

and he is convinced that there is a flow of hormonal codes from the pituitary to the brain.

It was considered necessary to include a brief review of the ventricular system in this section, because of its traditionally recognized clinical importance in certain conditions, such as hydrocephalus; the enlargement of the ventricles due to CSF blockage in the ventricles, or brain atrophy. More importantly, the inclusion of this system is crucial when it comes to speculations regarding cerebral function and the basis for cerebral processing in subsequent chapters.

PHYSIOLOGICAL, ELECTRICAL, AND CHEMICAL FACTORS RELATED TO ANATOMY

There are two types of cells in the CNS: *neurons,* which are responsible for "the functional characteristics of nervous tissue" according to Barr and Kiernan (1983, p. 13), and *glial cells,* which provide both structural and metabolic support to nerve cells (Kandel, 1985e). Neurons are specialized for the generation, conduction, and control of electrical impulses by the mechanisms of excitation and inhibition. Cerebral function is based on neurons and connections between them. Although neurons may seem to be simple structures, they are capable of extremely complex functions because of their enormous number and the complexity of neural connections, according to Kandel (1985a). In this section, a brief and simplified summary of electrical transmission in cerebral neurons is provided because of its contribution to function of the CNS and because some of the assessment methods reviewed later are based on electrical activity.

Other assessment methods are based on the brain's circulation of blood, such as angiography; still others use radioactive contrast agents, making use of the blood-brain barrier phenomenon: the way in which the brain keeps chemicals constant in its environment (Kuffler, et al., 1984).

Electrical transmission in the cerebral cortex

Electrical transmission in the cerebral cortex is based on the neurons, which are composed of three parts: (1) a dendrite tree, which receives the electrical input, (2) a cell body, which includes the functional organs of the cell responsible for protein synthesis and metabolic functions, and (3) an axon, which serves as the conduction unit of the neuron (Barr and Kiernan, 1983; Daube and Sandok, 1978; Kandel, 1985a; Netter, 1983). Some axons are covered with an insulating myelin sheath, which is important for increasing the velocity of electrical transmission. This sheath is interrupted in numerous places along the axon at points termed *nodes of Ranvier*. Fig. 2-14 shows the structure of a neuron (Kandel, 1985a).

During a resting state, electrical charges at each side of a neuronal membrane are different: they are negative on the inside and positive on the outside. This difference of electrical charge across the cell membrane has been termed *resting membrane potential*. The resting membrane potential is a result of a different concentration of sodium ions (Na^+), potassium ions (K^+), and chloride (Cl^-) in the intracellular fluid as compared to the extracellular fluid.

A suffucient reduction in the membrane potential results in a flow of ionic current across the cell membrane. This shifts the membrane resting potential to an *action potential*. The action potential is the mechanism by which a neuronal axon carries information from one end to another. (Kandel, 1985a; Kuffler et al., 1984; Netter, 1983). A discussion of membrane permeability to the different ions, which is the underlying factor for the

electrical conductance of nerve cells, is beyond the scope of this review.

Neurons contact each other via synapses. A synapse is usually composed of terminal fibers of a neuronal axon, dendrites of the adjoining neuron, and the gap between the two. During development and nervous system organization, neurons connect in a selective way. (Kandel, 1985b; Kandel and Siegelbaum, 1985). According to Kandel and Schwartz (1985), brain function depends on highly specific neuronal connections based on nerve cell "structure, biochemistry, and electrical properties" (p. 87). They further state that the "average neuron forms about 1000 synaptic connections and receives even more." Thus, based on the number of CNS neurons, "10^{15} synaptic connections are formed in the brain" (p. 87).

According to Barr and Kiernan (1983), most synapses in the CNS are based on chemical transport of messages across the synaptic gap. These chemical synapses are capable of more complex activity than the electrical ones. The axons of these presynaptic neurons are capable of releasing chemical agents called neurotransmitters into the synaptic gap. The neurotransmitters are either produced in the neuronal cell body and moved down the axon or produced at the presynaptic axon end. Release of a chemical agent into a synaptic gap occurs subsequently to an action potential in the presynaptic axon and is mediated by Ca^{++}. The transmitter diffuses across to act on the postsynaptic membrane. It binds to receptors of the postsynaptic cell, altering membrane permeability to ions, resulting in a depolarization of its dendrites if the transmitter had an excitatory function. Synaptic potentials can be either excitatory or inhibitory depending on the nature of the synapse (Barr and Kiernan, 1983; Daube and Sandok, 1978; Kandel, 1985a; Netter, 1983). The neurotransmitters of neurons are of different kinds, but the resulting electrical signals are basically the same, according to Kandel (1985a).

Kandel and Siegelbaum (1985) compare the presynaptic terminals of chemical synapses to endocrine glands, and chemical transmission to the action of hormones. According to them, both "re-

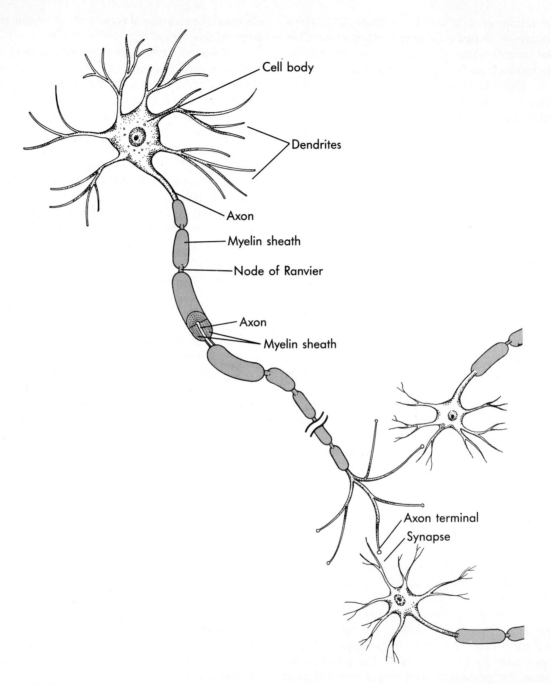

FIG. 2-14 A neuron. The main features of a typical neuron include a cell body, an axon enclosed in a myelin sheath, and dendrites. The terminal axon branches form synapses with other neurons. One part of the myelin sheath has been opened, revealing the axon that the sheath surrounds.

lease a chemical mediating agent" (p. 93). The advantage of chemical synapses, they argue, is the selectivity of the action and the closeness of operating sides, which increases the speed of the action. The difference between the two is the operating distance, although some neurotransmitters can act at distant sites, and some can even be released into the blood stream, where they act as hormones.

Neuronal processing depends on input from sensory pathways to pertinent cerebral reception areas, as well as complex inter- and intrahemispheric connections. The electrical activity along these pathways has been used, for example, by Berger, who developed the electroencephalogram (EEG), and later by Duffy (1982) in the assessment of cerebral function. Duffy's methods of spectral analysis and topographical mapping are based on the EEG and evoked potentials (EP).

Chemical factors

The blood-brain barrier is a chemical phenomenon; according to Eyzaguirre and Fidone (1975), it is the "degree of selectivity with which substances cross from cerebral blood vessels into the brain tissue" (p. 395). In other regions of the body, the exit from capillaries is less restrictive. The blood-brain barrier includes many different barrier systems, some related to the anatomical structure of cerebral capillaries, others to the physiochemical properties of cerebrospinal fluid (CSF) and blood. These mechanisms act together to maintain a constant cerebral environment (Rowland, 1985).

Different mechanisms are involved in transport across the blood-brain barrier. Water-soluble compounds seem to pass between the cells, whereas lipid-soluble compounds appear to pass through the cells. Glucose is thought to pass the barrier by a facilitated diffusion. Proteins do not cross the barrier, but amino acids seem to cross it easily, and no restriction appears to be present for water, oxygen, and carbon dioxide, according to Eyzaguirre and Fidone.

The blood-brain barrier mechanism makes certain assessment methods possible. These include angiography, where a radioactive substance does not cross the blood-brain barrier, and blood-flow measurements, including Positron Emission Tomography (PET) scans, where the radioactive substance crosses the barrier over to brain tissue. These assessment methods are described later, as are methods based on electrical and magnetic principles. Understanding the chemical or physiological basis for the different evaluation methods is therefore important.

NEURONAL PLASTICITY

The nervous system has a high level of plasticity, especially during early development. Genetic as well as environmental factors affect neuronal development. In addition to developing specific neuronal properties, appropriate connections with other nerves must be made, and these complex synaptic connections can be influenced by environmental factors acting upon the genetic properties of the neurons. There are critical periods for neuronal development and optimal cellular interactions. During the critical periods, neurotransmitters and hormones affect cerebral development. They help to "specify critical periods," both in respect to time and sensitivity to external environmental stimuli, according to Lauder and Krebs (1986, p. 167). Thus these factors can contribute to individual variations in nervous system organization. Any injury during development can also bring different factors into play, affecting axonal and dendritic sprouting or collateral rearrangement, synaptic formation, the excitability of neurons, "substitution of parallel channels," and "mobilization of redundant capacity" (Devor, 1982, p. 45). Because of this plasticity, one cannot expect any two brains to be structurally or functionally identical (Moore, 1986). Although the functional organization presented in this book does not apply 100% to all individuals, because of individual differences for whatever reasons, it is considered to be a useful guide to understanding the nervous system as well as some of the factors that underlie CNS dysfunction and subsequent deficits in the performance of tasks that are necessary if an individual is to function independently.

CHAPTER
3

Functions of the Cerebral Cortex

To assess a dysfunction and localize it within the cerebral cortex, it is necessary to have a thorough understanding of normal cortical functions. During the last century numerous studies have indicated that discrete anatomical areas of the cerebral cortex, as described in the previous chapter, are involved in specific functions. Studies of how brain damage affects behavior, as well as examination of the effects of electrical stimulation during surgery, have provided information that has become a foundation for localization maps. These localization maps originated by assigning specific motor and sensory functions to discrete cortical areas. The French physician, Paul Broca, was the first to report case studies indicating that functions were localized in the cerebral cortex. He made postmortem examinations of two patients who had right hemiplegia with aphasia. Broca's findings, reported in 1861, revealed a serious deterioration of brain tissue in a specific location of the left hemisphere. On the basis of his findings, Broca concluded that speech function was located in this particular region of the brain (Geschwind, 1979a and b; Kandel, 1985c; Lassen et al., 1978; Springer and Deutsch, 1981). He also concluded that a relationship existed between handedness and speech, suggesting that manual dexterity and speech were features of the left hemisphere in right-handed people. Broca was a pioneer in terms of introducing functional localization within the brain and the concept of cortical asymmetry (Kandel, 1985c; Springer and Deutsch, 1981).

Following Broca's discoveries, other investigators utilized postmortem examinations of patients with known functional deficits as a result of brain damage to study localization of cortical functions. One of these was Carl Wernicke. He provided major contributions to the localization maps by describing a comprehensive type of aphasia that resulted from localized cortical damage and, later, conduction aphasia resulting from a disruption of a pathway connecting the motor and the receptive language zones of the cortex. Thus Wernicke demonstrated not only that behavior and basic mental functions are mediated by specific cortical locals but also that these specific functional zones are interconnected. More complex mental functions are thus a result of interaction between several of the specific functional locales through interconnecting pathways, according to Kandel, (1985c). Kandel states that Wernicke's ideas provide a basis for localizing specific functions as well as serial and parallel processing in cortical functions.

Other methods also became available to explore and support specific cortical localization of functions. Penfield and his associates used electrical stimulation of the cerebral cortex during surgery on epileptic patients. The patients were conscious throughout the stimulation. Thus they were able to indicate verbally how the stimulation affected them, and the characteristics of the response could subsequently be determined. By this method the cortical sensory and motor areas could be mapped in further detail. A map forming a homunculus

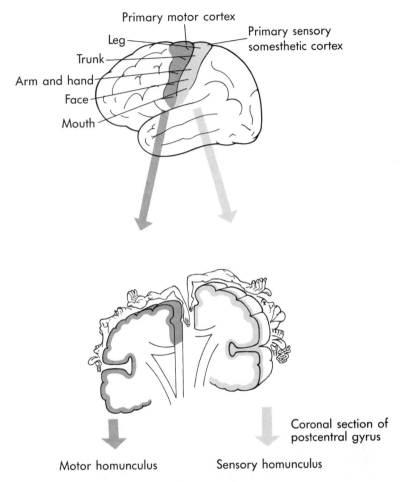

FIG. 3-1 Sensory and motor homunculi of the hemispheres. Topographical distribution within the motor and sensory cortex in the precentral and postcentral gyri. As indicated, different cortical sites within each homunculus can be associated with the body part they represent.

representing topographical distribution of body parts in the sensory and motor cortices, for example, was constructed, as shown in Fig. 3-1 (Kandel, 1985c). Further support for a relation between cortical areas and functions was established by subsequent localization studies performed by similar methods. The findings of the localization studies were later supported by many animal observations (Lassen et al., 1978). Heilman (1983) supported the use of animal studies for information gathering and the generalization of those findings to humans. He argued that, although animal brains may be

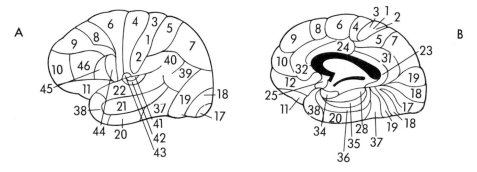

FIG. 3-2 Adaptation of Brodmann's cytoarchitectural map on the lateral, **A**, and medial, **B**, cortical surfaces. Some Brodmann's areas, which are referred to by numbers, are the primary motor area (4), the primary auditory cortex (41 and 42), Wernicke's auditory association cortex (22), the primary visual area (17), visual association area (18 and 19), the primary somesthetic sensory area (1, 2, and 3), the secondary sensory association area (5 and 7), the premotor area (6 and 8), prefrontal area (9, 10, and 46), orbitofrontal cortex (11), and the motor speech area (44 and 45).

organized differently from human brains, some neuronal systems may not be specific to species and that animal studies thus could become a valuable source for expanding knowledge in such instances. Kandel (1979) also supports the use of animal studies to study the human brain and behavior in cases where the appropriate similarities are present, as these could reveal common principles of behavioral patterns.

Others have attempted to divide the cerebral cortex into cytoarchitectural areas based on differences in its six identified molecular layers. These studies were performed in the hope of establishing a basis for structural and functional correlations. The most widely used of such maps is the one of Brodmann's areas, which was published at the turn of the century (Fig. 3-2). However, this method of differentiating between functional areas on the basis of molecular layers has been met with skepticism (Barr and Kiernan, 1983); therefore, reference to such localization will be made in this book only where original literature in the review requires it.

Heilman (1983) stated that several neuropsychological paradigms have been developed over the past two or three decades to study laterality. These paradigms include the delivery of selective stimuli or the production of selective responses in order to determine which hemisphere is processing responses. A tachistoscope, for example, is used to present brief visual stimuli to either visual field, and dichotic auditory tasks are used for simultaneous presentation of stimuli to both ears. According to Heilman, these paradigms are not sufficient to provide an understanding of intrahemispheric neuronal mechanisms. Recent advances in evoked potential studies, and measurements of cerebral blood flow have, on the other hand, turned out to be a promising paradigm with which normal subjects can be studied, according to Heilman (1983). However, he pointed out that activation of an anatomic area does not always reveal what the area is doing.

The information gathered from numerous localization studies can be used to construct functional maps of cerebral activity. These maps are divided according to the nature and complexity of the function that takes place in each area. It is common to consider three levels of functional complexity, which are commonly termed *primary, secondary,* and *tertiary cortical projection areas*. A primary area is concerned with direct processing of primary sensory and motor information. Primary areas include the primary sensory cortex, primary visual cortex, primary auditory cortex, and primary motor cortex. The cells in these areas respond primarily to information from a particular sense modality. Function in the primary areas is fairly symmetrical in both hemispheres; asymmetry increases in secondary and tertiary cortical areas.

All cortical areas, other than the primary ones, are association areas, which, except for the motor association cortex, receive information from the primary areas and integrate it with information from other areas. The secondary association areas are adjacent to primary cortical areas and connect with them. They are involved in more complex processing aspects of a single sensory or motor function. These areas include the visual association cortex surrounding the primary visual cortex, the auditory association cortex, the somatosensory association area in the superior parietal lobule, and the premotor cortex. The secondary association areas connect with each other and with higher order association areas, as well as with adjacent primary areas.

The tertiary, or higher order, association areas are involved in complex integration of information from many different cortical areas. There are three of these higher order cortical association areas: the prefrontal cortex, the limbic cortex, and the parieto-temporal-occipital cortex. The prefrontal association cortex is involved in complex motor functions. The limbic association cortex was described in the previous chapter on gross anatomy as the limbic cortex. As indicated earlier, it includes the orbitofrontal cortex in the frontal lobe, the temporal pole, the parahippocampal gyrus, and the cingulate gyrus. This area is concerned with memory as well as motivation and emotional aspects of behavior. The parieto-temporal-occipital cortex on the border of these three lobes is involved with complex sensory functions based on information from two or more of the secondary association areas of the three lobes. Fig. 3-3 illustrates functional organization of the cerebral cortex. Thus, there are connections between the secondary and tertiary association areas as well as between the different tertiary areas, (Barr and Kiernan, 1983; Kaupfermann, 1985a; Walsh, 1987). The various fiber connections between cortical areas were reviewed in Chapter 2.

From the preceding discussion it is evident that the localization of functions is not synonymous with the isolation of distinct functional areas. Luria (1973) differentiates between two definitions of *function:* it can refer to a function of a particular organ or cell, and it can also refer to a functional process that is concerned with the integration of information from many different areas. The sense of a functional process is in agreement with Kaupfermann's (1985a) view of the localization of functions. In his view, some localizable areas are more concerned with a particular kind of function than others; however, most functions are based on integrated action from different locales. In addition to the importance of information obtained from localization theorists, Luria (1980) gives additional credit to those he calls *antilocalizationists* (p. 19) for their contribution to knowledge development. He points out that although the brain is a highly

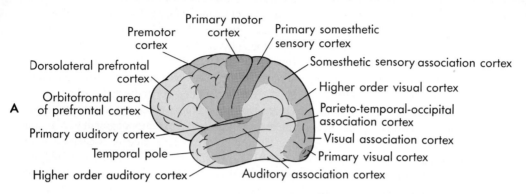

A

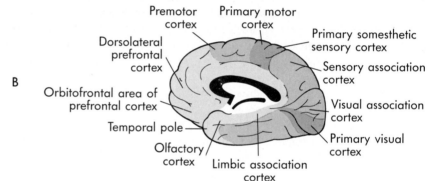

B

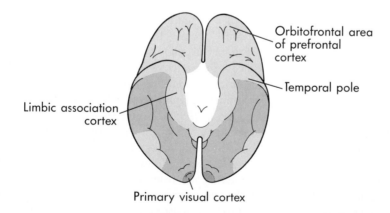

C

FIG. 3-3 Functional organization of the cerebral cortex. **A,** Lateral surface. **B,** Medial surface. **C,** Inferior surface. The different shades refer to primary, secondary, and tertiary functional areas of the cortex.

differentiated organ, it always functions as a whole. Further, its plasticity limits the degree to which functions can be localized in discrete areas. However, as Kandel (1985a) points out, neuroanatomy provides us with a "functional guide to localization" (p. 11). This guide is a mapping of behavior that can be used in the clinical examination of patients' behavioral performance to make inferences regarding the localization of the difficulties causing abnormal behavioral performance. This fundamental tenet and the following literature review are the basis for designing a guide for localizing dysfunctions that result in impaired functional performance during primary activities of daily living, as stated in the Introduction.

In summary, much of the knowledge about functional localization within the human cerebral cortex is derived from clinical observations of patients who have either had pathological cortical damage or lesions due to brain surgery performed as a remedy for neurological or behavioral disorders. Additional information has been provided by studies of primates, in which the effects of experimental damage were observed. A number of different imaging techniques have been developed, some of which are being used to study functional localization within the brain, such as the blood-flow measures of Lassen et al. (1978), and Duffy's (1985) brain mapping. The remainder of this section reviews the literature on functional localization within the brain. The traditional method of classifying behavioral information by lobes will be used.

FUNCTIONS OF THE FRONTAL LOBES

By using the categories of primary cortical areas and association areas mentioned previously, the frontal lobes can be divided into three areas: the primary motor cortex, the premotor cortex, and the prefrontal cortex. The flow of information in the frontal lobes or anterior cortex is from the tertiary association areas in the prefrontal cortex, through the secondary association area in the premotor cortex, to the primary motor area or cortex, contrary to what happens in the three lobes of the posterior

cortex. Each of these frontal areas can then be subdivided into different functional areas. According to Daube and Sandok's (1978) review of functional anatomy, the frontal lobes have seven functional areas: the primary motor cortex, the premotor cortex, the supplementary motor cortex, the frontal eye field, the motor speech area, the prefrontal cortex, and the orbitofrontal cortex (Fig. 3-4). Luria (1973) postulates that the frontal lobes are "responsible for the programming, regulation, and verification of human activity" (p. 187), including memory and intellectual functions, in addition to the execution of motor responses.

The primary motor cortex

According to Barr and Kiernan's review (1983), the primary motor cortex receives input from the premotor cortex and somesthetic cortex, as well as the ventral lateral and ventral anterior nuclei of the thalamus. Further, they reported that this area gives rise to about 60% of the motor fibers in the pyramidal tract. It is concerned with muscle contraction, mainly on the opposite side of the body and is responsible for the execution of movement and the maintenance of simple movements. In the primary motor area, most of the body is mapped; the body is inverted on this map as illustrated previously (Barr and Kiernan, 1983; Geschwind, 1979a and b).

The premotor cortex

The premotor cortex, anterior to the primary motor area, receives fibers from the ventral lateral and ventral anterior nuclei of the thalamus in addition to connecting with the other cortical areas (Barr and Kiernan, 1983). It has close connections with secondary sensory areas (Kaupfermann, 1985a) and gives rise to fiber pathways to the red nucleus, caudate nucleus, and reticular formation. These fibers coordinate movement and control gross or postural movements (Daube and Sandok, 1978). It also contributes to motor function by influencing the primary motor cortex as it develops programs for the motor routines necessary for skilled voluntary action; thus, it is important for motor sequences.

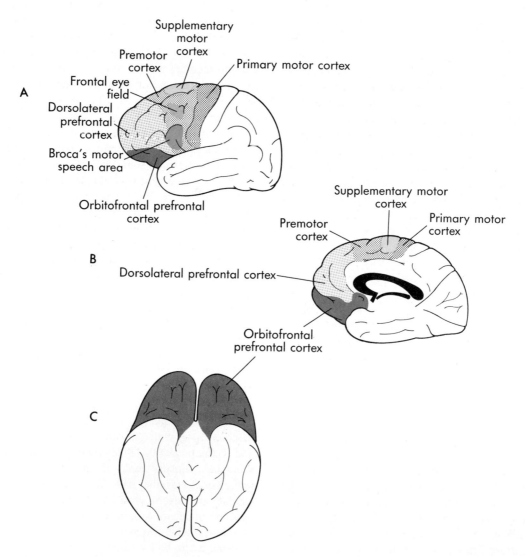

FIG. 3-4 Functional areas of the frontal lobe. **A,** Lateral surface. **B,** Medial surface. **C,** Inferior surface.

This contribution occurs both when a new program is formed as well as when previously established programs are altered. The premotor area, therefore, programs skilled motor activity and, in turn, directs the primary motor area in its execution (Barr and Kiernan, 1983).

The supplementary motor cortex

The supplementary motor cortex is located in front of the motor area on the medial side of the hemisphere (Barr and Kiernan, 1983; Daube and Sandok, 1978). It is a continuation of the lateral premotor cortex described previously. According to Stuss and Benson's (1986) review of the frontal lobes, this area seems to provide the drive for the initiation of movements, rather than being involved in the execution of movements. It is thought to coordinate internal needs with external demands in order to initiate motor programs. This coordination refers to both new and previously established programs, including motor speech. According to Barr and Kiernan, however, it may contribute to the upper motor neuron execution of motion.

The frontal eye field and the motor speech area

The frontal eye field, located anterior to the premotor area, is concerned with voluntary eye movements on the opposite side of the stimulation. The motor speech area is located in the inferior frontal gyrus of the left cerebral hemisphere. It controls the programming of speech (Daube and Sandok, 1978). This area receives numerous connections from the temporal and parietal lobes via pathways in the cingulum and the superior longitudinal (arcuate) fasciculus (Barr and Kiernan, 1983; Netter, 1983), thus gaining access to pertinent sensory experience.

The prefrontal cortex

The prefrontal cortex, or the tertiary cortical areas of the frontal lobe, can be divided into two functional areas. These are the dorsolateral frontal cortex, which is a part of the frontal association area, and the orbitofrontal cortex at the base and medial aspect of the frontal lobe. The orbitofrontal cortex is considered a tertiary association cortex of the limbic system, as indicated in the previous section. According to Luria (1980), in addition to being phylogenetically young, the prefrontal cortex takes longer to mature ontogenetically and to myelinize than other cortical areas. In addition to being the last to develop, these areas are more vulnerable than others to functional disturbances. Due to the late development, these areas are unique in the richness of their connections to all other cortical parts (see Chapter 2 for corticocortical connections) and to subcortical structures, including the brain stem, reticular formation, hypothalamus, and thalamus (Luria, 1973; Luria, 1980; Walsh, 1987). The prefrontal cortex is concerned with aspects of memory, emotion, and intellectual functions (Daube and Sandok, 1978). It monitors and controls behavior through higher mental functions, such as judgment and foresight (Barr and Kiernan, 1983). According to Luria (1973, 1980) the prefrontal cortex is important in the maintenance and control of cortical tone. It integrates information, both from the individual and the outside environment, and subsequently regulates the behavior of the organism according to the outcome of its actions. The prefrontal areas also select the appropriate responses among available possibilities. Thus, these areas regulate higher forms of organized conscious activity, be it voluntary movement, memory, or cognition.

Luria (1980) has described the way in which internal speech aids in monitoring the course of action by self-regulation throughout the performance of voluntary activity. According to him, action is first compared with the original plan. The results of this comparison are identified, and apparent errors are corrected. Subsequently, performance is either discontinued, or if the aim has not been achieved, activity is resumed. During this process, irrelevant actions that do not relate to the motor act are inhibited. The frontal lobes affect all complex forms of activity in this way. Thus, as stated by Walsh (1987) in his review of neuropsychology, in order for an activity sequence to be smooth and effective, continuous monitoring through feedback is essential, and adjustments need to be made according to the feedback. According to this review, this process also applies to thought processes, as thinking is considered to be a form of problem-solving behavior. Thinking involves the integration of events in time and space; it includes exploration, the search for a solution, testing possible solutions, comparison to previous memories, and an appropriate response in the form of action.

Ayres (1985), in her excellent review of developmental dyspraxia and adult onset apraxia, describes praxis as "one of the most critical links between brain and behavior" (p. 1). According to her, "Praxis is a uniquely human skill that enables us to interact effectively with the physical world" (p. 1). It serves the same role in the physical world as speech does in the social world; that is, it allows interactions and transactions. She goes on to describe the common features of speech and praxis, including integration of sensory input, planning, and motor expression. Ideation, or the generation of an idea, as well as concept formation are important components of praxis. Thus, the individual needs to know not only how to perform, but also what to do in order to perform. Ideation requires choice of an action plan, conceptual organization of the anticipated actions, and correct sequencing of the actions. In addition to organization and sequencing, the timing of the actions becomes important for successful performance. All these components of praxis are important in daily activities. Further, although praxis is commonly used for referral to motoric output, components common to praxis are important to all behavioral organization (Ayres, 1985). Many of these components are functions of the frontal lobes, including ideation, coordination of incoming information with memory traces stored in different cortical areas, planning, organization, sequencing, and timing of actions. Thus the function of the frontal lobes is crucial for segmental organization of praxis, as well as behavior in general, regardless of motor output.

Returning to the differentiation of the func-

tional areas of the prefrontal cortex, the dorsolateral cortex, or the prefrontal association cortex, has numerous connections to other cortical and subcortical areas, as mentioned previously, particularly the higher order sensory cortex. Thus the more abstract sensory information and perceptions affect the planning that takes place in the dorsolateral area (Kaupfermann, 1985a). The dorsolateral cortex is important in initiating and planning action. According to Walsh (1987), intellectual activity seems to be more associated with dorsolateral activity than with activity in the orbitofrontal areas. The orbitofrontal cortex houses functions that are important to consciousness or arousal; it contributes to the regulation of cortical activation, selectivity of functions, personality, emotions, and memory (Luria, 1980).

According to Barr and Kiernan (1983), memory traces are laid down in the different association areas throughout the cortex, over the years. These engrams, which probably produce molecular changes in the neurons involved, form the basis of learning at an intellectual level. Barr and Kiernan further state that the extensive connections throughout cortex permit memory traces to be combined in order to form ideas and allow abstract thinking. As stated earlier, the prefrontal cortex plays the role of an integrator in combining these memories and forming ideas. Table 3-1 summarizes the functions of the frontal lobes.

In summary, the frontal lobes are concerned with the execution of movement, motor control, and planning. They are also concerned with higher mental functions, such as intellectual functions, memory, and emotion. These functions are, according to Stuss and Benson (1983), subcomponents of personality, or the "sum of characteristics or qualities that make an individual a unique self and intelligent being" (p. 115).

FUNCTIONS OF THE PARIETAL LOBES

The parietal lobes have three functional areas that can be classified as primary, secondary, and tertiary zones on the basis of functional complexity (see Fig. 3-3). These are the primary sensory area, the

TABLE 3-1 Functions of the Frontal Lobes

Functional area	Location	Role	Direction of information flow within cortex
Primary motor area	Precentral gyrus	Execution of motor movement	
			↑
Secondary association area	Premotor cortex	Planning and programming of movement Sequencing and organization of movement	
	Frontal eye field (bilateral)	Voluntary eye movements	
	Broca's area in left inferior frontal gyrus	Programming of motor speech	
	Supplementary motor area (bilateral)	Intention of movement	
			↑
Tertiary association area	Prefrontal cortex	Ideation Concept formation Sequencing, timing, and organization of action and behavior Initiation and planning of action Judgment Abstract thought Memory Intellectual functions Emotion	

superior parietal lobule, and the inferior parietal lobule, respectively. The flow of information during neuronal processing is classic for the posterior cortex, that is, from the primary sensory area via the secondary functional area in the superior parietal lobule to the tertiary functional area in the inferior parietal lobule.

The primary sensory area

The primary sensory cortex, situated in the postcentral gyrus, is the primary receiving area for sensation. Fig. 3-1 showed the topographical distribution of sensory fibers in the primary sensory cortex. Each hemisphere receives sensory fibers, mainly from the contralateral body side. Areas are represented according to their sensitivity, where sensitive areas have larger topographical representation than less sensitive areas. The body is represented as inverted on this map. It should be noted that neither the primary sensory nor primary motor cortices have purely sensory or motor functions: there is some functional overlap between these two areas. The primary sensory cortex receives fibers from the thalamus. Its role is the detection of fine touch, proprioception, and kinesthesia. Electrical studies have indicated localized feelings of numbness and tingling sensations depending on the placement of the electrical stimulation.

The superior parietal lobule

The secondary area in the parietal lobe, the sensory or somesthetic association cortex, situated mainly in the superior parietal lobule, is responsible for integrating functions from multiple sensory sources (Barr and Kiernan, 1983; Daube and Sandok, 1978; Geschwind, 1979a and b; Werner, 1980). The sensory association cortex of the parietal lobes receives input from the primary sensory cortex. It also has reciprocal connections with nuclei in the thalamus (Barr and Kiernan, 1983) and with the supplementary motor cortex in the frontal lobe (Ghez, 1985). According to Daube and Sandok (1978) it "coordinates, integrates, and refines the perception of the external sensory input" (p. 392). It deals mainly with discriminative aspects of tactile sensation. These include tactile localization, and stereognosis, or the identification of objects by tactile discrimination based on size, shape, and texture (Daube and Sandok, 1978; Williams and Warwick, 1980).

The inferior parietal lobule

The inferior parietal lobe is a part of the posterior tertiary area, which combines information from the three posterior lobes: the parietal lobe, the temporal lobe, and the occipital lobe (Luria, 1980). The function of this tertiary area is thus complex, and according to Barr and Kiernan (1983), it is difficult to analyze it on the basis of input, output, and intrinsic organization. Complex functions that require the integration of the functions of different cortical areas take place in this zone. These include gnosis, praxis, and body image, which have been associated with the parietal part of the zone.

Gnosis refers to recognition beyond reception of sensory input, be it tactile, visual, or auditory (Bauer and Rubens, 1985). *Praxis*, as previously mentioned, includes, according to Ayres (1985), ideation, concept formation, planning, and motor execution. In terms of praxis, Heilman and Rothi (1985) hypothesized that the association cortex in the left parietal lobe contains motor engrams, which these authors call *visuokinesthetic motor engrams*. They include formulas for programs of movement sequences based on time and space that

are needed to perform skilled learned acts. According to Heilman and Rothi "one must place particular body parts in certain spatial positions in a specific order at specific times" (p. 135) in order to perform such acts. The nature of the act, as well as the shape, size, and position of the object with which body interaction is intended, determine the necessary spatial positions of the body and the required sequence of movements over time. This process requires integration from the parietal and occipital lobes, along with feedback about how the movement executed previously by the frontal lobes on the basis of such integration affected the environment. This process is in agreement with Ayres' (1985) view of praxic functions.

The *body scheme* defined by Siev, Freishtat, and Zoltan (1985) as a postural model related to the perception of one's own body position and the relationship of one's body parts is also based on the integration of visual and somesthetic information as well as language and feedback from the interaction of the body with the environment. (Table 3-2 displays the functions of the parietal lobe.)

In addition to the functions mentioned above, a part of Wernicke's speech area, or the auditory association cortex, which has to do with the interpretation of auditory stimuli, is situated within the left parietal lobe (Geschwind, 1979a and b; Williams and Warwick, 1980). It lies between the primary auditory cortex and the angular gyrus. The angular gyrus is thought to mediate between the visual and auditory centers of the brain, according to Geschwind (1979a and b). According to Kaupfermann's review of cortical function (1985a), studies have indicated that the right parietal cortical area, parallel to Wernicke's area on the left side, plays a role in nonsyntactic speech functions. These functions are concerned with interpretation of tone, loudness, and timing of words as well as modulating sound and verbal output.

FUNCTIONS OF THE OCCIPITAL LOBES

The occipital lobes have a primary sensory area and a secondary visual association cortex. The border area of the occipital, temporal, and parietal

TABLE 3-2 Functions of the Parietal Lobes

Functional area	Location	Role	Direction of information flow within cortex
Primary sensory area	Postcentral gyrus	Fine touch, sensation Proprioception Kinesthesia	↓
Secondary sensory association area	Superior parietal lobule	Coordination, integration, and refinement of sensory input Tactile localization and discrimination Stereognosis	↓

Tertiary association area	Inferior parietal lobule	Gnosis: Recognition of received tactile, visual, or auditory input
		Praxis: Storage of programs or visuokinesthetic motor engrams necessary for motor sequences
		Body scheme: Postural model of body, body-parts, and their relation to the environment
		Language:
		    Comprehension of words, interpretation of tones, loudness and timing of words
		    Sound modulation	

lobes contributes to the posterior tertiary association zone mentioned previously. The primary visual areas are located on the medial side of the occipital lobes around the calcarine fissure, identified as Brodmann's area 17 (Daube and Sandok, 1978). The images from the right half of space in both eyes are transmitted to the left visual cortex, whereas the left visual field from both eyes goes to the right hemisphere.

Adjacent to the primary visual areas are the visual association areas (Brodmann's areas 18 and 19), which synthesize visual impressions, integrate them with other sensory modalities, and aid in the formation of visual memory traces (Daube and Sandok, 1978). The area where parietal and occipital lobes meet is important for the perception of spatial relationships, including prepositional construction in language comprehension and speech (Luria,

1980). The role of this area in contributing to the formation of visuokinesthetic motor engrams has already been discussed in the section on the parietal lobes (Table 3-3) reviews the functions of the occipital lobes.

FUNCTIONS OF THE TEMPORAL LOBES

The temporal lobes have primary, secondary, and tertiary functional areas. They contain the primary auditory cortex, located in the superior temporal gyrus, or Heschl's gyrus (Brodmann's areas 41 and 42), which is concerned with the reception of auditory information (Daube and Sandok, 1978; Netter, 1983). Each auditory cortex receives input from both ears, but the connections to the contralateral side are stronger than the ipsilateral connections (Geschwind, 1979a and b). The dominant

TABLE 3-3 Functions of the Occipital Lobes

Functional area	Location	Role	Direction of information flow within cortex
Primary sensory area	Calcarine fissure	Visual reception	↓
Visual association area	Brodmann's areas 18 and 19	Synthesis and integration of visual information Perception of visual spatial relationships Formation of visual memory traces Prepositional construction in language comprehension and speech Formation of visuokinesthetic motor engrams	

temporal lobe plays a primary role in language functions (Daube and Sandok, 1978; Netter, 1983). The auditory association area surrounding the primary auditory cortex, Wernicke's area (Brodmann's area 22) is concerned with the interpretation of auditory information. Wernicke's area stretches over to the tertiary association cortex in the temporal, parietal, and occipital lobes. As mentioned earlier, Wernicke's area on the left side is involved with language comprehension, whereas its counterpart on the right side is concerned with tones, loudness, sound modulation, and timing, including the perception of music (Kaupfermann, 1985a). The angular gyrus probably mediates between visual and auditory centers of the left side of the brain (Geschwind, 1979a and b), and plays a role in language functions such as the naming of objects (Luria, 1980). In addition to language processing, the tertiary association area in the temporal lobe is concerned with some aspects of pattern recognition and higher visual coordination (Geschwind, 1979a and b).

The anterior part of the temporal lobe, the temporal pole, is a tertiary functional area and a part of the limbic association cortex. It is concerned with emotional behavior, as are the frontal lobes (Netter, 1983). According to Barr and Kiernan

(1983), the temporal lobes seem to have properties related to the highest level of brain function. They stated in their anatomical review that electrical stimulation of this region performed on conscious subjects has elicited recall of objects seen and music heard. It has further elicited other experiences in the past, indicating that this area plays a role in both recent and remote memory.

According to Kaupfermann (1985a), the tertiary association area in the temporal lobe is involved in learning and memory of higher order visual tasks and auditory patterns. Stimulation of the auditory cortex can even produce auditory illusions and hallucinations. Kaupfermann states that the inferior temporal lobe includes a higher order visual region that is concerned with the rate of learning visual tasks. Similarly the superior temporal cortex is involved with learning auditory patterns. The hippocampus, an extension of the parahippocampal gyrus in the tertiary limbic association area on the medial side of the temporal lobe, is important in long-term memorization. The right hemisphere is important for remembering patterns of spatial input, whereas the left side is involved in verbal memory (Geschwind, 1979a and b; Kaupfermann, 1985a). According to Kaupfermann, electrical stimulation of the anterior medial tem-

TABLE 3-4 Functions of the Temporal Lobes

Functional area	Location	Role	Direction of information flow within cortex
Primary temporal area	Superior temporal gyrus	Auditory reception	↓
Secondary association area	Wernicke's area	Language comprehension Sound modulation Perception of music Memory	
Tertiary association area	Temporal pole, para-hippocampus	Memory Learning of higher order visual tasks and auditory patterns Emotion Motivation Personality	↓

poral areas elicits emotional responses, including fear. Table 3-4 summarizes the functions of the temporal lobes.

Walsh (1987) states that the temporal lobes, because of their complicated connections with all the other cortical areas, play an important role in the integration of aspects essential to emotion and motivation. They further state that because of these connections, and connections to the limbic system, its limitations, both functional and morphological, are not clear.

FUNCTIONS OF THE LIMBIC LOBES

The limbic lobes are not discussed separately in this review. Their function is related to the medial aspect of the frontal and temporal lobes, as stated earlier. According to Daube and Sandok (1978), the limbic lobes are an integral part of the limbic system. They stated that the limbic lobes play an integral role in visceral and emotional activity. Further, according to them, the function of these lobes is more related to the function of subcortical structures than are the functions of other cortical areas.

Damasio and Van Hoesen (1983) stated that the limbic lobes seem to project to the association areas of the cerebral cortex in addition to the cortical and subcortical areas of the motor system. Similarly, a large proportion of the input to the limbic structures seemed, according to these researchers, to be from the cerebral cortex, particularly the association areas, as stated earlier. This input may thus contribute to memory, which is stored in the association areas. They further state that there seems to be structural support for connections between the hypothalamus and the subcortical limbic system. As the hypothalamus is an important control center for endocrine and automatic nervous activities, this structural link may have important influences on cortical function. Damasio and Van Hoesen further stated that the limbic system seems to make an important contribution to most activities that take place through discrete connections within the CNS. They stated also that the influence on functional areas within the brain and on symptoms seemed to be specifically affect-related. In addition, they claimed structural evidence for the selectivity in the limbic system output.

It should be kept in mind that the limbic system is very complex in terms of structure and function. Investigation methods that record electrical activity from the brain, such as computerized mapping of EEG, have detected only surface cortical potentials, not potentials from deeper or medial surfaces. Further, studies based on other imaging techniques, including blood-flow measures, have revealed more information on cortical activity than detailed subcortical activity because of technological difficulties. These limitations of functional investigation should be kept in mind.

After reviewing the different cortical lobes, keeping in mind the classification of primary, secondary, and tertiary functional areas, it is timely to remind the reader of the various connections between all of these areas as outlined in Chapter 2. All of the association areas in the three posterior lobes send information to the frontal association areas via the cingulum of the limbic system. A result of this, as stated by Barr and Kiernan (1983), is that "Complex and flexible behavioral patterns are formulated on the basis of experience, emotional tones are added, and overt expression may follow through the motor system" (p. 236).

FUNCTIONS OF THE THALAMUS AND THE HYPOTHALAMUS

According to Barr and Kiernan (1983), the thalamus is composed of a group of nuclei with different functions. Some of these nuclei receive incoming sensory information and transmit it to pertinent cortical areas. Some of the thalamic nuclei are important in pathways of the motor system, including the motor cortex and subcortical motor structures. Still other thalamic nuclei are concerned with complex mental processes and contribute to emotion and memory. A detailed discussion of functions of the thalamus is beyond the scope of this book, as are the functions of other subcortical structures, such as the cerebellum, the basal ganglia, and the brain stem.

According to Barr and Kiernan (1983), the hypothalamus plays an important role in maintaining homeostasis, or constant internal environment. Its autonomic control functions include regulation of body temperature and food intake, according to Barr and Kiernan (1983). It also contributes to emotional experience and related behavior, based on responses to emotional behavior. According to Kaupfermann (1985b), the hypothalamus is a control unit for the endocrine system. This control can be performed either by a direct or an indirect process. Neuroendocrine products are secreted into the circulation directly through the pituitary gland. Hypothalamic regulating hormones can also control the flow of anterior pituitary hormones into the general circulation in an indirect way, by secreting regulating hormones into the blood vessels that serve the anterior pituitary. The vascular connection of the hypothalamus to the pituitary is thus very important, as it mediates hormonal information from the former to the latter. The hypothalamus contains neurons with a dual function: they are capable of transmitting electrical information as well as secreting endocrine products into the blood stream. Various neurohormones or precursor peptides are synthesized in the cell bodies of these neurons. They are subsequently packaged in neurosecretory vesicles and transferred to the axon terminals for storage, awaiting stimulation for secretion. There are peptide neurohormones that control most hormones of the anterior pituitary. According to Kaupfermann, some hormones circulate extensively through the brain. However, only a few neurons may have receptors for a particular hormone; thus, while some hormones are in general circulation, specific hormonal action may affect only a restricted neuronal population. Kaupfermann further states that these hormonal effects are thought to play a role in modifying mood and behavioral states. They can also provide signals that result in complex motor patterns. Hormones and peptides are thought to be important in learning, and they may contribute to the arousal state of animals (Kaupfermann, 1985b).

FUNCTIONS OF THE CORPUS CALLOSUM

As stated in the section on the anatomy of the cerebral cortex, the cortical fiber connections play a crucial role in the functions of the brain. Therefore, the function of the corpus callosum, the largest bundle of such connections, is further outlined in this section.

Sperry (1964), in his review of the corpus callosum, reported that the commisural fibers, described previously, "form reciprocal connections between parallel centers in the two hemispheres" (p. 42). He considers the corpus callosum to be the most important of these fiber bridges. Although each hemisphere controls functions on the contralateral body side, to a considerable degree each hemisphere has a potential function as the "whole brain" (p. 42) according to Sperry. Because of this apparent ability, it had for a long time been difficult to support the idea that the corpus callosum had functional, as compared to purely structural, importance.

Sperry (1964) studied the behavior of people with split brains due to commisurotomy, or severance of the corpus callosum. Using specifically designed tests, he found that the split brain did not function in the same way as a normal brain does. According to Sperry, the training of one hemisphere did not transfer over to the other hemisphere. Further when different stimuli and learning procedures were presented to each hemisphere, the patients learned different solutions to the same experimental problems.

Similarly, in animal studies, Sperry (1964) reported that learning and memory transferred readily from one hemisphere to the other in animals with an intact corpus callosum. However, there was a failure of transfer when the corpus callosum was severed. Thus, when the two hemispheres received different training, there was conflict when the corpus callosum was intact, whereas no sign of conflict was observed when the corpus callosum was cut. Sperry concluded that the corpus callosum was important in the sharing of incoming information,

memory, and learning experiences of the two hemispheres. Thus one would expect it to contribute to the brain's ability to function as a "whole." On the other hand, when the corpus callosum is lesioned, learning that takes place in one hemisphere appears to be inaccessible to the other.

In humans, memory relating to language functions seems to be in the dominant hemisphere. Thus, a right-handed person with a lesion in the corpus callosum may adequately perform functions of the left hemisphere, which controls the right side of the body, but have difficulties in performance on the left side of the body when a task requires language functions and judgment, according to Sperry (1964). That person will also have difficulty in reading material presented in the left visual field, writing with the left hand, and carrying out commands with the left body side. The same person will not be able to name or describe objects held in the left hand when blindfolded, nor to describe things in the left half of the visual field. Sperry emphasized that most of the functional impairment resulting from disconnection of the hemispheres due to a lesion in the corpus callosum is not manifested in daily activities. Specific testing conditions, such as "blindfolding the subject," restricting movements to one hand, or "using quick-flash projection" (p. 47) to confine vision to one visual halffield, are required to detect dysfunctions.

Sperry (1964) proposed that attention played a role in performance. Thus, active attention required by a learning task presented to one hemisphere would, according to Sperry, dominate and interfere with the attention of the other hemisphere, although there was no apparent connection between the activities presented to each hemisphere.

Sperry's article emphasized the importance of functional connections within the CNS for optimal cerebral function. The importance of these and other connections will become more evident in the review of the processing of cerebral functions in the next section. In addition to the deficits mentioned above, one would question whether activities such as motor praxis would not be affected by lesions of the corpus callosum. According to Geschwind (1975) and Heilman and Rothi (1985), the motor engrams for movement are stored in the left hemisphere; thus severing the corpus callosum should deprive the right hemisphere of access to those memory engrams.

FUNCTIONAL HEMISPHERIC ASYMMETRY

According to the literature review regarding the functions of the different lobes, functional asymmetries between the two hemispheres do exist, as previously mentioned. These asymmetries are summarized more specifically in this section, which also reviews lateralization and the concept of cerebral dominance. As does functional location in general, laterality depends upon different factors. According to the excellent review of cerebral lateralization by Geschwind and Galaburda (1985, 1987), these factors are related to both genetic and environmental influences. Environmental influences can occur during fetal and early postnatal development. Damage to a particular area during pregnancy leads to excessive neuronal growth in adjacent areas in the same hemisphere, as well as in homologous areas in the opposite hemisphere, affecting functional location. Apparently the environmental factors with the strongest effects on neuronal development and the subsequent lateralization of function are hormonal and chemical agents, which have different consequences depending on the developmental stage upon which they act, keeping in mind that different functions have different "critical periods." The male sex hormone, testosterone, has especially been linked to impaired neuronal migration. According to Geschwind and Galaburda (1987), the left hemisphere develops more slowly than the right hemisphere, and these more slowly developing areas reach larger size in the mature brain than corresponding areas on the right side. Since the regions in the right hemisphere develop faster than homologous regions on the left side, harmful environmental factors are more likely to affect the development of the left brain.

Kimura (1973), in her review on asymmetry of the human brain, stated that each cerebral hemisphere is lateralized in terms of motor and sensory functions. The right hemisphere thus receives sensory information from the left, or contralateral, body side, and controls that side motorically. The opposite holds for the left hemisphere, in terms of sensory and motor functions. The auditory system, as stated earlier, is less crossed; each hemisphere receives bilateral input. However, according to Kimura, the crossed pathways are stronger than the uncrossed ones. Kimura states that the two hemispheres are interconnected by commissural nervous pathways, and agrees with Sperry (1964) that these pathways play an important role in coordinating the activities of the hemispheres.

Kimura states that the left hemisphere is superior in processing visual and verbal material, as well as spoken sounds, based on her observation of better responses when stimuli are presented to the right visual field and right ear, as compared to the left. The right hemisphere, on the other hand, is superior for the perception of some "fundamental visual processes" (p. 72), such as dot location and geometric forms. She also reported an asymmetry in tactile perception, having found that blind people perceive Braille patterns more rapidly with the left hand as compared to the right hand. She reported that the left arm is more accurate on tests of point localization with vision occluded, as compared to the right arm.

Speech is a function of the left hemisphere, according to Kimura. She suggested an overlap between language functions and functions controlling certain kinds of manual activity. She concluded that the left hemisphere might be particularly well suited for the execution of specific motor activity that partially relies on communication.

Geschwind and Galaburda (1987) emphasize that handedness, referring to the superior ability of one hemisphere to acquire programs necessary for executing unimanual fine motor functions, and language are dependent on different "neural substrates" (p. 69) and that these substrates might develop at different time periods. However, according to these authors, handedness and language are both functions of the left hemisphere under normal circumstances. Geschwind and Galaburda further differentiate between two kinds of motor learning and subsequently two separate neural substrates for motor movements. In addition to fine motor movements controlled by the contralateral pyramidal system, there is an axial movement system, which is concerned with the acquisition of programs for coordinated trunk and gross limb movements and for control of proximal girdle movements. The outflow from this system is represented by several brain areas that are bilaterally distributed. These authors consider the programs for axial learning to be located in the left cortex under normal circumstances, like many other complex cortical functions.

Memory functions are also reported to be lateralized, according to Butters and Miliotis (1985). They reported that the right temporal lobe is involved with the processing of nonverbal material, including geometric patterns and recognition of tonal patterns, as well as the learning of visual and tactile mazes. The left temporal lobe, on the other hand, is involved in memory and the learning of verbal material. Geschwind (1979a) supported this view.

Geschwind and Galaburda (1987) emphasize the role of the right hemisphere in survival. According to them, this hemisphere is dominant in certain spatial functions, including the orientation of body within the external space. It also plays an important role in emotional functions, attention, and certain automatic activities.

Geschwind and Galaburda (1987) speak of a "left-shift" factor in terms of cerebral "dominance" for language functions and certain motor skills. According to them, genetic influences are responsible for this shift, but many nongenetic components also play a significant role. The majority of people, according to these authors, exhibit the "standard dominance pattern" (p. 70), of left-hemisphere superiority for language and hand dominance; however, the "degree" (p. 67) of dominance varies between persons. Further, 30% of the population have what Geschwind and Galaburda have termed *random dominance* (p. 70) for either language or handedness, and occasionally for both. "Anomalous dominance" (p. 70) or diminished superiority of the left hemisphere in language and handedness functions, can be caused by pathological lesions, but more often they are related to delayed development of the left hemisphere. This usually results in more symmetrical brain function, and sometimes even in reversed function. Because language and handedness are due to different neuronal substrates, and so are pyramidal and axial motor functions, any of these can deviate from the standard left-hemisphere location separately from the others, as the critical periods for each probably differ. The result, according to Geschwind and Galaburda, will be a "mixed dominance," which in the motor system can be manifested by a person who writes with pencil on paper with the hand controlled by the dominant hemisphere for fine motor movements (pyramidal motor system) but uses the other hand to write with chalk on a blackboard, this hand being controlled by the dominant axial motor system. On the basis of the writings of Geschwind and Galaburda one can conclude that handedness is not an either-or phenomenon. Rather it can be considered as a degree of right- or left-sided use along a continuum reaching from strong right handers to strong left handers. The degree of dominance can vary in different neuronal substrates (Exhibit 3-1).

Further, in relation to hemispheric dominance, Geschwind and Galaburda (1987) claim that the classification of the two hemispheres as dominant and nondominant is outdated. Rather, each side is dominant for specific functions. In agreement with Geschwind and Galaburda, I refer to the hemispheres as right and left, rather than in relation to their dominance.

Semmes (1968) presented an interesting view of hemispheric dominance. She linked differences in neuronal organization to different functions of the two hemispheres. According to her, the left hemisphere has a "focal representation of elementary functions" (p. 11). These are the previously

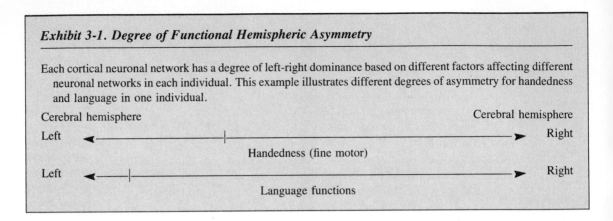

Exhibit 3-1. Degree of Functional Hemispheric Asymmetry

Each cortical neuronal network has a degree of left-right dominance based on different factors affecting different neuronal networks in each individual. This example illustrates different degrees of asymmetry for handedness and language in one individual.

Cerebral hemisphere   Cerebral hemisphere

Left ◄─────────────────────┼───► Right

Handedness (fine motor)

Left ◄──────┼──► Right

Language functions

mentioned language and fine motor functions. The right hemisphere, on the other hand, displays a "diffuse representation of elementary functions" resulting in the integration of dissimilar factors and specialization that requires multimodal functional convergence of, for example, visual, kinesthetic, and vestibular factors. According to Semmes, various spatial abilities depend on these abilities of the right hemisphere. This kind of asymmetrical neuronal processing is reflected in a deficit as a result of a small, crucial lesion in the "focally-organized" left hemisphere, whereas a similar lesion in the "diffusely-organized" right hemisphere will, according to Semmes, have "less or no effect . . . regardless of its location" (p. 19).

Luria (1973) agreed with Semmes (1968) regarding differences in functional organization within the brain. The right hemisphere is, according to him, much less differentiated than the left one. Similarly, he describes the frontal lobes as being much less differentiated than the posterior cortex. In contradiction to Semmes, who argued for the relativitiy of the concept of dominance, Luria labeled the left hemisphere as the dominant one.

Goldberg and Costa (1981) propose an interesting explanation of the reported gross anatomical asymmetry of the hemispheres (see Chapter 3) after an extensive review of the literature including studies which conclude that the right hemisphere has relatively more white matter or long, myelinated fibers and that the left hemisphere has relatively more gray matter or neurons and short, nonmyelinated fibers. They propose that the left hemisphere, possessing more secondary association areas, is concerned with unimodal processing, and that the right hemisphere, possessing more tertiary association cortex, is capable of intermodal integration. They suggest that the right hemisphere, which is better able to deal with informational complexity and with processing the many models of representation within the same cognitive task, is better able to process "novel stimuli" and that the left hemisphere is more capable of storage and utilization of "well-routinized codes." Thus, in terms of acquisition or what Goldberg and Costa call a "new descriptive system" (p. 144), they propose a "right-to-left shift of hemisphere superiority as a function of increased competence with respect to a particular type of processing" (p. 144). Thus they argue against a fixed hemispheral specificity for tasks suggesting a "gradient of relative hemispheral involvement in a wide range of cognitive processes, reflecting the degrees of their routinization" (p. 165). Further Goldberg and Costa support the idea that the right hemisphere is better able to "activate the entire cortex" than the left hemisphere is, based on its extensive interconnections and its greater ability to take over the role of the whole brain.

Bergland (1985), on the basis of his literature review, speaks of different processing patterns for each of the hemispheres. The left brain, according to him, utilizes sequential processing, whereas the right brain seems to process in a parallel fashion, focusing simultaneously on many interrelated things. Thus, Bergland agrees with Semmes that the left brain "considers one thing at a time," whereas "the right brain is committed to patterns" (1985, p. 108): it operates holistically. But Bergland goes further and implies in an interesting way that many of the world's geniuses, for some reason, utilized the "pattern recognizing" hemisphere more than the average person does. According to him, some of these exceptional individuals play a crucial role in evolution and are even responsible for some of the most significant paradigm shifts that have taken place, for example, in medicine and neurology. Geschwind and Galaburda (1987) also favor this view. They state that although some anomalies at the lower end of the curve, such as dyslexia, immunity disorders, and left-handedness, are related to defective neuronal maturation in the left hemisphere, there are superior talents at the upper end of the curve—talents that are not present in right-handed people, including some artistic abilities, some musical abilities, and some talents that are present in mathematically gifted people. However, Bergland does not believe that the "more harmonious use of the right and the left brain" (p. 56) is responsible for superior work; rather, it is the "pattern-dependent sense of beauty in the right brain" (p. 57) that is accountable. According to him this "hidden star" of the mind, referring to a "mental force" that results in "magnificent accomplishments," can only be seen when it is totally dark around it—when there has been injury or anomalous development that results in disability of some kind. This view, although having a different tone from the classical neurological literature, does not seem to disagree with the views of Geschwind and Galaburda (1987) and others who claim that at the time of a lesion, excessive cell death or retarded growth in one cerebral area leads to excessive growth of adjacent areas and contralateral homologous areas.

The cerebral hemispheres have also been reported to be chemically different, on the basis of information from animal studies. Biochemical asymmetries have been related, for example, to the neocortex, hippocampus, and thalamus (Geschwind and Galaburda, 1987). Some neurotransmitters have also been reported to act differently on the two hemispheres.

It is evident that the concept of brain asymmetry includes differences in both functional localization and processing patterns in the two hemispheres. These differences can be related to developmental factors of both a structural and chemical nature. The left hemisphere is specialized in focal functions of language and refined movement, whereas the right hemisphere utilizes holistic patterns and pattern recognition to direct complex spatial functions, as well as basic survival functions such as attention and emotion. The sequencing of maturation in the two hemispheres is thought to be related to their different functional roles, and developmental anomalies can disrupt the classical functional locations within cortex. Such disruption can apparently lead to impaired behavior, but it can also result in extraordinary talents. The difference in functional localization between the two hemispheres is important for attempts to localize dysfunction as well as for the formation of treatment strategies. In addition to lateralized cerebral differences in function of the cerebral cortex (see Exhibit 3-2), sexual differences have been related to brain function. Before moving on to other issues, reports of those differences should be reviewed.

SEX DIFFERENCES AND HANDEDNESS IN CEREBRAL LATERALIZATION

According to Springer and Deutsch's (1981) neuropsychological review of the brain, a variety of evidence suggests that females show greater bilateral representation for verbal and spatial abilities than do males, who display more strongly lateralized functions. According to Geschwind and Galaburda (1987), not only does the left hemisphere develop at a slower rate than the right one, but the male cortex develops at a slower rate than the fe-

---

Exhibit 3-2. Functional Hemispheric Asymmetry

LEFT HEMISPHERE	RIGHT HEMISPHERE
Movement of right body side	Movement of left body side
Processing of somesthetic sensory information from the right body side	Processing of somesthetic sensory information from the left body side (and some bilateral sensory processing)
Visual reception from right visual field	Visual reception from left visual field
Visual verbal processing	Visual spatial processing
Bilateral motor praxis	Contralateral motor praxis
Verbal memory	Nonverbal memory (geometric figures, tonal patterns, visual and tactile spatial information)
Bilateral auditory reception	Bilateral auditory reception
Speech	
Processing of verbal auditory information	Processing of nonverbal auditory information (tonal sequences, loudness, sound modulation)
	Attention to incoming stimuli
	Emotion
Sequential Processing Mechanism ?	**Parallel/Simultaneous Processing**

NOTE: Exhibit is based on hemispheric lateralization in most individuals, although it is recognized that the degree of asymmetry and functional localization of neuronal networks varies in different individuals. Processing comments are based on tradition.

---

male cortex. Thus it seems that the faster the development, the less focal functional location within the brain.

On the basis of developmental studies, Kelly (1985a) reported that steroids affect neuronal organization within the CNS. Prenatal steroids affect both the pattern of neuronal connections, and the responsivity of the CNS. He also claims that sex steroids affect growth differently in males than in females. This difference may affect axonal differentiation rates and subsequently synaptic organization and patterns of neuronal circuitry. Kelly also reported that studies had indicated the previously mentioned potential for bilateral representation of spatial processing in females, this potential lasting longer than in males. Males showed more focal right-hemisphere representation at earlier ages on the same spatial tasks. On the basis of these findings, he suggests that females have a greater cortical plasticity than do males, and that this plasticity lasts longer in females than in males. He supports this view with reports of clinical findings showing

that young females have a greater potential for transferring language functions over to the right hemisphere after a lesion in the left one than do males. This plasticity may also be reflected in the lower incidence in females of developmental disabilities after left hemisphere lesions. Similarly, in adults, the association of verbal functions with left-hemisphere lesions and nonverbal functions with right-hemisphere lesions is much weaker in females than males, suggesting diminished asymmetry of the female cortex.

Earlier researchers have provided information that is reflected in the preceding views. Kimura (1973), for example, in considering male-female differences of cerebral lateralization, reported that males tended to exhibit superiority of the left visual field in some spatial relation tasks. She proposed that the right hemisphere had a greater degree of such specialization, with regard to specific visual-spatial tasks, and that this was more eminent in males than females. She also reported females to have greater "verbal fluency," although this finding did not point to more asymmetry with regard to verbal functions in females. She did, however, point out that speech lateralization might develop earlier in females. This suggestion is consistent with Geschwind and Galaburda's (1987) finding that the female brain may mature faster, at least during pregnancy and early prenatal periods. Kimura concluded that some intellectual functions of the brains of males and females appeared to be differently organized. Kimura's findings thus support the idea of different processing mechanisms in males and females.

Tucker (1976) studied male and female processing differences by EEG analyses during visuospatial tasks. His results showed sex differences in cortical function, including lateralized as well as specific regional differences. On the basis of his findings, Tucker suggested that females used more differentiated functions of the entire hemisphere during visuospatial performances, while males used more focal and specialized functions. Females, for example, used the occipital region of cortex for both complex visual processing and simple visual perception. This study is thus in agreement with the view of sex differences in cerebral lateralization mentioned above.

McGlone's (1978) findings also agree with the previously outlined view of sex differences in cerebral lateralization. She, in agreement with Kelly (1985a), reported that in a comparative study of differences in verbal and nonverbal intellectualized abilities in males versus females, following lateralized lesions only men showed specific verbal or nonverbal deficits that related to which hemisphere was lesioned. Women "had less severe" and "less specific" (p. 126) deficits when compared to men. These findings were found to support the notion that right-handed men had greater cortical asymmetry of function than females. This accounted most clearly for verbal processes, but it also accounted for nonverbal processes.

Piazza (1980) studies sex differences and handedness in hemispheric specialization of verbal and nonverbal dichotic listening and tachistoscopic tasks in 16 subjects. She found that hemispheric specialization was affected by handedness and "familial sinistrality" (p. 163). In agreement with subsequent reports of Geschwind and Galaburda (1987), she reported that left-handedness was associated with lack of right-hemisphere dominance in language and fine motor functions. Thus, either left-hemisphere dominance or bilateral specialization was associated with left-handedness. Speech functions were more lateralized in males, whereas the processing of "nonspeech auditory stimuli" had stronger lateralization in females. However, visual processing was not influenced by sex in this study. Piazza's study thus provided empirical support for sex-linked processing differences.

Hécaen De Agostini and Monzon-Montes (1981) studied the cerebral lateralization of left-handers. They analyzed both verbal and spatial performances of 141 left-handed and 130 right-handed patients who had sustained unilateral hemispheric lesions. Their results confirmed the previously established relation between left-handedness and familial sinistrality, and decreased functional localization within cortex, including language functions. These researchers claimed such relationships to exist in both left- and right-handers, but to a lesser degree in right-handers. However, this type of organization does not exist for spatial functions, according to the researchers.

Hécaen et al. pointed out, in agreement with previously mentioned clinical findings, that left-handers recover language more quickly and more thoroughly than right-handers. They also reported a difference in the scores of right-handers and left-handers, depending on anterior-versus-posterior location of the lesion within the hemisphere. Thus, there seems to be less focal functional representation in the cerebral cortices of left-handed individuals. Unlike some of the previously reviewed authors, Hécaen et al. considered it impossible to determine the influence of sex on cerebral organization, although they acknowledged some influence.

In summary, most of the findings reviewed above suggest the presence of sex differences and effects of handedness on functional organization and neuronal processing within the brain. Males are considered to have more lateralized functions in terms of verbal and spatial abilities, as opposed to greater bilateral representation in females. The findings also suggest that males have more focal and specified brain function, compared to females. These differences have been related to differences in the timing of maturity, the male brain taking longer to develop than the female brain, just as the left hemisphere has been reported to take longer to mature than the right one, which results in a focalized left hemisphere, as compared to a holistic right hemisphere. According to this review, information regarding handedness and gender in relation to cerebral organization is important when considering localization of cerebral dysfunction and processing disturbances. It may also prove to be important for treatment considerations.

SUMMARY

In summary, the frontal lobes are concerned with the execution of movement, motor planning, and control, as well as higher intellectual functions, memory, and emotion. The functions of the parietal lobes include primary somatic sensation and interpretation of that sensation, gnosis, praxis, body scheme, and involvement in language comprehension. The main function of the occipital lobes is processing visual sensations and integrating those sensations. The temporal lobes are concerned with auditory processing of information and its interpretation, as well as memory and some behavioral and emotional aspects. In addition, the corpus callosum plays an important role in communicating information between the hemispheres regarding what is occurring in each one. It, as well as other fiber connections within the CNS, plays a crucial role in processing and the integration of cerebral activity by relaying information between the two hemispheres, the different lobes and different areas within each lobe, as well as the subcortical structures. Most specialized functions of the cerebral hemispheres are lateralized; that is, certain func-

tions seem to be handled more effectively by one side of the brain than the other. Details regarding specialization and lateralization are summarized in the localization table in Chapter 12.

Localization of cerebral function is used in this book for the purpose of simplification. However, specialization of the hemispheres should not be overstated, because many behaviors require that the two hemispheres work together. In addition, behavior often depends on the synchronization of processes in different locations within each hemisphere. In addition to structural and chemical differences between males and females, according to the literature review, males seem to have more specialized cortices than do females, and right-handed individuals have more focal and specialized cerebral function than left-handers. Further, the hemispheres have different schedules for maturity; the left hemisphere takes longer than the right and develops a more focal representation of functions than the right. This leads to structural differences between the hemispheres and may be related to hormonal and chemical effects of CNS development.

Knowledge and understanding of the localization of a lesion that produces specific impairments is important in terms of identifying the problems that interfere with functional performance. It is also important for treatment considerations. Therefore, the Árnadóttir OT-ADL Neurobehavioral Evaluation (A-ONE) instrument was designed to have the potential of making speculations regarding such predictions, keeping in mind the variations in functional location. However, cerebral localization is just a road map showing where certain functions take place. Functions of the brain do not occur in isolation; often many different areas of the CNS contribute to a function. Thus it is not just the specific function of the lesioned area that matters, but also how the lesion affects the traffic that travels along the roads of cortical connections in order to contribute to different functions. Chapter 4 reviews some examples of neuronal processing during activities.

CHAPTER
4

Neuronal Processing Related to Cerebral Function

Cerebral localization, as described in Chapter 3, is one way of looking at the nervous system. This localization can be compared to a map, which shows the location of the work that will be performed by the cortex. Structure and structural abnormalities relating to anatomy can be detected by CT scans, as described in Chapter 6. However, CNS functions are based on the combined activity of many different cerebral regions. This activity is a physiological phenomenon that takes place as electrical impulses travel along different interhemispheric and intrahemispheric connections, in addition to connections with subcortical structures. This physiological phenomenon of electrical activity, an indication of neuronal processing during CNS function, has sometimes been compared to traffic, traveling along roads on the map, between the various locations. These electrical impulses can be detected by technological evaluation methods such as electroencephalography (EEG), evoked potentials (EP), as well as computerized mapping of EEG (CMEEG), all of which are described in Chapter 6.

Brain activity at certain locations can also be detected by the examination of oxygen and glucose utilization and of blood flow patterns by use of regional cerebral blood-flow studies (rCBF) and positron emission tomography (PET) techniques, both of which are also outlined in Chapter 6. These methods trace function in a more holistic way than the methods depicting only isolated structural localization, such as postmortem studies and CT scans.

This chapter reviews a few studies that have used the above-mentioned techniques to trace neuronal processing of the CNS during functional activities and proposes processing models. However, without the localization map, following such processing would be difficult; thus, the study of anatomy and cerebral localization, as outlined in Chapter 3 is a valuable foundation for the study of neuronal processing, which is the basis for neurobehavior. This chapter focuses on processing and therefore should aid the reader in understanding the CNS to obtain more complete patient assessments, and have a better basis for choosing effective treatment. It is recognized that present knowledge of the CNS is rapidly changing. Although one can trace functional processing to some extent by today's methods, this does not imply that we know the underlying mechanisms for the functions. Although electrical activity, for example, indicates that some function is taking place, the extent of this activity and what causes it is not yet known in any detail. Further, as recognized by Heilman (1983) knowledge of activation of a particular area does not "always" indicate "what this area is doing" (p. 3).

Before looking at specific studies of the evaluation of cerebral processing, it is worthwhile to

55

look for a few moments at Luria's (1973) contributions to the development of a theory regarding neuropsychological processing in the CNS. He encouraged a new look at the classical localization of mental functions in the cortex. According to Luria, elementary functions can be localized precisely in particular cell groups. However, mental functions cannot be localized in narrow zones of isolated cell groups. Rather, they must be organized in systems of working zones. Each of these zones, in turn, performs its role in a *"complex functional system . . . which may be located in completely different . . . areas of the brain"* (p. 31). Luria proposed that the localization of these higher mental processes is not static; it shifts during development and training.

Luria (1973) stated that external aids "are *essential elements in the establishment of functional connections between individual parts of the brain,* and that by their aid, areas of the brain which previously were independent become the *components of a single functional system"* (p. 31). Thus, "historically formed measures for the organization of human behavior tie new knots in the activity of man's brain" (p. 31). During such development, the cerebral organization changes and the location of activity will depend on the location of what Luria calls a *working zone.* Luria thus tried to analyze which cerebral areas are involved in an activity, what their contribution to a complex functional system is, and how the relationship between these working parts of the brain, when performing complex mental activity, changes throughout development. In the occupational performance frame of reference, life-space influences become synonymous with what Luria terms "external aids." This view of cerebral function refers to processing, which is based on cooperative function of different areas; it is this processing that the studies reviewed in the remainder of this chapter attempt to describe.

The concept of external aids certainly brings to mind the potentials in therapy for using an activity-oriented external evaluation to examine the integrity of the CNS, as well as activity-oriented treatment to influence further organization, or re-

organization, of the nervous system after CNS dysfunction. Could daily tasks, for example, be used to activate what Geschwind (1979a and b) calls *dormant cerebral areas?* These areas, which are outlined in more detail in Chapter 8, are capable of resuming, to some extent, lost functions of damaged cortical areas, according to Geschwind. Thus CNS processes, as well as the external activities incorporated in the treatment media must be analyzed and then combined, so that they meet the goal of improving function. In an ADL assessment the components of daily activities, and the objects used for performance, can be considered as complex environmental stimuli that provoke neurobehavior, as will be outlined toward the end of this chapter. Throughout the chapter, the information in each section is summarized in a processing illustration. These illustrations are intended as simplified summaries only and should be viewed as such.

VISUAL PROCESSING

Before the processing of neuronal activity during functioning is described, the visual and auditory pathways will be described briefly, as they contribute to more diffuse cerebral functions, such as visuospatial perception and language. According to Kelly (1985b) the visual fields are "the way in which the visual world is projected onto the retina" (p. 357). There are left and right hemivisual fields, which project to temporal and nasal hemiretina fields. Fig. 4-1 shows the visual pathway. According to Kelly, *"The visual field is the field of view of the external world seen by the two eyes without movement of the head"* (p. 357). Stimuli from the peripheri of each visual field project to the nasal retina, whereas stimuli from the middle part of the visual fields project to the temporal retina. Further stimuli from the superior part of each visual field project to the inferior part of the retina, and stimuli from the inferior visual field project to the superior part of the retina. Fibers from the retina form the optic nerves on each side. The optic nerves meet in the optic chiasma, where fibers from the nasal hemiretina cross over to the opposite side. The

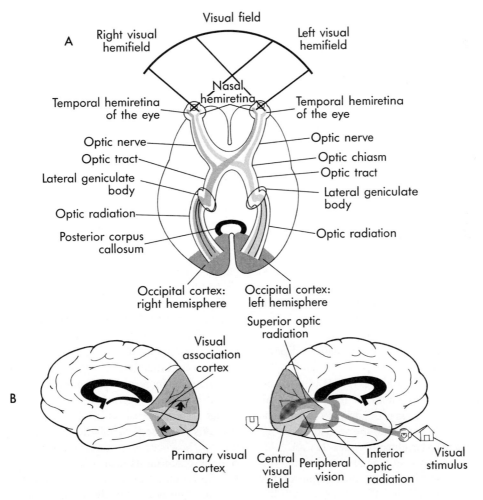

FIG. 4-1 The visual pathways. **A,** Inferior view depicting flow of information from the visual fields to the visual cortex. **B,** Medial view of components of the visual cortex and visual processing.

optic tract on each side, which is continuous with the optic chiasma, thus carries fibers from ipsilateral temporal hemiretina (the inner visual field) and contralateral nasal hemiretina (the outer visual field). The optic tract on each side projects to the lateral geniculate body of the thalamus. The optic radiation then carries visual information from the lateral geniculate body to the calcarine cortex in the occipital lobe (Daube and Sandok, 1978; Kelly, 1985b). In the radiation, the fibers fan out the upper part of the bundle carrying information from the lower visual field, running posteriorly in the parietal lobe. The lower part, with information from the upper visual field, loops around the temporal horn of the ventricles in the temporal lobe, on its way to the inferior visual cortex. Note that stimulus in the superior visual field is projected to the inferior retina, resulting in an inverted image. Because of this inversion, the information from the superior visual field is carried by the inferior optic radiation. The image is then carried on to the cortex, inverted. In the primary visual cortex around the calcarine fissure (Brodmann's area 17), the occipital pole is concerned with vision from the central or middle visual field, whereas peripheral vision is taken care of by a more anterior part the medial occipital cortex. The association areas (Brodmann's areas 18 and 19) receive information from the primary visual cortex. They integrate this information with previous experiences and information from other sensory modalities, and they also form visual memory traces (Daube and Sandok, 1978).

Kandel (1985d), in his review of visual processing, describes a hierarchy of increased visual abstraction. Further, cells in the primary visual cortex (Brodmann's area 17) and the secondary visual association cortex (Brodmann's area 18) are "the early building blocks of visual perception" (p. 381). These cells "operate by a principle of increasing convergence" (p. 381). Thus at each hierarchical level, the cells "see" more than cells at lower levels in the hierarchy. However, according to Kandel, the hierarchical structure has a limit. In addition to hierarchical processing, a pattern of parallel processing contributes to function. This means that cells in different cortical areas—for instance, in the posterior parietal cortex, the inferior temporal cortex, and the visual cortex in the occipital lobe—are simultaneously working on a particular stimulus aspect. Thus one aspect of vision may be lost during specific cortical dysfunction although other aspects are intact. Two major intercortical visual pathways are proposed for processing different aspects of visual stimuli, according to Kandel. These are a pathway from the primary visual cortex to the inferior temporal lobe, involved in perception of form and color, and a pathway from the primary visual area to the posterior parietal lobe, involved in attention to stimulus components and perception of movement. The two pathways are connected at different levels, providing a basis for almost endless analysis of vision.

Stone and Dreher (1982), are in favor of the parallel processing model for visual information. They differentiate between three different types of ganglion cells. According to them, the primary visual cortex (Brodmann's area 17) receives input from all three types of cells. However, the association area adjacent to the calcarine area, (Brodmann's area 18) receives input from one type of ganglion cells, and the association area adjacent to it (Brodmann's area 19) receives input from another type. According to them, the different classes of ganglion cells contribute to parallel processing.

Phelps et al. (1981a) used PET scans (described in Chapter 6) and glucose metabolism to map cerebral metabolism in humans during visual stimulation. Increased metabolic rates were detected both in the primary visual cortex and the visual association cortex as the complexity of the stimulus increased. Metabolic rate increased more rapidly, however, during increased stimulus complexity, reaching its peak while subjects observed the environment of a park. During simple visual stimuli, however, only the primary visual cortex was activated. This supports the role of the visual cortex in processing visual stimulation and the idea that the involvement of both the primary visual cortex and association cortex is variable according to stimulus complexity. Phelps et al. (1981b) suggested that the discrimination for the simplest task occurred mainly at the lateral geniculate body of the thalamus and the superior colliculus before the visual information reached the cortex.

Roland and Skinhøj (1981) studied the involvement of cortical areas outside the primary visual cortex during a visual discrimination task in humans. The task involved two forced choices of shape discrimination. Flow increases were detected in the visual association cortex including the lateral occipital cortex, superior occipital cortex, and the inferior temporal cortex, and also in the superior parietal area, parieto-temporo-occipital area, the frontal eye fields, the superior prefrontal cortex, and the lateral prefrontal cortex. These authors proposed that the parietal involvement was related to spatial analysis, whereas the visual association cortex performed visual analysis. The frontal cortex was, on the other hand, thought to be involved in task organization, information retrieval, decision making, comparison, and figuring out sampling strategies, as well as directing the eyes to the visual stimulus. This study thus suggests that, depending on the requirements of a visual task, different cortical areas that are not primarily involved with vision may be brought into play.

Kimura (1966) used a tachistoscope to investigate processing differences during verbal and nonverbal stimuli. Kimura tested 20 right-handed normal subjects and found that verbally identifiable forms, such as letters and words, were identified more accurately in the right visual field, whereas nonalphabetical stimuli, such as dots, where perception of shape was not required, were more accurately identified when presented in the left visual field (the left visual field information being processed by the right hemisphere). Her conclusion was that the left posterior cortex "plays an important role in the identification of verbal-conceptual forms" (p. 275), while the corresponding cortical area on the right side plays an important role in registration of nonverbal stimuli. Thus, input from the right visual field may be more directly transmitted to the left occipital lobe than input from the

left visual field. According to Kimura, the field differences probably indicate function of the occipital, rather than the temporal lobe.

Srebro (1985) studied the localization of cortical activity following visual recognition of objects in humans. He used a topographical analysis of EPs. The potentials were recorded from subjects observing differently illuminated pictures of human faces and simple embedded shapes. The cortical activity measured localization to both of the temporal lobes, with some extent of increased right hemisphere lateralization in right-handed subjects. Measurable differences were obtained between right temporal lobe activities, depending on association with face recognition and association with simple shape recognition. Based on these findings, Srebro suggested that the right posterior temporal lobe may contain a surface map related to shape, important for visual recognition, which is analogous to the visual field map that has been described on the surface of the occipital lobe. On the basis of animal studies, the parietal lobe has been associated with spatial localization of visual stimuli, whereas the temporal lobe has been associated with visual recognition of objects.

Srebro located this surface mapping in the posterior part of the temporal lobe. His suggestion that visual memory traces are stored in the temporal lobe for visual recognition is supported in Butters and Miliotis's (1985) review of amnesic disorders and in Walsh's review (1987) of neuropsychology. These reviews further supported the left hemisphere's superiority in verbal memory functions and the storage of language engrams. Walsh, for example, states that the middle temporal gyrus is important for verbal memory.

According to Friedman and Albert (1985) reading ability is based on connections between the calcarine areas in the occipital lobes and the angular gyrus in the left hemisphere. The lingual gyrus and the fusiform occipital gyri (also termed the *medial occipitotemporal* gyrus) are important in this respect, and connections in the corpus callosum are necessary for information from the right occipital lobe to reach the left hemisphere. Figs. 4-1 and

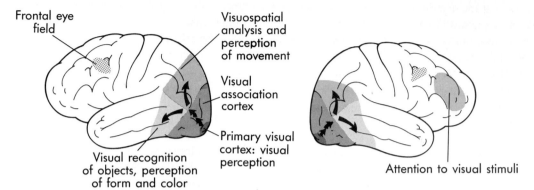

Frontal eye field

Visuospatial analysis and perception of movement

Visual association cortex

Primary visual cortex: visual perception

Visual recognition of objects, perception of form and color

Attention to visual stimuli

LEFT HEMISPHERE : processing of verbal conceptual forms

RIGHT HEMISPHERE : processing of nonverbal information

FIG. 4-2 Cortical visual processing. Parallel processing has been reported in the primary and secondary visual cortices in the occipital lobe. The frontal eye fields are also simultaneously involved in attending to the stimulus. The posterior temporal cortex is involved in object recognition and the recognition of forms and color. The posterior parietal cortex plays a role in visuospatial analysis. The different processes can occur at the same time. The left hemisphere is thought to be involved in processing verbal conceptual forms such as letters, whereas the right hemisphere is concerned with processing nonverbal information related to visual spatial perception.

4-2 illustrate the visual pathways and intercortical connections for the processing of visual information.

AUDITORY PROCESSING

The cochlear nerve, also called the auditory nerve, carries auditory information from the organ of Corti in the cochlea to the cochlear nucleus. Information is then carried to the medial geniculate body of the thalamus via several relay stations. From the medial geniculate body, the auditory radiation carries auditory information to the cerebral cortex of the temporal lobe (Brodmann's areas 41 and 42). Along the auditory pathway there are a number of commissural connections, so that information reaching the cortex is both ipsi- and contralateral. The contralateral information is, however, stronger (Barr and Kiernan, 1983). Thus, as stated by Walsh (1987), auditory fibers from either ear are represented "bilaterally but unequally" (p. 174) in the two temporal lobes. Along the auditory pathway,

information is processed and refined before it reaches the cortex. Further, there are different feedback connections from the cortex to the thalamus and cochlea (Barr and Kiernan, 1983).

According to Kelly (1985c), because of the bilateral representation of auditory information, the perception of sound frequency is not affected by unilateral cortical lesions. However, sound localization in space will be affected. The auditory cortex on each side is primarily concerned with localizing sound from the contralateral side, (e.g., the left hemisphere is concerned with localizing sound from the right side). For the localization, according to Kelly, comparison of differences in sound intensity and in the arrival times from each ear are used. As reviewed by Walsh (1987), the order in which stimuli are reported to the ears is important, the first stimuli being more successful, whereas later ones are subject to short-term memory decay. Anatomical explanations have been given for the arrival time difference according to

Springer and Deutsch's review of left and right hemispheric differences (1981). The authors report that in people for whom the left hemisphere is "dominant" for language, information from the left ear needs to go first to the right hemisphere, and from there through the corpus callosum to the left language-comprehension area. From the right ear, on the contrary, information travels directly to the left hemisphere.

From the auditory receptive area there are connections to the auditory association area, which is important for auditory discrimination and comprehension. This process will be expanded upon in the next section on language processing.

LANGUAGE PROCESSING

Larsen et al. (1978) considered the following pattern of neuronal activation during speech to be the fundamentally correct approach to locating speech functions. They measured regional cerebral blood flow (rCBF) during rest and during an automatic speech test, which consisted of counting to 20 or repeating the weekdays (see Chapter 6 for further details on this evaluation method). They used 18 normal, right-handed subjects. For the mapping, they recorded decay of radioactivity from 254 regions in the left hemisphere of half the subjects and the right hemisphere of the other half.

The authors established a normal resting pattern for rCBF for both hemispheres for comparison. This pattern showed high flow values in the frontal regions, up to 12% over the hemispheric mean in the upper part. The flow in the parietal lobes was average, whereas the flow in the temporal lobes was below the mean. The pattern revealed no difference between the two hemispheres. When the flow pattern during speech was compared to this normal pattern, consistent differences were found. During speech, the rCBF was increased in the upper premotor area in the left hemisphere, probably representing the supplementary motor area. The rCBF was also increased in the sensory-motor mouth area on the left side, and in Wernicke's speech area. No increase was found in Broca's area. In the right hemisphere, the same three areas

showed increased rCBF as on the left side, with less marked premotor activation however.

These findings of bilateral hemispheric involvement during speech are, according to the authors, in keeping with earlier findings of Penfield and Rasmussen (1949), which were obtained by electrical stimulation of the cortex. However, Larsen et al. did not detect activation of Broca's area. They suggest that this discrepancy may be due to the fact that Broca's area is also active during rest; studying the difference from the resting pattern as they did would not reveal activation of that area.

Larsen et al. concluded that their results supported the involvement of the supplementary motor area, and the Rolandic face area, as did the findings of earlier studies of cortical electrical stimulation. These areas are considered to be involved in motor performances of speech. The researchers interpreted the finding of activation in the superior temporal region as being due to activation of the auditory cortex, because the subjects had been listening to their own voices.

According to Larsen et al., several areas of the cortex, rather than one specific locale, are involved in the processing of speech, a fact that should be kept in mind when impairments in the language area are observed and predictions made regarding localization and pertinent treatment methods. The fact that Broca's area did not show up on the mappings in this study indicates that imaging methods that detect neuronal processing need to look at earlier localization maps to fill in the gaps in their findings in order to explain the results. Although the two-dimensional blood-flow method has yielded to other methods, this may still hold.

Nishizawa, et al. (1982) studied cerebral blood flow during the task of listening to words. They measured blood flow in the right hemispheres of seven subjects, and the left hemispheres of another seven subjects. In addition to general activation of a hemisphere, as indicated by increased blood flow, focal flow also increased. A much higher increase was thus detected in the superior temporal regions (Brodmann's areas 41, 42, and

22), prefrontal, and orbitofrontal regions. These increases were found in both hemispheres but were substantially higher on the left side. This was found to support the dominance of the left hemisphere in detecting verbal auditory information. The results of these studies were found to contradict results from a previous study performed by the same authors, in which the right hemisphere was found to be dominant for nonverbal auditory signals, supporting the notion of different lateralization for speech and nonspeech auditory processing. Focal increases in primary and secondary auditory areas were found to be related to audition. Orbitofrontal increases were related to corticocortical connections between that area and the superior temporal area. The uncinate fasciculus connecting these areas has previously been related to attention mechanisms, short-term memory, and auditory discrimination. Flow increase in the prefrontal area was thought to be related to attention, and increases in the frontal eye field were related to either auditory activation or involuntary eye movement. The supplementary motor area, which is thought to be important during movement and exhibited activation in the study reported by Larsen et al. (1978) on speech, was not activated according to the study by Nishizawa et al.

Geschwind (1979a and b) suggested that the language areas of the brain have been investigated in greater detail than any other cortical functional areas. The language areas to which he refers include Broca's motor speech area in the frontal lobe of the left hemisphere and Wernicke's area in the temporal lobe. Broca's area, as stated in Chapter 3, is involved in motor speech functions, and Wernicke's area in auditory comprehension and speech feedback.

Geschwind (1979a and b) stated that it has become evident that Broca's area and Wernicke's area are connected by the arcuate fasciculus for language processing, which supports the importance of neuronal processing and communication between localized functional areas of the brain during language functions. Thus, neurobehavioral deficits could be considered in relation to that processing pathway. He further stated that Wernicke's

area probably mediates between the visual and auditory centers of the brain. The processing proposed by Geschwind is related to the older localization maps.

The language model described by Geschwind (1979a and b), based on Wernicke's original ideas, is associated with sequential processing in different cortical areas, dysfunction being related to "disconnection." Brown and Perecman (1986) suggest an alternate conceptual framework for the processing of language. This framework is based on three theoretical statements: (1) sequential brain levels contribute to evolutionary processing; (2) simultaneous or parallel processing of language takes place in two systems located in different cortical divisions, anteriorly and posteriorly; and (3) pathways between the two divisions have a temporal role of phase maintenance only.

The first statement proposed by Brown and Perecman regarding evolution assumes that the limbic mechanisms play a role in early language representation, whereas the neocortex, including Broca's and Wernicke's areas, is concerned with final processing stages. The so-called posterior and anterior language areas are related to the function of the limbic mechanisms. The anterior language area includes, according to these authors, the anterior cingulate gyrus, the supplementary motor area, and the left premotor area, including Broca's area. The posterior language area, on the other hand, houses Wernicke's area. Language in each of these neocortical areas is progressively specified during development. Wernicke's area, for example, deals with phonological processing, while the surrounding area is concerned with mediation of semantic processing. This framework has been termed the *microgenic approach*. According to this approach, language is not a single nervous system activity. Rather, it is composed of functions involving two separate activities — movement and perception — which are located in different cortical areas. These activities branch from the same primary level, and each activity passes different levels of processing during development. The pathways connecting the locations of the two systems serve a temporal function regarding phase maintenance at the different

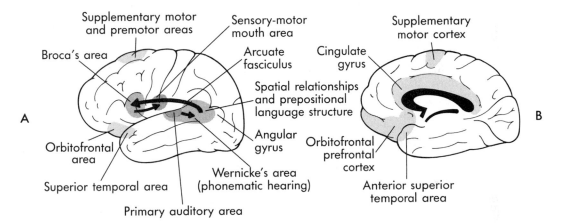

FIG. 4-3 Language processing. **A,** Function of the left hemisphere during speech and comprehension. The primary auditory area receives auditory information. The information is analyzed by Wernicke's association area. The angular gyrus connects the visual and auditory cortical areas (see also Fig. 4-2) for mediation of information from the visual cortex. The arcuate fasciculus connects the auditory comprehension area in the posterior cortex to the motor speech areas in the frontal lobe. Broca's speech area is situated in the frontal lobe. It connects with the sensory-motor face area in the pre- and postcentral gyri. The supplementary motor area is thought to play a role in attention and intention. The orbitofrontal, prefrontal area and the anterior, superior temporal area, which have been reported to be active during language functions, are considered to play a role in internal speech or ideation, short-term memory functions, and auditory discrimination. **B,** The cingulate gyrus (especially its anterior portions) is associated with limbic mechanisms and the supplementary motor cortex on the medial aspect of the hemisphere; these have also been identified by some authors as active cortical areas during language functions.

locations, while the systems perform processing independently of each other, according to these authors.

This model supports the earlier localization maps regarding the traditional speech and comprehension areas, although it explains the functions of cortical connections differently from Geschwind (1979a and b). It further supports Lassen et al.'s (1978) cortical blood flow maps of glucose utilization during language functions, including involvement of the supplementary motor area. It is evident that to use imaging such as blood-flow studies to examine whether processing is sequential, as suggested in earlier studies, or parallel, as suggested in this study, major technological refinements related to the timing of events are necessary. In addition, this study stresses the importance of limbic and subcortical structures in language functions.

Fig. 4-3 illustrates proposed language processing, based on the information reviewed in this section. Bilateral activation occurs for many of the areas shown, although during language comprehension and speech the left hemisphere is more active, especially in the primary speech and comprehension areas. For perception of nonverbal auditory signals and music, the right hemisphere appears more active than the left one. The connecting pathways have been thought to serve a sequential role in the flow of information by some authors, and a temporal role of phase maintenance by others.

PROCESSING OF PRAXIS

Geschwind (1975) proposed a processing model of movement based on his clinical experience, as well as papers written by Liepman and previous descriptions from Liepman's chief, Wernicke. He suggested that when a person is ordered to carry out a movement with the right hand, the stimulus goes to Wernicke's area in the left hemisphere through the arcuate fasciculus in the lower parietal lobe on its way to the left premotor region. The left premotor cortex in turn controls the precentral motor cortex on that side, which sends information through the pyramidal tract to the right hand. Geschwind implied that when a person receives a command to move the left hand, the instruction also travels through Wernicke's area to the left premotor region, and from there via the corpus callosum to the premotor region of the right precentral motor cortex, controlling the left limb. It is also possible, but less likely, according to the author, that a command to move the left hand will go from Wernicke's area across the corpus callosum to the right angular gyrus, and from there to the right premotor and primary motor cortex. Thus, according to Geschwind, apraxia is a result of a disconnection of Wernicke's language-comprehension area from the premotor cortex. With this model, Geschwind provided support for the neuronal processing necessary for movement, and intra- and interhemispheric functional connections.

Heilman and Rothi (1985) criticized Geschwind's emphasis on Wernicke's area and language influence on praxis. They pointed out that patients with comprehension difficulties could have problems performing on command, but those problems would not necessarily be related to praxis. Patients with such dysfunctions should also be able to perform when instruction was not required. Further, despite the possible existence of connections from the visual cortex to the arcuate fasciculus that carries visuomotor information necessary for the imitation of movement, this could not explain clumsiness during object use in spontaneous motor tasks.

Heilman and Rothi thus suggest an alternative hypothesis to account for the flaws they perceived in Geschwind's model. They suggest that the dominant parietal lobe stores visuokinesthetic motor engrams, and that these engrams are necessary for movement. According to them, Wernicke's area and the visual cortex are both connected to the angular gyrus, which in turn connects with the supramarginal gyrus, both of which are located in the inferior parietal lobe on the left side and are responsible for storing visuokinesthetic motor engrams. From the inferior left parietal area, information goes to the premotor area, which programs movement before the information gets released to the primary motor cortex on the left side, controlling the right side of the body. The premotor area on the left side connects with the premotor area on the right side via the corpus callosum, and in turn relays the visuokinesthetic motor information over to the right hemisphere. The right premotor cortex programs movement and instructs the primary motor cortex on the same side regarding execution of movement in the left side of the body. Both comprehension difficulties and visual perceptual problems can influence performance, depending on the method of instruction during testing for apraxia, because both areas for these functions connect with the angular gyrus. However, according to this model, neither accounts for all types of clumsiness, or what is referred to as *ideomotor praxis* by Heilman and Rothi. This model thus does not consider praxis of ideational origin (recall from Chapter 3 that praxis is composed of three components: ideation, programming, and motor execution).

Ingvar and Philipson (1977) studied the distribution of rCBF in the left hemisphere during motor ideation and motor performance in six patients. They obtained recordings from the patients while at rest, while imagining movement without motor performance, and during actual movements of the right hand. At rest, the dominant hemisphere showed the classical flow increase in the frontal regions, indicating frontal activity at rest. According to the authors, the area responsible for the programming of behavior thus seemed to be more active at rest than other regions such as the parietal lobe, where sensory and memory functions are located.

During motor ideation, in which patients attempted to imagine rhythmic cleansing movements of the right hand, an increase in mean cerebral blood flow was recorded, especially in the frontal lobe, including the premotor and orbitofrontal cortices. Increased flow was also detected in parietal and temporal structures around the lateral fissure. The involvement of the area around the lateral fissure points to the possible use of inner language in ideation, as mentioned in Chapters 3 and 7. The patient might use this inner language to program the movement (i.e., to straighten or clench the fist and to sequence the movement). Thus it might inform the subject what to do and how, in order to perform. Ingvar and Philipson suggest that storage for memory engrams may be located in this region, and that these must be mobilized for the conceptualization of movement. The prefrontal cortex, including the orbitofrontal area, has been associated with short-term memory, among other factors. This might contribute to the order of sequencing of the hand clenching. During actual hand movements, flow increase was only seen around the pre-

and postcentral sulci, or the primary motor and sensory areas.

If a more complex motor act than repetitious hand clenching had been used, one would expect, on the basis of Ayres' (1985) outline for praxis components, that activation of the cortical sides concerned with ideation would have been seen prior to the actual execution, and that the posterior parietal lobe would have been active prior to and during movement. This method of blood-flow measurement shows that cortical areas are involved in praxis, but does not necessarily reveal information on timing and sequencing of activation of the different cortical areas.

This study and others of its kind have provided a unique contribution to the research on behavioral mechanisms. It supported the importance of the ideation component in movement, and also suggested the important contribution of memory components to the planning of movement. Such information could only have been speculative without evaluation techniques such as rCBF. It certainly could not have been detected by postmortem studies. This study provided important knowledge for understanding the CNS and neurobehavior. It also stressed the importance of using behavior to record and learn about CNS functions. Intention of movement has been associated with the function of the supplementary motor areas by subsequent studies.

Roland et al. (1980) studied the role of cortical areas, including the supplementary motor area, in the organization of voluntary movement. They measured rCBF in 28 subjects. The studies were performed during rest, planning, and execution of previously learned voluntary hand movements. They found increases in cerebral blood flow in the supplementary motor area during ideation as a result of internal programming of the finger movements. During execution of the finger movements, these researchers detected equivalent flow increases in both right and left supplementary motor areas, whereas only the contralateral motor area was activitated during the execution of the movement. In addition, the authors reported modest increases in the contralateral sensory hand area, which could be a result of sensory feedback. They further reported bilateral increase in the premotor and orbitofrontal regions, in agreement with Ingvar and Philipson's (1977) results. Repetitive fast flexions of one finger, similar to the clenching movements in Ingvar and Philipson's study, raised only contralateral flow in the primary motor and sensory areas, in agreement with Ingvar and Philipson. Sensory discrimination of object shapes involving no voluntary movements was also tested. This revealed no supplementary motor activity.

Roland et al. concluded that the primary motor area and its projections were capable of controlling ongoing simple movements, but a sequence of isolated finger movements required involvement of the supplementary motor areas for programming movement. They suggested that the supplementary motor areas programmed movement by forming a "queue of time-ordered motor commands" (p. 118) before execution of voluntary movements. Further, it was speculated that the inferior frontal lobe involvement was related to the anatomical closeness of the basal ganglia, or internal speech.

This study supported the frontal lobe involvement in the previously reviewed models of movement, as they did not report visual involvement or visual motor connections; this study excluded imaging of the occipital lobes, most likely because these are supplied by the vertebral arterial system. Therefore, the occipital areas do not show up in carotid angiography. Further, task presentation may not have required the use of occipital connections because previously learned movements were used during the recordings. It is interesting that no focal flow increases were reported in the left inferior parietal lobe, which was associated with storage of visuokinesthetic motor engrams by Heilman and Rothi (1985).

Foit et al. (1980) measured rCBF in seven subjects during peripheral nerve stimulation and during voluntary movement. They recorded somatosensory evoked potentials (SEP) simultaneously over the primary cortical projection areas during median nerve stimulation. Focal rCBF changes were observed under both conditions in the primary sensory and motor areas of the hand in the pre- and postcentral gyri. Additional rCBF changes were seen during voluntary movement in the supplementary motor area. During nerve stimulation, additional flow changes were detected in the contralateral auditory association cortex. The authors concluded that activation of the primary sensory and motor cortices, as well as the sensory association cortex, were due to early components of the SEP, whereas the premotor activation would more likely be involved in the electrical activity that precedes voluntary movement.

The authors argued, on the basis of their results, that the precentral gyrus was active during sensory input, and that sensory feedback to the postcentral gyrus may have a functional role in the organization of motor patterns. Thus the functions of these areas were considered to be interrelated. The involvement of other frontal areas is in agreement with results of the previously reviewed blood-flow studies, and thought to be related to motor planning.

These findings support the idea of the localization of sensory and motor areas of earlier maps. In addition, they suggest involvement of additional areas, such as the supplementary motor area and a secondary sensory area, similar to the results of the previously reviewed studies. Further, they indicate a sequencing order of activation based on the observations. Foit et al. combined use of biochemical and electrophysiological studies of the CNS. They seem to find agreement between the results from both methods.

Busk and Galibraith (1975) analyzed EEG signals recorded from four scalp electrodes in 15 subjects who engaged in three visual-motor tasks, varying in complexity. The electrodes recorded activity from visual, primary motor (left and right), and premotor areas. Their findings supported the importance of visual-premotor and premotor-motor pathways in visual motor integration. It further indicated significantly lower visual-motor electrode-coupling levels than did recordings from electrodes located at the visual and premotor areas. Further, electrode coupling of the right and left primary motor areas was significantly lower than all other electrode combinations. This may, according to the authors, suggest that these areas may not be connected by callosal fibers. Further, the results suggested stable visual input to the premotor area during the type of visual-motor learning used in the experiment. However, the premotor-motor pathways manifested decreased interaction as learning took place.

The limitations of EEG recordings, which include difficulty in obtaining subcortical activity and activity from the cortex adjacent to the electrodes (the electrodes only representing four cortical points), must be kept in mind when interpreting results from studies like this one. The results emphasized the existence of the anatomical connections between premotor and motor areas, as well as visual and premotor areas, whereas connections were not detected between the two primary motor areas. These findings do not contradict the views of Heilman et al. (1982) and Geschwind (1975) that the two premotor areas on the right and left sides of cortex are connected, as well as the premotor and primary motor areas. Heilman et al. also suggested visuomotor connections between the visual cortex and the angular gyrus, which subsequently connects with the premotor area. This may be consistent with Busk and Galibraith's visuo-premotor coupling results.

The literature reviewed above has been synthesized into a processing model. Fig. 4-4 illustrates possible processing areas for praxis. Additionally, according to Ayres' literature review (1985), the basal ganglia have been reported to play a role in storing engrams for automatic actions. In Fig. 4-4, *A*, the kinesthetic-visuomotor engrams are stored in the left inferior parietal lobe. This area receives input from visual and auditory association areas, as well as from the somesthetic sensory association cortex. These secondary association areas are not directly involved in praxis, but their functions are important for interpretating information presented in praxic tests. They contribute to the initial formation of engrams but not to retrieval of the engrams. The premotor area plans

movement sequences based on the memory engrams. The supplementary motor area is important for intention, preparation of action, and timing of movements. The movement is then executed by the primary motor cortex of the left hemisphere if the right body side is to be moved. Such movement provides somesthetic sensory feedback to the postcentral gyrus. The left premotor area connects with the right premotor area via the corpus callosum. This connection is important if the left body side, controlled by the right hemisphere, is to be moved, as it provides access to the visuokinesthetic motor engrams that are thought to be stored in the left inferior parietal lobe. The right premotor area then connects with the right primary motor area, which carries out the movement that provides somesthetic feedback to the right postcentral gyrus. This pathway accounts for praxis. The supplementary motor areas, orbitofrontal areas, and the superior temporal area have been reported to play a role in ideation, which is a prerequisite for motor praxis. These areas may involve programming by internal speech, memory engrams for conceptualization of movement, and short-term memory related to sequencing of the needed movement patterns. It should be kept in mind that the premotor area is important for organizing and sequencing movements, whereas the prefrontal cortex is important for organizing and sequencing action steps.

The transverse view of the pathway in Fig. 4-4, *B*, begins in the left inferior parietal lobe and travels via the left premotor area to the right premotor area or the left primary motor cortex for execution of movements on the right body side. The left hemisphere is important for bilateral praxis, whereas the corpus callosum and the right hemisphere are only involved in praxis performed by the left body side.

PROCESSING INVOLVED IN ATTENTION

Heilman and Van Den Abell (1980) suggested a processing pathway for attention or orienting response. This pathway runs from the reticular formation via the limbic system to the cortex. The authors suggest that there is one such pathway for

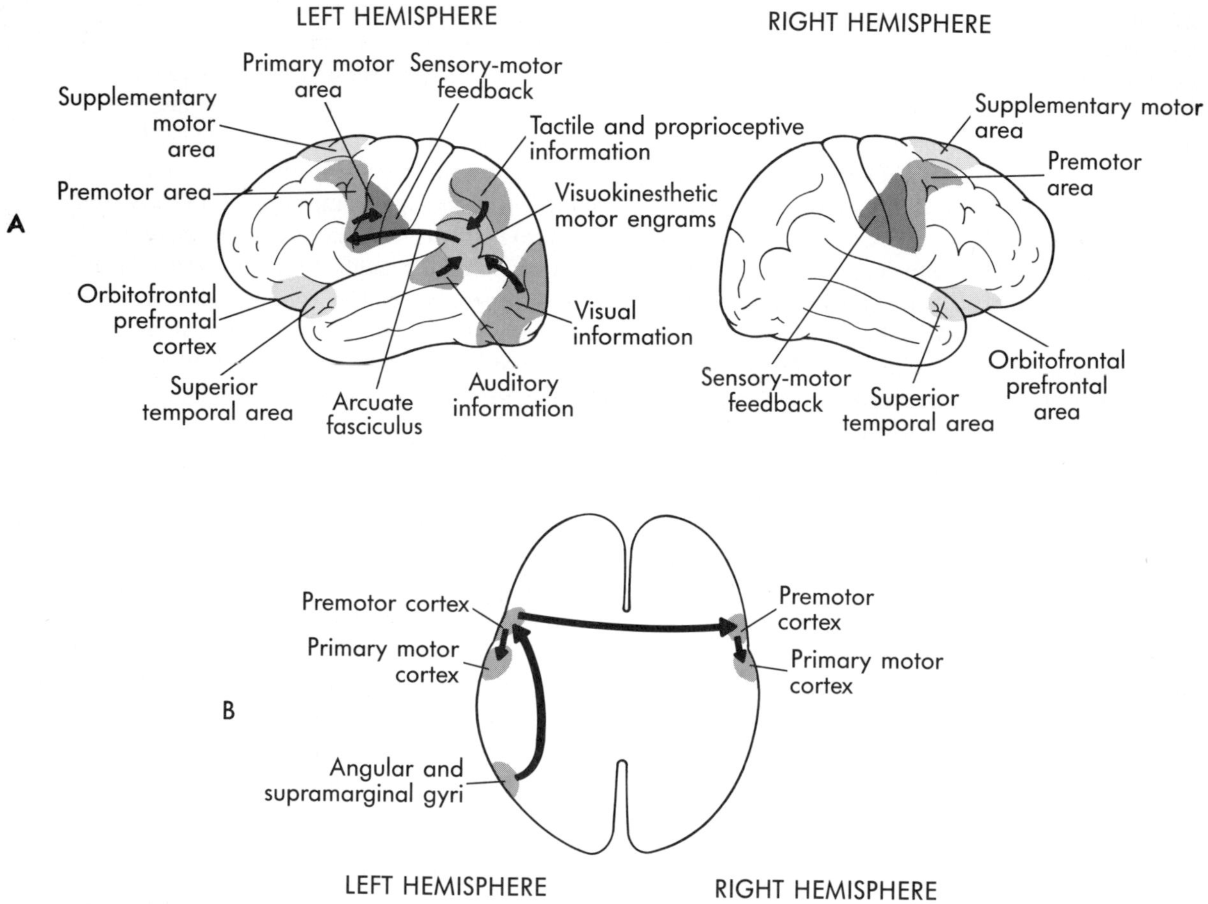

LEFT HEMISPHERE

RIGHT HEMISPHERE

Supplementary
motor
area

Primary motor   Sensory-motor
area   feedback

Tactile and proprioceptive
information

Premotor area

Visuokinesthetic
motor engrams

Supplementary motor
area

Premotor
area

Orbitofrontal
prefrontal
cortex

Visual
information

Superior
temporal area

Arcuate
fasciculus

Auditory
information

Sensory-motor
feedback

Superior
temporal area

Orbitofrontal
prefrontal
area

A

B

Premotor cortex

Primary motor
cortex

Premotor
cortex

Primary motor
cortex

Angular and
supramarginal gyri

LEFT HEMISPHERE   RIGHT HEMISPHERE

FIG. 4-4 Processing of praxis. **A,** Active functional areas of the left and right hemispheres during praxis. **B,** Transverse view of the most commonly accepted sequential processing model of motor praxis.

each hemisphere, but that the left parietal lobe attends to stimuli to the right side, whereas the right hemisphere attends to stimuli to both the left and the right sides. On the basis of their findings, they conclude that the parietal lobe of the right hemisphere is dominant for attention.

Heilman et al. (1985) propose a processing pathway for attention and arousal. This pathway

originates in the reticular activation system, which receives input from the different sensory modalities, including visual, auditory, and somatosensory input. From the reticular activating system, sensory information is relayed via thalamic nuclei (ventral posterolateral, medial geniculate, and lateral geniculate) depending on the nature of the activation on the way to the specific cortical areas. The nucleus reticularis in the thalamus can inhibit the thalamocortical flow from the specific thalamic nuclei if the nucleus itself has not been previously inhibited by the reticular formation. The reticular formation also receives direct input from the sensory modalities, according to this model. Its dopamine system mediates intention, whereas its acetylcholic system mediates behavioral arousal. This input is thought to be transmitted to diffuse cortical areas influencing the processing of sensory stimuli. Thus there are two ways for sensory information to affect the cortex. One is direct activation of primary sensory areas via the specific sensory nuclei in the thalamus. From the primary sensory areas information reaches the association areas. The other route influences both primary sensory and association areas and the cingulate gyrus of the limbic system. The cingulate gyrus in turn influences the association cortex in the inferior parietal lobe, as well as the prefrontal cortex and the superior temporal cortex. The limbic system's influence on the frontal lobes is important in determining the significance of a stimulus and the needs of the individual, which play an important role in goal-directed behavior. The inferior parietal lobe has reciprocal connections to the limbic association cortex in the frontal and temporal lobes, as well as to the limbic system. When considering this processing model, it is evident that different cortical areas are involved in sensory perception, as well as in attention to the different sensory stimuli to determine their significance according to the need of the individual, all of which affects intention. See Fig. 4-5 for a simplified processing model for attention.

Heilman et al. (1985) have suggested dopaminergic pathways mediating intention from the reticular formation through the anterior cingulate gyrus to the prefrontal cortex, including the orbitofrontal area. They state that the dorsolateral frontal cortex containing the frontal eye field, which is important in orientation to a stimulus, may play a role in mediating a response to a stimulus that a subject is attending to. It has connections to the limbic system, reticular formation, and sensory association cortex. Thus the sensory cortex may inform the dorsolateral cortex regarding external sensory information, whereas the limbic system plays a role in mediating motivational information. By combining the different information, the dorsolateral frontal cortex is in a unique position to "execute" a response as a reply to stimulus attention (Heilman et al. 1985).

In Gronwall's (1987) review of advances in the assessment of attention, attention was referred to as a "slowed rate of information processing" (p. 365). According to her review, in agreement with Heilman et al. (1985), some authors relate attention and attentional deficits to functions of the reticular formation in the brain stem. A dysfunction was related to lowered arousal of this system, which is important for the operation of the cortical part of the attentional system. These authors thus agree that the reticular formation and the frontal lobe are important functional units in attention. Further, a distinction has also been made between tonic alertness, which refers to arousal, and phasic alertness, which includes interest and intentions. Attention does, according to Gronwall, refer to different subcomponents. These include divided attention to more than one aspect at a time, sustained attention over time, selective attention (keeping out irrelevant stimuli), and focused attention regarding subject matter.

Buchtel (1987) points out the role of frontal cortical structures in modulating the activity of lower visual structures, such as the superior colliculus. This modulating function is considered important in deciding on the importance of stimuli, as well as for attention to visual stimuli and organization of eye movements.

Before leaving the subject of attention, some thought should be given to motivation. Kaupfermann (1985c) claims motivation to be important in arousing and directing voluntary behavior. Further, motivation and drives (urges that impel people to action) arise from an internal state of the organism; they cannot be completely correlated with stimuli from the external environment. These complex mechanisms controlled by multiple stimuli are, for example, responsible for the regulation of

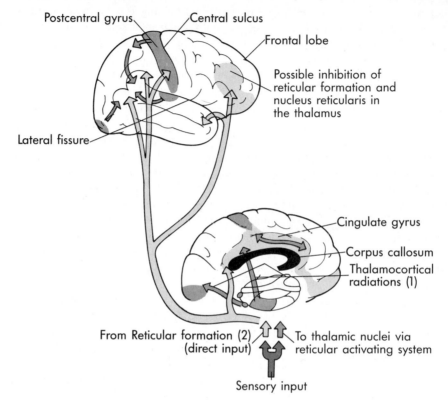

FIG. 4-5 Attention and processing. Sensory input reaches the cortex via two routes. Sensory transmission occurs as a result of input from the reticular activating system via the thalamus to primary sensory areas, and subsequently to the sensory association areas. The nucleus reticularis in the thalamus can inhibit thalamocortical flow from specific thalamic nuclei. Cortical arousal occurs, on the other hand, as a result of sensory input reaching cortex from the reticular formation directly. This leads to a flow of information to the limbic system, prefrontal cortex, superior temporal cortex, pertinent cortical sensory reception areas, and sensory association areas, as well as the nucleus reticularis in the thalamus. The right hemisphere has been considered "dominant" in attention mechanisms. (Adapted from Heilman, Watson, and Valenstein, 1985, Fig. 10–8, p. 255.)

body temperature and feeding behavior. The mechanism is thought to involve the concepts of homeostasis, feedback, and adjustment to control systems relating to a particular variable, such as temperature.

According to Kaupfermann (1985c), pleasure plays an important role in the control of motivated human behavior. The mechanisms involved, although poorly understood, are thought to involve brain and hypothalamic functions relating to reward and reinforcement of learned behavior. Kaupfermann states that arousal includes both peripheral and central arousal, which is important in improving behavioral efficacy. These actions might even relate to substances such as hormones, which act on both sites. Hormones from the pituitary gland have been reported to enter the brain via blood flowing from the pituitary vessels. By providing the same messages both centrally and peripherally, responses could be directed toward the same behavioral goal. The role of the hypothalamus in motivation, in addition to different other sites, such as the medial forebrain bundle, has been supported by stimulation that results in a drive state, as well as activation of symptoms that, according to Kaupfermann, are normally activated by a reinforcing stimulus. Further reinforcement is thought to involve different transmitters.

In studying motivation and its relation to CNS sites and hormones, one cannot overlook a daily, seemingly apparent behavioral example as support for the idea that these factors may be functionally related. A cat that has been castrated stops playing and running and prefers to take it easy, lying down most of the day and gaining weight. Similar behavior is observed in many head-injured patients with frontal lobe damage. These patients prefer to stay in bed and are not motivated to participate in ordinary daily activities, except eating. This can be related to the prefrontal damage, or disrupted pathways between the frontal lobe, which provides control, for example, over primitive drives, and the hypothalamus, including the center for controlling food intake, which surrounds the third ventricle. The hypothalamus also plays an important role in motivation. It is possibly also related to hormones, which act both centrally and peripherally, and thus affect these functions. As a result, the environmental stimuli that motivate the individual are more primitive and evolve around drives, such as food intake.

EMOTION AND PROCESSING

Bryden and Ley (1983) studied hemispheric specialization for emotion by different methods. In one study, a tachistoscope was used to present drawings of human faces that showed different emotions. They found that the subjects' identification of those emotions was more accurate when presented in the left visual field than when presented in the right visual field. In another study of 20 subjects, they used a dichotic listening measure of auditory stimuli. Bryden and Ley developed tonal sequences that were considered to be different

in affect. These stimulus sequences were paired dichotically and presented to subjects who judged the affective value of the stimulus presented to a particular ear. The "affective value" of the "attended stimulus" was found to be "correctly identified" much more frequently when the subjects attended to the left as opposed to the right ear.

Bryden and Ley also used "speech studies" in which 31 subjects listened to a sentence presented to a particular ear and reported the content of the sentence. Subjects were asked to categorize the affect of the sentence they heard, and report its contents. This study indicated that subjects' accuracy in judging the emotional tone of sentences was greater when listening with the left ear, but they were more accurate regarding content when listening with the right ear. According to Kaupfermann (1985a), the inferior parietal lobe has been associated with perception of the emotional tone of incoming information. This refers to timing, loudness, and tone.

These authors suggested that the right hemisphere has a special and dominant influence on the reception and expression of emotions in normal subjects. According to their report, men showed more predictable and stable hemispheric localization than women. This is in keeping with findings mentioned in the section on sex differences and lateralization in Chapter 3, which indicate that males have more focal and lateralized CNS functional localization than females.

Although no specific processing path was indicated by these studies, different sensory information contributes to the reception of information with "emotional tones" in normal subjects. Thus, one would assume that fibers from auditory, visual, and even somatosensory association areas all contribute to the perception of information with emotional content. Further, different aspects of incoming sensory information are stored in different memory compartments connected with the association areas. This information affects emotional reactions to different situations at a later date. The orbitofrontal cortex and the temporal lobe have both been associated with emotion. These areas, in addition to being connected anteriorly by the uncinate tract (Kolb and Whishaw, 1980), are connected by the parahippocampus, hippocampus, and the cingulum, as stated in Chapter 2. The association areas from all the sensory modalities receive input from and contribute information to this pathway. Emotional experiences, such as fear and anger, as well as the expression of emotion or emotional behavior depend on the integration and coordination of motor and endocrine responses, which take place in the hypothalamus, according to Kaupfermann (1985b). Further, electrical stimulation of the lateral hypothalamus is reported to produce anger, but a lesion produces the opposite effect: emotional placidity. Kaupfermann states, in agreement with the previous review, that the hypothalamus projects information to the forebrain via the medial forebrain bundle, a fiber pathway belonging to the limbic system. It continues rostrally as the cingulum, connecting the orbitofrontal areas to the parahippocampal gyrus in the temporal lobe. According to Kaupfermann, the forebrain suppresses emotional responses according to the significance of environmental stimuli. Further, it is responsible for the conscious experience of emotion, and provides the motor mechanisms necessary for responding to the emotional experience. The forebrain thus acts as a feedback mechanism between the external and the internal environments. In patients with frontal-lobe damage, emotional flattening and lack of emotional control are often reported.

This review indicates that the processing of emotion is based on the functions of the hypothalamus and its connection with the limbic cortex of the cerebral hemispheres (Fig. 4-6).

PROCESSING AND MEMORY

Little (1987) comments on the complexity of human memory and describes different types of memory deficits. These include immediate, short- and long-term storage, in addition to modality-specific memory, and material-specific memory. Further, memory deficits may be associated with the encoding, storage, or retrieval of information. The immediate form of memory storage refers to sensory memory, and can be subdivided according to

stimulus type into visual memory (sometimes referred to as *iconic* memory), auditory *(echoic)*, or tactile *(haptic)* memory. This sensory memory is of very short duration. Short-term memory lasts from a few seconds to a few minutes, whereas long-term memory refers to retention over a longer period of time (over 15 minutes), the length of which has been controversial.

Baddeley et al. (1987) comment on the sensory memory systems mentioned above. According to them, deficits resulting from dysfunctions of these systems would manifest as impaired perception, rather than memory deficits. In their view, the sensory memory systems convey information to a temporary storage system that has been given different labels, including *short-term memory, primary memory,* and *working memory*. They believe that the terms *short-term memory* and *primary memory* have conceptual limitations and that their definitions are controversial, leading to a conceptual confusion. These authors point out that the term *working memory* includes integration of different subsystems, whereas the other two terms refer to a unitary storage.

According to Baddeley et al., working memory refers to "the temporary storage of information necessary for the performance of such cognitive tasks as reasoning, comprehending, and learning" (p. 296). They distinguish between two systems of working memory: a "general concept of working memory" and a "specific model of the structure of working memory" (p. 296). The model implies that there is a *"central executive system,"* which coordinates and integrates different subsystems. According to the author, the best-known subsystems are the *"articulatory loop,"* which stores and manipulates phonological and verbal information, and the *"visuospatial sketchpad* which is involved in visuospatial imagery" (p. 296). Further, if storage of information is needed for more than a brief period of time, passage into the long-term memory system is necessary.

According to Little (1987), memory can also be classified according to modality specificity. The most common differentiation is between verbal and visual information, but this classification also in-

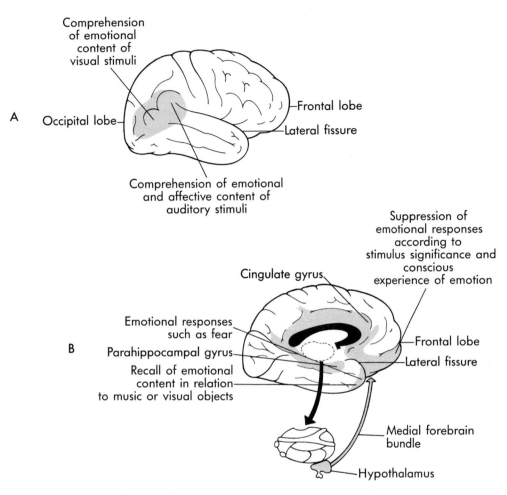

FIG. 4-6 Emotion and processing. **A,** Lateral surface of the right hemisphere, which is considered to be dominant in processing emotional and affective information, regardless of its type. **B,** Medial view of the cerebral hemisphere and its connections via the medial forebrain bundle to the hypothalamus, which plays an important role in emotion. The cingulate gyrus and its different connections with the cortical association areas, hippocampus, parahippocampus, temporal pole and orbitofrontal cortex all play a role in processing emotion and expressing emotional responses.

cludes motor learning and procedural learning. Fig. 4-7 indicates where these modality-specific functions can take place, based on information from Chapters 3 and 7. Visual memory storage has been related to the inferior temporal lobe, according to Kaupfermann (1985a). He states that lesions of this area interfere with the acquisition and retention of visual memory tasks. Further, the superior tem-

poral gyrus has been associated with auditory memory (Kaupfermann, 1985a), and the inferior parietal lobule with storage of visuokinesthetic motor engrams necessary for motor memory or praxis (Heilman and Rothi, 1985).

Little (1987) further differentiates between *semantic* memory, referring to the knowledge of facts, and *episodic* memory which refers to per-

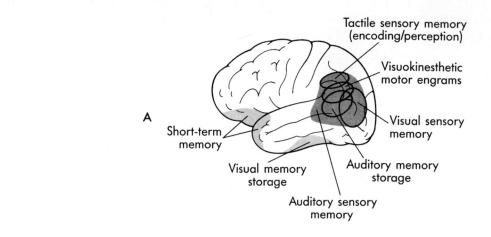

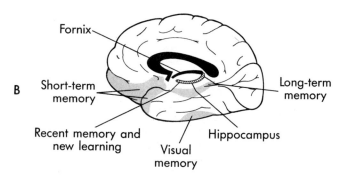

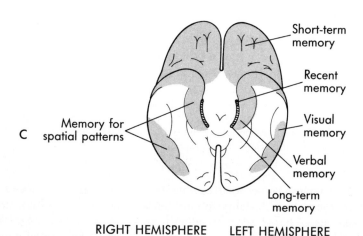

RIGHT HEMISPHERE   LEFT HEMISPHERE

FIG. 4-7 Memory and processing. Both hemispheres: **A,** Lateral view. **B,** Medial view. **C,** Inferior view. Shading indicates sensory memory, which refers to encoding or perception of different types of incoming stimuli, as well as areas important for the storage and retrieval of different types of memory engrams. The right hemisphere is considered to be primarily involved in memory of spatial patterns, whereas the left hemisphere is more involved with verbal memory.

sonally experienced events. Baddeley et al. (1987) claim that long-term memory seems to be less modular than short-term memory. However, according to them, some conceptual distinctions have been made, including the distinction between semantic and episodic memory. They also refer to another distinction between *procedural* learning, including the "acquisition of perceptual, motor, and intellectual skills" (p. 297), and *declarative* learning, referring to discrete information, be it semantic or episodic.

The hippocampus and the medial sides of the temporal lobes have been related to memory processes (Geschwind, 1979a and b). According to Butters (1979), lesions of the anterior temporal lobe result in anterograde amnesia, or a deficit in recent memory and new learning. Conversely, lesions of the posterior aspects of the temporal lobe produce retrograde amnesia, or an inability to recall events that happened prior to injury. Kolb and Whishaw (1980) report that the hippocampus has been associated with memories of visual and auditory nature. However, they point out that controversies have arisen regarding whether the temporal stem should be held responsible for this, rather than the hippocampus. According to them, the term *temporal stem* refers to a pathway that connects temporal lobe structures to the dorsomedial thalamus, basal ganglia, orbitofrontal cortex, and temporal lobe of the other hemisphere. The orbitofrontal cortex has been associated with short-term memory, whereas the temporal lobe has been associated with long-term memory. The left hemisphere has been associated with memory of verbal material, whereas the right hemisphere has been associated with memory of patterns such as faces or geometrical forms. Others (Goldberg et al. 1981) suggest that structures in the reticular activating system, specifically the ventral tegmental area, play a role in the consolidation and retrieval of long-term memory. This area projects to the medial forebrain bundle, the medial septum, hippocampus, and mammilary bodies.

As mentioned in Chapter 3, the modality-specific association areas provide information to higher order association areas of the limbic cortex via the limbic system connection on the medial sides of the hemispheres. Refer again to Fig. 4-7 to review the possible sites for memory processing.

NEURONAL PROCESSING DURING DAILY ACTIVITIES

The previously reviewed processing samples are either theoretical models based on clinical studies correlated with anatomical findings, or controlled studies of isolated events by a new technology. These and other experimental studies have provided isolated models for different cortical functions. During daily activities, of course, cerebral function is not divided into isolated components; many processing events take place simultaneously in a very complicated fashion. Although under experimental conditions simple events can be studied at a few locations in a reductionistic way, we are far from being able to evaluate all our patients by such technology, and the technology is far from being able to handle complicated daily situations. However it is possible to synthesize information from the available studies so that it can be related to task performance in daily activities, and then analyze the stimuli used and the behavioral responses to speculate regarding CNS function and dysfunction. This is the methodology on which the A-ONE is based. It attempts to evaluate signs of CNS dysfunction through a holistic evaluation of task performance during complex but "natural" activities, as opposed to structured experimental conditions. The resulting information may not be as detailed, but it will be informative in terms of the functional abilities of the particular individual, and it can be utilized directly in the formation of treatment goals by therapists.

It should be emphasized that although knowledge regarding brain function has expanded exceedingly in recent years through new imaging and electrical techniques, we still have far to go to understand what is "really" happening. We may, for example, be able to see different illuminated areas during specific tests indicating function at different cerebral locales during blood-flow studies. However, this does not necessarily tell us the sequence of events, or the connections that lead to increased oxygen uptake by certain areas, although we may be able to subdivide tasks and perform two studies, one for ideation and another for execution of movement. Conversely, such studies indicate, as do electrical measures, that function is taking place, but they do not reveal the mechanisms that caused the cerebral activity. Images can appear as connected parallel "happenings," and we might sometimes be able to point to anatomical pathways that could connect the different parallel areas, but can we explain why these "happenings" take place?

Following is an activity analysis of the self-care task of a subject combing the hair, from a neurobehavioral viewpoint. This analysis is based on current information of CNS function. Performance of daily activities is observed on a regular basis by occupational therapists working with neurological patients. Therapists should be able to use this kind of analysis to evaluate the behavior, detect a dysfunction (if any), and relate it to CNS mechanisms. This can be done without any fancy equipment at any location (Fig. 4-8).

A patient is sitting by a sink for hygiene and grooming activities, and a brush is located by the sink. There are three possibilities for sensory information in order for the patient to attend to the brush. The patient attends to the brush visually, and the visual information travels through the visual pathway to the primary visual cortex, where it is synthesized and further analyzed by the association areas. Memories are brought into play, along with ideational processes, resulting in the subject getting the idea that she is to brush her hair. (See previous illustrations for attention, vision, memory, and ideation processes.) Another example of visual information, which may be given if a patient does not understand what to do, is imitation of the activity for her; she must then visually process that information. Similarly when the subject is verbally instructed to brush the hair, auditory information is attended to, and the auditory input travels over the auditory pathway to the primary cortical auditory area in the temporal lobe, where it is processed by aid of the association areas and compared to information in memory stores, which

leads to the formation of an idea based on the auditory information.

The third pathway that comes into play during this situation is the somesthetic one. A patient who grasps a brush, or is handed one, receives tactile and proprioceptive information, which, after it reaches the primary sensory cortex in the parietal lobe, is analyzed by the association areas and integrated with prior experiences. If this is not enough information, it might be necessary to take the patient through the motions (guiding), which also provides tactile and proprioceptive sensory input.

Information from all three modalities goes to the pertinent primary receptive areas "more or less" simultaneously, depending on the sequence and timing of stimuli presentation, if the subject's CNS is working adequately. From there it travels to secondary and tertiary association areas, where further processing takes place. Attentional processes are brought into play, as well as memory processes, emotions, and higher order thought. The sensory information is integrated with previous experiences, and responses are planned that can be both emotional and motoric, resulting in different processing mechanisms, depending on the nature of the response. Simultaneous processing of information takes place as information from the secondary association areas is fed into the limbic system, the tertiary association areas in the prefrontal lobe, and the temporal pole, where higher cognitive functions take place, including emotion and memory. Different fiber connections within a hemisphere, between hemispheres, and between the cortex and other CNS structures play important roles in processing.

During processing, ideation, the intention to perform an action, and the preparation of a sequenced plan of action occur, all of which result in a flow of information to the primary motor cortex and ultimately in the functional response of picking up the brush. This process requires praxis. The intention to perform is related to the frontal lobes and supplementary motor areas. From the lower parietal lobe, housing visuokinesthetic motor en-

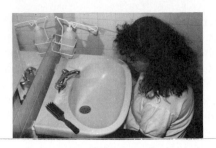

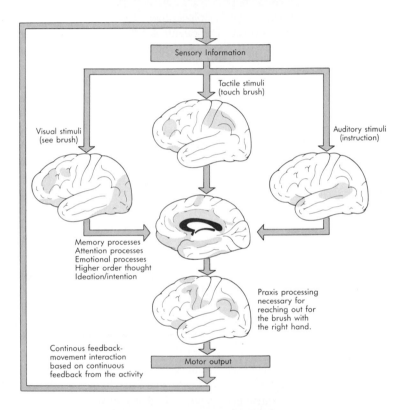

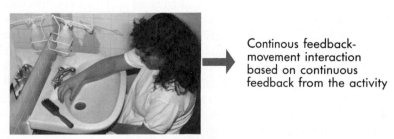

Continous feedback-
movement interaction
based on continuous
feedback from the activity

FIG. 4-8 Processing during a daily activity. A person sitting by a sink preparing for grooming is asked to brush the hair. Note that three types of sensory stimulation can lead to performance.

grams, information travels to the left premotor cortex, which is responsible for planning and sequencing of the movement, on its way to the middle part of the primary motor cortex of the frontal lobe in the left hemisphere, which is responsible for movement performed by the right hand. A series of feedback-movement interactions and readjustments follow, based on continuous sensory information from the activity. During the complex process of performing what we may consider to be a simple activity, other responses, such as emotional and verbal ones, may be elicited.

If the response had been verbal instead of motoric, language information, including ideation and internal speech, would be activated in Wernicke's area and the arcuate fasciculus. Information regarding praxis of mouth movements would "travel" from the visuokinesthetic motor area in the inferior parietal lobe to Broca's areas in the prefrontal lobe and subsequently to the mouth area in the right and left primary motor cortices. Fig. 4-8 illustrates some of the processing components that take place both simultaneously and in sequence during the brushing activity. As will be evident in the following chapters, this process and the resulting neurobehavior can reveal substantial information regarding dysfunctions of cerebral processes. Using this kind of analysis, we can not only observe neurobehavioral deficits but also analyze and control the sensory input that may be important when forming treatment goals.

Inspecting functions from a neurobehavioral viewpoint underlines the importance of Kandel's (1985c) statement: "What is localized to discrete regions in the brain is not a set of elaborate faculties of the mind, but a large family of elementary operations often carried out in parallel" (p. 11). He goes on to propose that "more elaborate faculties derive from the interconnections of several, even many, brain regions" (p. 11). Kandel believes that slow acceptance of the idea of cerebral localization in the previous decades was in part due to lack of awareness of the complexity of functions, the possibility of subfunctions, and the existence of parallel processing in addition to the serial processing.

Kaupfermann (1985a) gives credit to the approach of reducing nervous system activities into discrete anatomical components, as this has provided information necessary for understanding the function of the "whole" nervous system.

Moore (1986) contrasted the classic cortical maps of discrete structural and functional territories with the new metabolic maps, which show brain function and plasticity. She stated that electrophysiological research has shown that CNS components such as basal ganglia, the cerebellum, inferior olivary nuclear complex, prefrontal lobes, sensory-motor and associative cortices, and thalamus all contribute to an *"anticipatory and preparatory circuit"* (p. 460), which fires before movement takes place. Thus she questioned if the traditional brain maps, which show that the motor cortex governs "fine motor coordination, speed, and precision of movement," are still viable. She stated that the new metabolic maps are not consistent with "traditional techniques" and previous perceptions of the CNS and its functions, dysfunctions, and recovery of functions. She predicted that "new atlases" would soon become available and that the recently available evaluation techniques would provide a different picture of the CNS in the near future.

So far, it has been difficult to perceive a holistic functional picture of the CNS. CT scans reflect structure in "slices" of different CNS units, but they do not reveal function. Magnetic resonance imaging (MRI) and PET scans, which will be reviewed in Chapter 6, are technical evaluation methods that can reflect this kind of information in a more functional way, but they are currently only beginning their course. The two-dimensional rCBF studies have been able to reflect only cortical activity and potentially some activity from deeper structures; they have revealed localization information that generally does not conflict with already existing localization maps, and it has even added to them. However, when experimenting with these new investigation methods, the researchers using them compared their findings with the traditional localization maps. The discrepancies between the newer findings and those older maps provoke questions that when answered will increase our knowledge not only of the CNS but also of the capacities and limitations of the newer methods.

EEG studies and topographical imaging of electric activity currently reveal only cortical activity; direct measurements from subcortical structures, therefore, are not yet possible. As will be apparent in Chapter 6, which reviews technological evaluation methods, these methods are generally used to localize focal cerebral dysfunctions. They have also been used by some researchers to show the spread of electrical activity during functional tasks, but only over the scalp, reflecting cortical processing and localization. The validity and the replicability of these studies are still questionable, as will be evident in the section on technological evaluation methods. Evoked potential measures record the spread of electrical activity from peripheral nerves via the brain stem and cortical structures, but they give only a crude localization of conduction impairment at specific levels.

Occupational therapists should use cortical localization maps to gather information regarding potential sites of dysfunction, which could be used to speculate on patterns. An understanding of processing is based on localization, or some reference points. These maps will evolve as our knowledge does; further improvement is grounded in current understanding of the nervous system. In other words, today's knowledge is needed to build on. Occupational therapists can contribute to the evolution of the maps by using existing knowledge and methodologies. My view is in keeping with the view of paradigms described by Kuhn (1970), that paradigms evolve to include new views of the world that change people's thought processes, but the new paradigms must include knowledge from preceding paradigms, which in this case would be the knowledge compiled by localization studies of the cerebral cortex.

Bergland (1985), in his radical and extraordinary publication *The Fabric of Mind,* argues that the brain is a gland and that hormones "are the stuff of thought" (p. 3), as opposed to the current notion

accepted by many that the brain is an "electrically driven computer" (p. 93). Thus hormones in a holistic way are the "prime moving forces of the brain" (p. 5). According to Bergland "holism" will replace "reductionism in a new paradigm that gives human thoughts qualities that are warm, soft, wet, colourful, qualitative, timeless, communal and united" (p. 93). After having previously stated that the reason we observe function at various cortical locales during, for example, imaging studies is yet unknown, it will be interesting to view Bergland's "new paradigm" in further detail. His "new hormone-based paradigm for the mind, acknowledges that electricity does flow from nerve to nerve and can be measured on the surface of the brain, or on the membranes of individual nerves" (p. 108). However, he states that the superficial electrical "signals are little more than dry echoes of deeper molecular events going on within the cell" (p. 108). Bergland describes the new evolving paradigm based on the current belief of scientists that understanding of the brain is to be found in intracellular molecular events rather than in "superficial electrical signals" as follows:

> Although this is a new paradigm, nearly all of the early experiments demonstrate that regulatory hormones join in holistic patterns that may be understood by organs other than the brain. The mechanisms of the mind are thus released from the conceptual confines of the reductionistic left brain. The mechanisms that drive thought are found all over the body and, wherever they live, they function at their highest level by recognizing the molecular patterns of the combination of hormones that modulate thought (p. 109).

Upon scientists' acceptance of this new paradigm, "the primary mechanisms of intelligent thought must be viewed differently. The mind is made pattern dependent and comes to share in the ubiquitous secret of evolutionary survival: pattern recognition" (p. 109). Bergland goes on in supporting the importance of pattern recognition by reminding the reader of "the DNA/RNA interactions, . . . antigen-antibody reactions, [and] pattern recognition" as the basis "to all the hormone/ hormone receptor interactions of cell regulation" pattern recognition being "the highest form of thought" (p. 109). He claims that "it is the synchrony, the synergism and the spatial juxtaposition of whirling hormonal forces that give life to the human soul" (p. 109).

Stuss and Benson (1986), in commenting on the holistic versus localization approaches to understanding the CNS, stated that "neither view is entirely correct, and neither is entirely wrong" (p. 4). Valuable information regarding the CNS stems from both approaches. They suggested that belief in one approach, as opposed to the other, is dependent on and varies with "current modes and fashions" (p. 4). I share the perspective that valuable and necessary information arises from both approaches. In reviewing some of the literature regarding both localization and processing of cortical functions presented during the last century in the Western world, I have envisioned the different approaches as different paradigms, one preceding the other, as described earlier, but both necessary for the evolution of knowledge.

CHAPTER
5

Causes of Cortical CNS Dysfunctions

The causes of dysfunctions of the cerebral cortex that result in neurobehavioral deficits are diverse and include vascular disorders, trauma, infections, toxins, tumors, and degeneration of the nervous system (Cummings and Benson, 1983; Daube and Sandok, 1978). This chapter outlines the most common causes of dysfunction. This should indicate in which patient group the neurobehavioral deficits potentially occur. The Árnadóttir OT-ADL Neurobehavioral Evaluation (A-ONE) should be suitable for these patient groups, although one should expect different performance patterns on the assessment in some of the diagnostic subgroups. It should be kept in mind that the prognosis for a particular dysfunction is related to its cause, and the resulting neurobehavioral impairments depend upon the localization and the extent of the lesion (Cummings and Benson, 1983; Daube and Sandok, 1978; Jennett and Teasdale, 1981).

VASCULAR DISORDERS

Two major types of cerebral vascular dysfunction cause neurologic lesions. These are *ischemia,* referring to insufficient blood suppply to the brain, which is responsible for 80% of all strokes according to Caplan and Stein (1986), and *hemorrhage,* or bleeding, due to a ruptured blood vessel, which accounts for the remaining 20% of strokes (Brust, 1985; Daube and Sandok, 1978; Caplan and Stein, 1986).

In ischemia, brain structures are deprived of glucose as well as oxygen, and the removal of potentially toxic metabolites is also prevented according to Brust (1985). The deprivation can result in temporary deficits that clear without tissue damage. However, it can be prolonged, resulting in tissue death (Brust, 1985; Daube and Sandok, 1978). The vessel affected by infarction may be large or small, which results in a focal destructive lesion. The severity of impairments depends on the location of the lesion (Daube and Sadok, 1978; Werner, 1980). Ischemia can be further divided into two groups according to its origin. These are thrombosis and embolism. *Thrombosis* refers to an obstruction caused by a process within one or more blood vessels. This leads to changes in the vessel wall, or the formation of a blood clot within the vessel, which narrows the lumen of the artery. Thrombosis is most commonly caused by atherosclerosis and usually affects the larger arteries supplying the brain. Smaller intracranial vessels are, on the contrary, affected by hypertension. In *embolism* the cerebral blood-flow obstruction is caused by material that is formed at a distant part of the vascular system, such as the heart or proximal vessels, and carried to the cerebral arteries. Swelling and edema may accompany the acute phase of brain and vascular injuries (Caplan and Stein, 1986; Daube and Sandok, 1978).

81

Hemorrhage can be divided into two subgroups: *subarachnoid* hemorrhage, which occurs at the surface of the brain, and *intracerebral,* or *intraparenchymal,* hemorrhage, which refers to bleeding within the cerebral tissue. Subarachnoid hemorrhage is usually due to a ruptured vessel associated with aneurism, arterio-venous malformation, or trauma. Intracerebral hemorrhage on the other hand, is usually due to hypertension and subsequent leakage from small intracerebral vessels. The resulting blood clot produces swelling of adjacent brain tissue, and may be responsible for disconnection of cortical fibers (Brust, 1985; Caplan and Stein, 1986; Daube and Sandok, 1978).

The reader is referred to the discussion of cerebral blood flow in Chapter 2 for arterial supply to the different cortical areas. Occlusion of the middle cerebral artery may vary depending on which of its branches are affected. If the dysfunction affects its upper trunk, which supplies the frontal and parietal lobes, this may result in contralateral hemiplegia, especially of the face and upper extremity, and hemisensory loss, including both tactile and proprioceptive information. Impairment of the visual field and conjugate gaze may be present. Unilateral neglect of space or body may be manifested, as well as spatial-relation dysfunction, and anosognosia, especially if the right hemisphere is affected. Further, attentional deficits and impaired organization of behavior may be present, as well as lack of judgment. If the left hemisphere is affected, speech and language functions may be impaired, and apraxia may be present (Brust, 1985; Caplan and Stein, 1986). In lesions of the lower trunk of the middle cerebral artery, there may be a visual-field defect, and Wernicke's aphasia. Some spatial relation problems may be evident if the right middle cerebral artery is affected, as well as constructional apraxia. Further, some behavioral abnormalities, such as paranoia and violence, may be manifested. When the obstruction affects both divisions of the middle cerebral artery, all these symptoms can be expected (Brust, 1985; Caplan and Stein, 1986). Dysfunctions due to the occlusion of branches supplying deep cerebral structures are beyond the scope of this review. The reader is

referred to Chapters 7 and 8 for more details regarding impairments and their location.

During dysfunction of the anterior cerebral artery, manifestations of paralysis and sensory loss are greatest in the leg, especially the foot. Unilateral apraxia may manifest as a result of dysfunction of the anterior part of the corpus callosum. Speech disturbance, or inertia of speech, can be related to dysfunction of the supplementary motor area. Urinary incontinence may also be present. A bilateral impairment of the anterior cerebral arterial territory may lead to behavioral disturbances due to dysfunction of the orbitofrontal cortex and limbic structures (Brust, 1985; Caplan and Stein, 1986).

Impairments accompanying infarction of the posterior cerebral artery include homonymous hemianopsia, with sparing of macular vision. A lesion of the left side may result in alexia without agraphia, and associate visual agnosia, whereas bilateral lesion will produce cortical blindness. Left-side lesions may result in transcortical aphasia with naming difficulties. Further, discrimination of left and right body sides may be difficult. Finger agnosia may be present as well as some spatial-relation difficulties, acalculia, agraphia, and memory problems. Dysfunction of the posterior cerebral artery can also affect subcortical structures such as the thalamus, if the lesion occurs proximally in the artery (Brust, 1985; Caplan and Stein, 1986).

ANOXIA

Conditions other than vascular diseases may also produce an anoxic dysfunction of the cerebral cortex. These include cardiopulmonary arrest, carbon monoxide poisoning, anemia, anesthetic accidents, and strangulation. These conditions normally result in a diffuse cerebral dysfunction (Daube and Sandok, 1978; Cummings and Benson, 1983). These conditions affect the border zones in the periphery of the major cerebral arteries most seriously. These zones are termed *watershed regions* (Fig. 5-1).

HEAD INJURY

Head injuries may manifest with focal or diffuse symptoms. Focal head injuries located at the point of impact occur as a result of severe local defor-

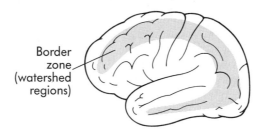

FIG. 5-1 Watershed regions. The areas most vulnerable for anoxic impairment are those at the distal branches where the main cerebral arteries meet.

mation, such as skull fracture, according to Jennett and Teasdale (1981). According to Grafman and Salazar (1987), penetrating brain wounds occur in less than 10% of head injuries. They claim that head injury creates acceleration and deceleration of the head, which produces movement and distortion of the brain within the skull. Further, in a closed head injury, the force of the blow is relatively more important than its location. It can cause what has been termed *coup,* or trauma due to cortical contact with bone directly under the blow, and *contrecoup* lesions resulting in brain damage due to brain-bone contact oppposite the impact force, usually at the frontal and temporal tips, as well as diffuse sharing of axons (Fig. 5-2). Jennett and Teasdale (1981) agree with Grafman and Salazar. They state that the contusions following head injury are usually multiple, bilateral, and asymmetrical. According to Daube and Sandok (1978), the initial manifestation of impairments after head injury is often diffuse, presenting as an extensive physiologic dysfunction of the CNS. This condition, which reaches its peak at onset or shortly after, usually improves to a state where the deficits become more focal manifestations of anatomic damage, due to contusions, lacerations or hematomas.

Jennett and Teasdale (1981) differentiated between impact damage and secondary damage as a result of head injury. Impact damage refers to skull fractures and contusions of the gray matter with possible intracerebral hemorrhage, according

to these authors. White-matter lesions, on the other hand, result from the tearing of nerve fibers at the onset of injury, or they may develop as secondary to necrosis, hemorrhage, internal herniation, edema, or raised intracranial pressure. The resulting secondary damage, including raised intracranial pressure and hydrocephalus, hematoma, and hypoxia may manifest as ischemic brain damage, and contribute to prolongation of coma. According to Jennett and Teasdale, increased intracranial pressure from hydrocephalus affects in particular the hippocampal gyri, cingulate gyri, medial occipital cortex, and the structures surrounding the ventricular system. Ischemic brain damage affects the hippocampus and the calcarine area, as well as the basal ganglia and cerebellum. Further, the previously mentioned watershed regions on the lateral surface where the three major cortical arteries meet were reported to be common sites of anoxia in this kind of lesion. Ischemic lesions due to anoxia were usually found to be bilateral.

Hemorrhage as a result of head injury may be of a different nature. It includes subdural hematoma, subarachnoid hemorrhage, or intracerebral hemorrhage. The reader is referred to the section on vascular disorders earlier in this chapter for more details regarding hemorrhage.

Jennett and Teasdale (1981) agree with Grafman and Salazar (1987) in concluding that contusions manifest most frequently on the inferior surfaces of the frontal and temporal lobes, as well as

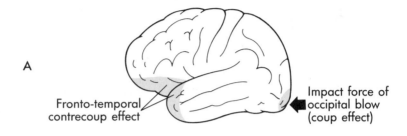

A

Fronto-temporal
contrecoup effect

Impact force of
occipital blow
(coup effect)

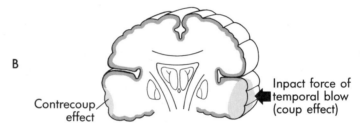

B

Contrecoup
effect

Inpact force of
temporal blow
(coup effect)

FIG. 5-2 Coup-contrecoup effect of head injury. **A,** An occipital blow leading to a considerable contrecoup effect in the temporal pole and in the orbitofrontal area. **B,** Coronal section of coup and contrecoup effect of a unilateral temporal blow.

the anterior temporal poles, regardless of the site of impact. This can occur, for example, as a contrecoup effect resulting from an occipital blow. These contusions have been related to more irregular surfaces on the inside of the skull at these areas. Further, unilateral skull fractures of the vault are reported to be accompanied by more marked contusions on the same side of the brain, except for the case of occipital fractures, which produce more marked frontal contusions. However, bilateral contusions are reported by the same authors to be common in humans and to frequently manifest with more severe damage of the hemisphere opposite the skull fracture.

Several factors are important in contributing to the outcome of head injury, in addition to the actual injuries identified in the neurological examination, according to Eisenberg and Weiner (1987). These include the mechanisms of injury, age of the subject, and duration of coma, in addition to some of the already mentioned secondary factors resulting from the injury.

INFLAMMATORY DISEASE

Certain diseases may influence cerebral states or mimic cerebral lesions; inflammation is one such disease. Foreign substances may produce inflammation in nervous tissue. These include microorganisms and toxic chemicals. Immunologic reactions can also result in inflammatory response, which is a complex series of events. CNS infections are usually diffuse. They occur either in the meninges and cerebral spinal fluid, or in the brain tissue, resulting in encephalitis. Infections can also be focal, however, affecting a specific brain area. Such lesions result in abscess formation, which can expand and produce a mass effect, with compression of the adjacent structures (Daube and Sandok, 1978).

TOXIC AND METABOLIC DISEASES

In addition to inflammatory diseases, toxic and metabolic diseases may influence cerebral status or mimic cerebral lesions. Such diseases can be caused by endogenous as well as exogenous chemical agents. Manifestations of neurological dysfunction in such cases are usually distributed in a diffuse manner, but their effects may be acute, subacute, or chronic. The resulting pathological changes may vary; they include ischemia, edema, and demyelination (Daube and Sandok, 1978).

BRAIN TUMOR

Brain tumors result from neoplastic changes in cells within the nervous system, according to Daube and Sandok (1978). They report that these changes include unrestrained proliferation of cells, which may be triggered by genetic, infectious, or chemical factors. Such changes can occur in any cell type within the CNS. However, neurocytomas are rare because the capacity of neurons to undergo cell division is limited, and this capacity is correlated with the potential to undergo neoplasic change, according to the authors. Daube and Sandok state that astrocytomas are the most common primary CNS tumors. This is because astrocytes are more reactive than other cells in the CNS. Tumors have focal and progressive effects in the nervous system,

according to Daube and Sandok. They produce functional alterations of the area in which they are located, and may further cause compression of adjacent structures or be accompanied by edema, resulting in functional alterations of adjacent structures.

BRAIN ATROPHY

Atrophy of the brain is manifested in *dementia,* which refers to a progressive deterioration of mental functions, including cognitive abilities, emotion, language, memory, personality, and spatial relations (Cummings and Benson, 1983; Côté, 1985). Dementia is associated with aging, but its exact etiology is unknown. Several types of microscopic changes accompanying aging in humans have been associated with dementia, according to Côté. These are the accumulation of lipofuscin granules in the cytoplasm, accumulation of granulovacuolar organelles within the cytoplasm of degenerating nerve cells of the hippocampus, accumulation of neuritic plaques within the hippocampus and neocortex. Further, there is an accumulation of neurofibrillary tangles, which are typical for Alzheimer's disease, and changes in cell bodies and dendrites that result in loss of dendrites, which in turn reduces the neurons' capacity to process information. The dendrite changes result in a decrease in the number of dendrites and synaptic interactions, this affecting information processing within the CNS. Further, gross anatomical changes may be seen, such as enlargement of the ventricles, shrunken gyri, and wide sulci. However, many of these structural changes occur in normal aging, and the changes may not parallel the severity of clinical symptoms. Some of the impairments caused by dementia have further been associated with altered function of neurotransmitters and their receptors (Côté, 1985). Cummings and Benson (1983) agree with Côté in that findings of enlarged cortical sulci and ventricular enlargement detected by neuroimaging techniques are not reliable predictors of dementia. However, they point out that these changes become more prominent as the disease advances.

The impairments caused by dementia vary in

severity in accord with the state of the dementic process. Dementias are commonly classified into two subgroups: cortical and subcortial dementias. The cortical dementias include Alzheimer's and Pick's disease (Cummings and Benson, 1983; Daube and Sandok, 1978). The deficits associated with cortical dementias are focal, and do not affect all cortical areas evenly. According to Côté (1985), Alzheimer's disease accounts for 70% of dementias, and about 15% are a result of multiple infarcts. According to Cummings and Benson, Alzheimer's disease only accounts for 20% to 50% of progressive dementia cases evaluated in hospital-based settings, and Pick's disease is about 10% to 15% less common than Alzheimer's disease.

Alzheimer's disease can affect people of different age groups, spanning the outdated terms of *senile* and *presenile* dementia, according to Cummings and Benson (1983). They describe the progress of deterioration in three stages, related to the severity of impairments. The first state includes memory disturbances and impaired judgment, as well as spatial and temporal disorientation. Anomia may be present, and so are emotional changes, such as apathy and sadness or depression. During the second stage, memory becomes more severely impaired, including both recent and remote memory changes. Ideational and ideomotor apraxia; aphasia including paraphasias, anomia, and impaired comprehension; agnosia; and restlessness are manifested. In the last stage all intellectual capacities are impaired, and so is motor performance, which is marked by extrapyramidal rigidity or spasticity. The language changes at this stage may include echolalia, perseverations, disarthria, or terminal mutism. There is a progressive deterioration in concentration, reasoning, abstraction, and judgment, which reaches a peak in the final stages. Personality and social behavior are, however, reported to remain relatively intact until the later stages of the disease. Incontinence also becomes a problem in the later stages.

Cummings and Benson (1983), in reviewing studies on dementia, report reduction of regional cerebral blood flow (rCBF) in Alzheimer's patients, especially in posterior temporal and parieto-occipital regions. The association cortices in the posterior temporal, parietal, and frontal lobes have also indicated marked blood-flow reductions on PET scans, as indicated by the same authors. Further, the reduced blood flow in the frontal lobes seems to correlate with symptoms in the late stages of the disease, such as echolalia, mutism, and impairment of spontaneous speech.

Electrical changes have also been associated with Alzheimer's disease, according to Cummings and Benson (1983). These include amplitude reduction on EEG and slight slowing of alpha activity in the early stages. In later stages irregular theta activity, frontal delta activity, and loss of fast activity are manifested. Abnormal delays have further been reported in auditory and visual evoked potentials, indicating disturbed attention and decision-making processes.

Postmortem studies of the brains of Alzheimer's patients have indicated reduced weight and atrophy, especially in the temporo-parietal and anterior frontal regions. The primary sensory and motor areas in the frontal, parietal, and occipital lobes are often spared. The earlier mentioned neurofibrillary tangles occur in the hippocampus, amygdala, and pyramidal cells of the neocortex. Senile plaques representing tissue deterioration are present in the cerebral cortex, hippocampus, amygdala, corpus striatum, and thalamus. The histological changes that affect the neocortex are specific, including primarily the temporo-parieto-occipital association area, temporo-limbic area, and the posterior cingulate gyrus. The anterior cingulate gyrus as well as primary motor and sensory areas are spared (Brun and Gustafson, 1978; Cummings and Benson, 1983). The nucleus basilis is thought to be involved in the reduction of cholinergic neurons affecting transmitter-related proteins (Côté, 1985). According to Cummings and Benson (1983), the nucleus basilis has diffuse projections to the neocortex, which may explain some of the cholinergic deficits evident in Alzheimer's disease.

Pick's disease is also a progressive form of dementia, where impairments manifest at three different stages of the disease, according to Cummings and Benson (1983). The first stage is characterized by personality changes and emotional alterations, such as apathy, irritability, depression, and euphoria. Emotional blunting, including loss of fear and diminished affective responses, is present, along with impaired judgment, lack of insight, and socially inappropriate behavior. Language abnormalities include anomia, and circumlocution may also be present. In the second stage, aphasia is more prominent, including comprehension deficits. During the final stage, all intellectual areas show impairment. Patients may become mute and incontinent, and extrapyramidal deficits progress. Further, deterioration includes memory deficits, and impaired visuospatial skills (Cummings and Benson, 1983).

In contrast to Alzheimer's patients, patients with Pick's disease show structural and blood-flow changes that indicate impairment of the frontal and temporal association areas, according to Cummings and Benson (1983). They state that the anterior medial temporal areas, including the parahippocampus and the orbitofrontal cortex are most commonly affected. The lobal distribution of atrophy varies: 25% of brains show primarily frontal involvement, 25% primary temporal, and 40% to 50% combined frontal and temporal atrophy. Further, although symmetrical distribution of impairment is common, a left-side predominance of dysfunction is more common than either bilateral or right-sided dysfunction. Neuronal loss also affects the basal ganglia, thalamus, and subthalamic nuclei, whereas no selective involvement of transmitter systems has been reported, according to the same authors. See Fig. 5-3 for distribution of topographical impairment of cortical dementia as presented by Brun and Gustafson (1978). Brun and Gustafson state, on the basis of microscopic neuropathological investigations, that anterior cortical regions are the most commonly involved sites in Pick's disease. These include anterior limbic areas and the orbitofrontal cortex.

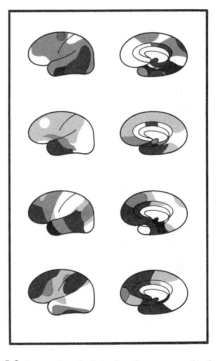

FIG. 5-3 Areas of cortical dysfunction as a result of Alzheimer's and Pick's disease based on histological studies. **A,** Cortical dysfunction in an Alzheimer's patient, emphasizing posterior cortical involvement. **B** to **D,** Examples of cortical dysfunction in patients with Pick's disease, emphasizing involvement of the anterior association cortex, including temporal, frontal, or temporal and frontal lobe involvement. (Adapted from "Limbic Lobe Involvement in Presenile Dementia," by A. Brun and L. Gustafson, 1978, *Archives of Psychiatry and Neurological Sciences,* 226, pp. 79-93.)

SUMMARY

The review of the literature in this chapter suggests patient groups for which A-ONE would be suitable. Neurobehavioral deficits may result from different causes. These are vascular diseases, including hemorrhage, and ischemia; anoxia; trauma; inflammatory diseases; toxic metabolic diseases; neoplasia; and brain atrophy. The manifestations of deficits can be either focal or diffuse. Cortical dementia is usually more focal than global and can be related to either the anterior or posterior association cortices. In terms of CVA, it is possible to classify deficits and relate them to the distribution of the three major arteries that supply the cerebral cortex. Similarly, neoplasms, or tumors, often result in deficits that could be confined to more specific areas of the cortex. The dysfunctions associated with head injuries, on the other hand, are generally more diffuse and asymmetrical; thus it is harder to confine those to limited areas of the cerebral cortex, although such instances certainly occur. Cerebral anoxia usually leads to more diffuse dysfunction. Thus, it would be harder to confine it to limited cortical areas. Because toxins and some infections are often associated with deficits that manifest diversely, it is more difficult to limit them to any specific areas of the cortex.

In conclusion, the information in this chapter gives the reader an idea of the classes of patients for whom the A-ONE would be suitable. It should also be valuable for those who are interested in using Part II of the A-ONE (see Chapter 12) to aid in forming a hypothesis regarding the location of a dysfunction that causes neurobehavioral impairments within the CNS. This is because patterns of CNS dysfunction were reviewed in relation to the different possible diagnostic groups that produce such deficits.

When choosing research samples to provide further development of the instrument, as was done in Part II, this information becomes useful. In some research situations it is desirable to have a homogeneous sample (for example, during neuroimaging comparative studies), and then one could select, for example, a sample with focal disorders due to a specific diagnosis. In other situations it may be more desirable to use a heterogeneous sample. This was done during the interrater reliability studies in Part II. Further, the progress of neurobehavioral deficits related to specific diagnosis should also be taken into consideration during research studies.

CHAPTER
6

Selected Evaluation Methods

A wide spectrum of evaluation methods is presently used to detect structural and functional disorders in patients having a potential for neurobehavioral impairment. Some of these evaluation methods have provided a part of the information that has been presented throughout the literature review in this book. This chapter describes the most common assessment methods currently used, in addition to neurological examinations by a medical doctor. For convenience, these methods have been divided into two categories: (1) neurobehavioral assessment tools, including those used in occupational therapy and neuropsychology assessments, and (2) technological investigation methods, which make use of modern technology for assessment purposes.

NEUROBEHAVIORAL ASSESSMENT METHODS

The neurobehavioral assessment methods reviewed in this chapter are those used in the disciplines of occupational therapy and neuropsychology. Such instruments, as compared to many of the neuroimaging techniques reviewed later, are noninvasive, and do not present risks of mortality or morbidity to the patients evaluated. As the cardinal issue of this book is an occupational therapy evaluation instrument that assesses the domain of activities of daily living, several common ADL evaluation tools will be examined, in addition to cognitive-perceptual evaluation instruments.

Occupational therapy evaluation instruments

As previously noted, there is presently no occupational therapy evaluation instrument known to me that is sensitive to both the level of independence in primary activities of daily living and the neurobehavioral deficits that interfere with functional performance. Such an evaluation tool would be valuable for determining both functional disability and the kind of impairment that results in the functional disability. Further, the lack of reliability and validity of the evaluation methods used in occupational therapy has been pointed out. Detailed standardized evaluation methods with normative samples for comparison are rarely available. Some available evaluations in the field, addressing the primary topics in this section, will be reviewed. The review considers important evaluation aspects, such as purpose, or intended use, of the assessment; reliability; validity; standardization procedures, including norms for comparisons; other psychometric qualities; scoring methods; methods of interpretation; and meaning of the data, as well as administrative requirements, where this information is available.

Cognitive-perceptual occupational therapy evaluation tools

Reports of evaluation tools originating within the discipline of occupational therapy that measure neurobehavioral dysfunctions are rare in the literature. Therapists seem to use cognitive-perceptual evaluations and ADL evaluations separately to assess patients with neurobehavioral dysfunctions. This section includes an overview of some of the available evaluation tools used and studies performed by occupational therapists in recent years, relative to neurobehavioral impairments.

Siev et al. (1986) published a literature review of the evaluation and treatment of perceptual and cognitive dysfunctions in adult stroke patients. The review described cognitive and perceptual dysfunctions, and related them to localized areas within the cerebral cortex. It presented several tests for assessing such dysfunctions. Many of the tests, such as tests for agnosias, apraxias, body scheme, and spatial relations, are similar to, or the same as, some of the subtests used by neuropsychologists. The purpose of the tests is to detect whether cognitive or perceptual deficits are present. However, they do not reveal how these deficits affect general functional performance. Several of the tests in the review were reported to be subjective, using qualitative scoring, rather than objective, including quantitative scoring criteria. The validity and reliability of many of the tests had not been examined. Further, according to the authors, only a few of the tests "have been standardized for adult populations" (p. 5). However, some had been "standardized for children" (p. 5). Because of the reported lack of validation for many of the tests, the authors suggest that a minimum of two tests be used to evaluate each impairment. However, they also recognize the time and the cost factors inherent in such testing, pointing out that it may not be possible for practical reasons to evaluate all the different impairments. The authors also indicated that because of deficit overlap, it may be necessary to administer specific tests in an attempt to differentiate between deficits. In many of the tests, scoring only implies whether a patient can, or cannot accomplish a task, but not to what degree it was accomplished, or why. Thus, for example, in terms of constructional praxis, a deficit may indicate perseveration, a spatial relation problem, or spatial neglect, without any of these deficits being identified.

Siev et al. reported a lack of research to correlate test scores from cognitive and perceptual assessments with functional performance of patients, and they claimed this to be the reason that some therapists rely solely on functional tests, such as dressing, rather than formal perceptual tests. The authors stated, however, that functional tests cannot always distinguish why a patient is having problems performing an activity. They suggested that reasons based on the results of the functional tests should be hypothesized, and then tested with formal perceptual tests. Such a combination of functional and perceptual tests would be very useful for occupational therapists in evaluating patients with CNS damage. Clearly, Siev et al. have made a considerable contribution to the awareness of neurobehavioral deficits in occupational therapy by their literature review.

Each of the tests which Siev et al. suggested that occupational therapists use is focused on a particular deficit, for example, constructional apraxia or somatoagnosia. The fact that a failure on a constructional test may be a result of many different impairments, such as perseveration or visual neglect, is not taken into consideration. With the evaluation method suggested by Siev et al., many tests must be administered to cover all the deficits, and these tests indicate only impairment, not functional level of independence, necessitating that separate studies be performed to examine the relation of these test results to function. This further requires that therapists should be aware of the results of these studies and use that knowledge. This process appears to be much more cumbersome than the one used in the A-ONE, which is less time-consuming and relates specifically to functional performance in daily activities. However, it is recognized that it may be necessary to use specific tests to differentiate between questionable deficits, just as suggested by Siev et al. for the tests in their review.

I suggest a completely different approach, emphasizing the importance of examining a primary functional ADL activity and observing all possible neurobehavioral deficits during that specific activity, rather than testing for each deficit separately. It is important for occupational therapists to develop their own theoretical frames for evaluation to reflect their unique approaches, not to test deficits separately by methods that might be considered as "borrowed" from the field of neuropsychology. After the evaluation of primary activities of daily living, some secondary ADL activities (for example, writing or preparing a meal) might be considered as a further evaluation if the patient's condition allows for it, although such an evaluation is beyond the scope of the A-ONE. Again, interpreting all the possible deficits that could appear during the same activity would be the approach. Siev et al. noted the lack of research correlating test scores to functional performance, with the result that therapists sometimes rely solely on functional tests, rather than neurobehavioral assessments; thus, their work supports the need for a functional instrument that is sensitive to neurobehavioral deficits. The A-ONE was designed with that need in mind.

Zoltan et al. (1983) published a manual for their Perceptual Motor Evaluation, which was designed for head-injured and other neurologically impaired adults. The evaluation includes the following subtests: Gross Visual Skills (Visual Attentiveness, Ocular Pursuits, Visual Fields, and Visual Neglect); Praxis; Constructional Praxis (Graphic Praxis, Block Designs, and Parquetry Board); Body Scheme (Draw a Person, Body Parts Identification, and a Body Puzzle); Depth Perception (Wands Depth Perception Test, and Skiing Picture); Form Perception; Size Discrimination; and Part-Whole Integration.

The test format used in the Perceptual Motor Evaluation is similar to the one recommended by Siev et al. One or more items are used to test each category of dysfunction, rather than observing behavior in general, and simultaneously detecting several deficits as in the A-ONE. Body scheme, for example, is tested by drawing a person and scored on a scale from 0 (intact) to 3 (unable to perform the task). The manual provides a list of possible indications for dysfunction which is valu-

able, but these possibilities are not checked off or included in the score. Each item is scored separately from 0 to 3, but it is questionable how informative these scores are from a functional viewpoint, and subsequently how informative they are for other team members. A summary sheet for a written description of performance is included. A direct evaluation of neurobehavioral impairments through "functional" activities would provide more useful and direct information for goal establishment in therapy, and for other team members, than do, in general, cognitive-perceptual tests with "neuropsychological" items. However, such an evaluation might be followed up by items like those in the Perceptual Motor Evaluation, which in some cases tests separate items more specifically.

Zoltan et al. stated that the manual can be used as a supplement to observations of ADL, and that it should be used to structure treatment goals. Results from the A-ONE, however, should be more effective in forming ideas for treatment approaches and suggesting appropriate treatment methods and rehabilitation goals, because this evaluation is geared more towards detecting those deficits that interfere with functional independence specifically, and the CNS sources of the behavioral dysfunctions. In other words, with the A-ONE, deficits are not only detected but can, by using Part II of the A-ONE, be related to specific CNS locations or processing dysfunctions. This enables the therapist to address the cause of the dysfunction, and provides a potential for speculation regarding the potential of utilizing the remaining CNS processes to a greater extent than does deficit identification alone. This, in turn, should provide the possibility of more precise treatment approaches and, in turn, better treatment.

It is possible, as mentioned previously, to use items from the Perceptual Motor Evaluation after the ADL assessment for further differentiation and determination of specific deficits, if necessary. The strength of the evaluation is that considerable effort has gone toward standardizing the instructions. Content validity of the Perceptual Motor Evaluation was provided by a literature review. The manual states that interrater reliability was established for all subtests, although the authors do not report its value in the manual. The internal consistency of the test was established by use of alpha item analysis, according to the test manual, although this value is not reported either. This evaluation has more of a research background than most evaluations used in occupational therapy for adult patients with neurobehavioral dysfunction.

Sørensen (1978a), a Danish occupational therapist, developed a Cognitive Test, which includes subtests in the areas of language functions, gnosis, praxis, body scheme, memory, abstract thinking, psychomotor speed and vigilance, as well as construction and task performance for geriatric patients. The Cognitive Test uses a 100-point scale that includes paper-and-pencil tasks, block designs, instructions for physical and abstract tasks, and memory tasks. The purpose of the test is to provide understanding regarding CNS dysfunctions, and it should be used as an aid in increasing the patient's independence, according to the author. Further, it was intended to aid in treatment and placement decisions. The test items were chosen to provide practical information regarding the patient's functional abilities, such as reading newspapers, managing money, keeping time, obeying light signals, and administering medication. The scores are added up, and a score that is less than 75% of the maximum total score is claimed to indicate that a person is unable to live alone (Sørensen, 1978a; Sørensen, 1978b).

Some of the tests used by Sørensen (1978a) are based on methods similar to those used in neuropsychology, in agreement with the approach used by Siev et al. (1986). However, Sørensen must be complemented on the functional and practical flavor in many of the subtests. Unfortunately, the scores are added up, instead of providing guidelines for therapists to interpret the information in relation to activities of daily living. It is unfortunate because some therapists have had difficulty relating the "functional" meaning of the scores from the subtests to the specific impairments, and to what this would mean in functional terms. Further, the scoring criteria only consider the ability to perform on a specific test, not why the person cannot complete the task, which makes it difficult for therapists to interpret the results, both in cognitive and functional terms. It is evident that a patient has difficulties writing if she scores low on a writing task, but why does she not succeed in performance? Is it because of motor apraxia, lack of an idea of how to write the different characters, motor perseveration, spatial-relation difficulties, and so on, which leads us back to the main problems with so many similar tests. Rather than dividing impairments into categories, and testing for each one separately on a pass/fail basis, which does not succeed completely in differentiating the various impairment components, I recommend the method of detecting many impairments from one activity. Further, the Cognitive Test lacks areas necessary for complete neurobehavioral evaluation, such as frontal lobe dysfunction. Factors such as emotional aspects and motivation can affect performance on cognitive tests, and these factors have to be given credit in the evaluation, or the scoring. Further, the test results give no indication regarding which cerebral functions are responsible for an impairment; thus, they do not allow direct speculation regarding how CNS processes can be affected by treatment. In addition, the reliability and validity of the evaluation are not reported in the test manual. The only sign of content validation is a comment from a doctor who read the test, stating it was a good test, but not referring specifically to its purpose.

Thus, although many of the subtests of Sørensen's Cognitive Test could be used to test for specific deficits, I recommend a different approach: first to use ADL activities to detect neurobehavioral dysfunctions and their effects on functional independence and second, if secondary ADL tasks such as writing are used for further neurobehavioral evaluation, to interpret them directly in terms of different neurobehavioral deficits for each activity rather than in terms of scores, which may hinder the therapist's and others' understanding of the exact meaning of the test and the subsequent score in terms of neurobehavior. An occupational therapy neurobehavioral evaluation instrument should also indicate the possible origin of the dysfunction within the CNS. That is, the therapist should, after performing the evaluation, be able to understand the dysfunction and be able to form a treatment plan on that basis, if pertinent, in addition to compensatory impairment reduction. It is recognized that the strategies emphasized by the A-ONE require training and practice for the average therapist.

Thus, although it is important to evaluate outcome status and placement of patients, as is done in the Cognitive Test, we must also detect impairments that interfere with independence, and determine, on the basis of that evaluation, how we will treat the patient before we consider the eventual placement. The A-ONE can be used to evaluate patients' performance early in the treatment process, even before table-task activities can be assessed. It provides specific information regarding neurobehavioral impairment that can be incorporated into treatment aims and rehabilitation. However, the emphasis on independence upon discharge and placement in Sørensen's evaluation is certainly relevant at the time of discharge for the population it was designed for, that is, geriatric individuals, but the evaluation is used, like many other evaluations, indiscriminantly by therapists for other patient groups than it was originally designed for. The summation of scores from different cognitive subtests addressing different deficits is a questionable method for the purposes of treatment consideration.

Sørensen (1983) attempted to combine results from what she terms *practical cognitive tasks* and ADL performance. She used three forms of cognitive evaluations, all based on the previously mentioned Cognitive Test. She presents three different versions of the cognitive assessments, which all include similar items, but are of different length: the Practical Total Status (30 points), which is intended to be the main version; Practical Mental Status (25 points), which is used when intellectual reduction is suspected, as in dementia patients; and the Cognitive Test–50 (50 points), which is used when cognitive perceptual problems are suspected, such as in CVA. One of these evaluations is then chosen for combination with results from the Barthel Index Activities of Daily Living (ADL) scale,

which according to Sørensen was designed for physically handicapped patients only. Physical handicaps, however, are not the only obstacle to independence according to her. Mental and perceptual factors must also be considered in placement determination. By combining the two evaluations, Sørensen thus established a functional quotient for geriatric patients to aid in decision-making regarding realistic future placement. The Barthel Index, reviewed in more detail later in this section under ADL evaluations, is a 100-point scale including items on feeding, dressing, bathing, toileting, transfers, wheelchair mobility, walking, and continence. According to Sørensen, all three test versions of cognitive function are equally effective in determining desirable types of placement. She uses graphic charts to combine test results and classify patients according to whether they are able to live alone, live with others, or need to be institutionalized. Unfortunately, no reliability studies are reported on the cognitive versions of the manual, nor are results from content validation provided. However, a follow-up study of patient groups evaluated by one of three different combinations of cognitive and ADL factors, upon discharge, provide a form of validation and criteria for determining suitable placement (Sørensen, 1983; Sørensen, 1984).

The combination of an ADL scale and a cognitive test is a good idea because it reveals more functional information; however, as stated earlier, the use of Sørensen's (1983) ADL test component is different from that in the A-ONE instrument. Her purpose is to provide information regarding future placement, not to identify specific impairments that interfere with independence in planning treatment. Sørensen also correlated functional and neurobehavioral scores, rather than using ADL observations directly to detect neurobehavioral function. As stated previously, it is preferable for occupational therapists to obtain information regarding neurobehavior directly from ADL observations rather than performing two different tests.

Ottenbacher (1980) conducted a study in an attempt to identify the areas most frequently included in the formal cerebral vascular accident

(CVA) evaluation forms used by occupational therapists. He also classified the most commonly used levels of data by examining the evaluation forms. He found that most of the data gathered were descriptive, which he considered the "least reliable level of measurement" (p. 269). ADL activities were included in 21 of the 35 evaluations (60%). This was the fourth most common evaluation group of 11 identified areas. Ottenbacher considered this an underestimation of ADL evaluations used with CVA patients, possibly because separate ADL evaluations might be used by some centers, and these might not be considered CVA evaluations specifically. The most commonly used evaluation forms were those for motor function, followed by sensory perception and hand function. Visual perception followed ADL forms in frequency, then came cognitive functions, apraxia, behavior or affect, oculomotor control, and language and aphasia; the least frequently used were sensory-integrative forms. It is interesting that motor function is the most commonly used form (97%), and one wonders whether it is in part because these measures are more "obvious" or straightforward than are the more indirect measures of cognitive, perceptual, and behavioral processes. At any rate, according to Ottenbacher, ADL assessments are among the most frequently used forms for evaluating patients with cerebral dysfunction. It should be possible to adapt the ADL assessments for the purpose of simultaneously detecting neurobehavioral impairments, but such an evaluation would need to be more objective and more reliable than the current methods.

Van Deusen Fox and Harlowe (1984) performed a factor-analytic study to identify various factors and constructs that were assessed by the 33-item Occupational Therapy CVA Evaluation used at St. Mary's Medical Center in Madison, Wisconsin. They used 100 subjects for the analysis and identified five factors, including self-care and perception. Self-care was composed of washing the face, drinking from a cup, dressing the upper extremity in an outer garment and the lower extremity in shoes, combing the hair, and performing a peg

test with the right hand. Perception included the following areas: body scheme, figure/ground, position in space, spatial relations, and stereognosis of the left hand. The A-ONE includes all these items, except the peg test, and tests for many additional neurobehavioral deficits that interfere with function. It also includes more ADL items than those used in the St. Mary's evaluation, because I considered it impractical to choose only one subcomponent of an activity such as eating for evaluation rather than to evaluate all the subcomponents like the A-ONE does. Such valuable indications of neurobehavioral deficits as sequencing, organization, and planning of an entire activity can be lost by evaluating only one subcomponent of an activity.

Harlowe and Van Deusen (1984) performed a construct validation of the St. Mary's Occupational Therapy CVA Evaluation in terms of the perceptual means previously mentioned. They found that the perceptual factors measured characteristics related to the discharge disposition of patients. These findings are in agreement with Sørensen (1983). However, Boys et al. (1988) criticized the chi-square statistical method used for the analysis, which does not reveal the degree of association between the variables studied, and also noted that the degree of impairment was not examined. As mentioned before, it is preferable to measure neurobehavioral deficits directly through functional activities, thus providing all the information by using one evaluation, rather than testing for specific deficits with tests that are not necessarily informative in relation to daily activities and then having to perform other studies to relate test results to functions.

Farver and Farver (1982) used an analysis of covariance to yield information regarding performance of normal older adults, on tests designed to measure parietal lobe function. Their test battery included arithmetic, block constructions, clock settings, drawings, finger identification, left-right discrimination, map localizations, stick designs, visual discrimination tasks, and visual organization tasks. The test items are thus similar to those used in other tests available in occupational therapy for evaluating cognitive perceptual deficits. They do not reveal functional deficits directly, nor how these deficits affect functions, such as dressing. The idea of testing for specific cerebral dysfunction by occupational therapy measures is interesting and in agreement with the method of the A-ONE. However, one has to evaluate the functions of more than one lobe and keep in mind that neurobehavioral deficits do not necessarily relate to one specific lobe only, especially not when measured by activities that are not more sensitive to specific deficits than, for example, block constructions are. Some of the items chosen by Farver and Farver to detect parietal function can thus be related to dysfunctions of other lobes, in addition to the parietal lobe, although most of them can be related to deficits resulting from an impaired parietal lobe function. During error analysis, the authors themselves point out that perseverations were noticed during performance of the stick-designs test. Perseverations, in turn, are a result of a frontal lobe dysfunction. Thus, we need more detailed information on the patients' performance to be able to locate the functional dysfunction within the CNS that causes the deficit more accurately. Further, the tasks need to span the functions of more of the CNS than the parietal lobe, because dysfunctions of, for example, the frontal and temporal lobes result in the lack of motivation, lack of attention, and memory deficits, which can all seriously interfere with independence in self-care activities. However, the findings of Farver and Farver (1982) of significant age-related changes on tests for neurobehavior are very important when interpreting results from such tests. Thus, this kind of standardization is important for every instrument used. A normative study was performed for the A-ONE, and its results are reported in Chapter 11.

Baum and Hall (1981) studied the relationship between constructional praxis and dressing in 37 adults with head injuries. They used three constructional measures, including "graphic, two-dimensional, and three-dimensional abilities" (p. 438). For the constructional praxis evaluation,

they used sections of a hemiplegic evaluation developed at the Massachusetts Rehabilitation Hospital. The graphic skills of copying drawings were timed, with a time limit for completion of each task. Observations including alterations in spatial relations, fractuation, overshooting, perseveration, poor planning, scrawlings, spatial neglect, and verticality were clinically rated. The grading was 0 (intact) to 3 (unable to perform). Two- and three-dimensional measures were broken down in a similar way. Dressing included putting on/off a slip-over shirt, a skirt, a pair of slacks or underpants, a bra, a pair of socks or stockings, and shoes. Manipulation of fastenings such as buttons, zippers, and a belt was also included, as well as getting clothes from a closet or a drawer. The scale used for rating a patient's performance was specifically created for the study. The Pearson product-moment correlation coefficients were calculated to detect correlation. The findings revealed a significant relationship between scores of mean dressing ability and the scores of constructional praxis, suggesting, according to the authors, "that a portion of inability to dress is perceptual, not motor, in origin in individuals with severe head-injuries and that constructional praxis re-training has functional significance for the patient" (p. 438).

This study suggested, like many of the previously reviewed studies, a perceptual component of ADL. Therefore, it should be possible to use ADL observations to detect neurobehavioral deficits. Such an evaluation is preferable to the method used by Baum and Hall (1981), who tested neurobehavioral impairments and ADL separately and then correlated the scores.

In my view, the results from Baum and Hall's study point out the danger that therapists may be misled by comparing the results of cognitive tests to functional outcomes. The correlation between dressing and constructional praxis does not reveal a cause-effect relationship. Rather it suggests a common component that affects both dressing and construction, but does not imply that by using constructional treatment sessions, one could improve dressing function. The common component must be isolated and an effort made to understand it, in order to hypothesize regarding treatment. Assuming transfers of training or transfers of constructional skills over to functional skills in ADL activities is risky, and has so far had no empirical support. Such support cannot be obtained without looking behind the functions to the CNS mechanisms. Even so, I doubt that the results will be promising for this type of therapy, that is, "transfer of training," even though one could look beyond functions to CNS mechanisms. If one is to teach patients splinter skills, it would be better for those skills to be related directly to the patient's independence; therapists should avoid the block construction or even computerized cognitive retraining programs when a limited time is provided for treatment, and concentrate on training for independent living, or on those skills that patients will need for survival.

Warren (1981) studied the relationship of constructional apraxia and body-scheme disorders and performance of dressing in adult CVA patients. Performance on the perceptual tests was additionally related to the patients' ability to dress upon discharge. Dressing performance was rated on a 4-point scale for putting on and taking off a front-opening pullover shirt. According to the authors, the findings revealed "that both constructional apraxia and body scheme dysfunction contribute to failure in achieving upper extremity dressing" (p. 431). However, body-scheme performance was found to be a "better predictor of dressing ability" (p. 431). Further impairments, such as visual field deficits and aphasia, were found to influence the subject's performance, as did the presence of medical complications. Thus, this study also tended to support the perceptual component of ADL. Like the other studies reviewed, it used the approach of measuring ADL functions and neurobehavior separately and then correlating the scores. Again, I would not conclude that constructional apraxia "contributes" to dressing disability. Rather, there is an association between constructional apraxia and dressing disability, which could be related to the same underlying CNS dysfunction.

Boys et al. (1988) conducted a study to examine some psychometric qualities, including the validity of the Ontario Society of Occupational Therapy (OSOT) Perceptual Evaluation. According to the authors, in terms of psychometric characteristics, only face validity had been established, despite extensive use of the evaluation. The 28 subtests are divided into six categories: *"Sensory Function, Scanning and Spatial Neglect, Apraxia, Body Awareness, Spatial Relations, and Visual Agnosia"* (p. 94). Further suggestions for preliminary evaluation of additional factors, such as activities of daily living, hearing, mental status, and vision, are reported to be included in the evaluation. Interrater reliability of the measures was reported to be 93.1% across items. Internal consistency was examined, and high item-total correlations were reported for most items within respective functional areas. The six areas were all found to be moderately intercorrelated. Thus, all contributed independently to a score of perceptual dysfunction. The evaluation was also found to be valid in differentiating between neurologically impaired patients and "neurologically normal" individuals, by use of a *t*-test. A cutoff score for dysfunction was also established.

The OSOT Perceptual Evaluation is reported to be composed of items based on perception and neurodevelopment. Thus, the test items seem to be based on foundations other than occupational therapy to a considerable degree, like so many of the previously reviewed perceptual evaluations. Boys et al. suggest that results from the evaluation be correlated with ADL performance in a later study, thus keeping up with the "traditional" idea of using two different occupational therapy evaluations for CNS patients and studies of correlation to combine the two. Further, many neurobehavioral deficits that play a role in independence do seem to be excluded from the evaluation.

Carter, Oliveira, Duponte, and Lynch (1988) concluded from their literature review that ADL outcome in CNS patients is related to cognitive skills performance. They conducted two studies to examine this relationship. First, they examined improvement scores in ADL on the *Barthel Index* in two groups of CVA patients who received the same rehabilitation program, except that one group additionally received a 3-week cognitive retraining program, including training of visual scanning, visual-spatial perception, and time-judgment skills. Significant improvement of total scores was found in the ADL areas of personal hygiene, toilet activities, and bathing. On the basis of their findings, the authors concluded that there is a "likelihood of an important causal relationship between the improvement of three cognitive skills . . . and the improvement of three self-care skills" (p. 451). Secondly, a separate study was conducted on a different patient sample, where scores for cognitive-skill improvement were compared to ADL improvement scores, measured by the revised *Kenny Self-Care Evaluation*. The cognitive skills were evaluated by pre- and post-tests from *The Thinking Skills Workbook*. Training programs included both ADL and cognitive retraining for 3–4 weeks. A statistically significant positive correlation between ADL improvement scores and cognitive-skill improvement scores was reported to be .37. Overall performance on the pretest for cognitive skills was found to correlate significantly with post-test ADL performance, where the auditory-attention cognitive tasks showed the strongest correlation. The conclusion supported the view that ADL performance depends partially on cognitive function.

Neistadt (1988) reviewed the literature on current research related to the effectiveness of perceptual training with the aim of providing suggestions for future research. Her article raises many valuable points worthy of consideration when contemplating treatment efficacy and research designs. She comments on the usefulness of the present efficacy studies as an aid in treatment choice for therapists, and states that "no definitive decision can be reached because all of the relevant studies have failed to examine several variables that could be significant to research and treatment outcomes" (p. 436). According to Neistadt, among these variables are "exact definition of the perceptual dis-

order," "standardized assessment of changes in ADL status," and "the client's central nervous system processing style" (p. 436). Comments regarding the faults of present studies include that, while information regarding the "patterns of errors" is lacking, it is not possible to make conclusions regarding the perceptual problems indicated by the test scores. Further, tests need to be standardized on adult populations, and subjects have to be matched on the basis of conceptual deficits, because different impairments may respond differently to the various treatment remediations. Neistadt also commented on the need for standardized ADL instruments to measure treatment outcome, and suggested that such instruments could be used across studies, in order to increase applicability and contribute to a uniform data base about the treatment methods used to remediate perceptual problems.

I agree with Neistadt (1988) that error analysis is important when considering neurobehavioral deficits and how they interefere with task performance. Further, it should be possible to study the direct effects of neurobehavioral dysfunctions on functional tasks, such as ADL, by using a combined evaluation, which is the purpose of the A-ONE. The scoring criteria of the A-ONE also give some indication of the processing style that the CNS-damaged patients use for ADL performance.

Van Deusen (1988) supports the need for occupational therapy research in which instruments measuring unilateral neglect are related to "functional activities of all types" (p. 443). In contrast, the A-ONE allows direct detection of how different neurobehavioral deficits interfere with ADL performance by a single evaluation: a more direct method of information gathering for therapists. Van Deusen, in her article, further supported the development of a new behavioral skills test to detect "unilateral neglect." She also supported the use of single-subject research design as a method to record functional improvement. I also support the use of a single-subject recording format to study the different variables in the A-ONE evaluation.

With a collection of such studies, it may be possible to eliminate variables that contribute most frequently to a lack of independence. Thereby, important information for outcome considerations may evolve. Further, after identifying a variable such as ideational apraxia as an important component of dependence in specific ADL activities by using a controlled stimulus, the effects of different treatment approaches on this variable may possibly be studied. In such studies, matching of type and severity of all items (variables) not under study is crucial. The reader is referred to the literature on single-system designs for further information (Ottenbacher and York, 1984; Ottenbacher, 1986; Ottenbacher et al., 1988).

ADL evaluation tools

Gresham et al. (1980) studied the relative merits of three standard ADL indexes. They scored independence in ADL in 148 patients by evaluating how the observations were classified by the Katz Index of ADL, the Barthel Index, and the Kenny Self-Care Evaluations.

The Barthel Index, which was also used by Sørensen (1983), mentioned earlier in this review, is a numerical scale revealing percentages of functional independence. Ten functions, including "feeding, wheelchair/bed transfer, grooming, toilet transfer and usage, bathing, walking (or propelling a wheelchair), using stairs, dressing, controlling bowels, and controlling bladder" (p. 357) are evaluated. The researchers stated that the index was developed for patients in a chronic-disease hospital. They also stated that this assessment requires total independence for maximum scores in each category, and it "weights each function separately and arbitrarily" (p. 357). The scores, according to Gresham et al., range from 0 as totally dependent, to 100 as totally independent.

Avlund (1988) states that the scoring of the Barthel Index is based on need for assistance, including the time it requires. Because of this, 30% of the points refer to toileting, including continence. Grooming and hygiene are, on the contrary, only devoted 5%, and bathing another 5%. Feeding and dressing each are devoted 10% of the points. Walking independently 50 yards is devoted 15%, whereas maneuvering independently the same distance in a wheelchair only counts for 5% of these 15%. This is especially interesting, since walking with assistance receives 10% of the points. The item of walking stairs counts for an additional 10% by itself (Mahoney and Barthel, 1965). According to Sørensen (1983), the criteria for scoring only reveal whether a patient is able to perform without help, with some help, or unable to perform, not what kind of help is needed. For example, a patient who needs help with changing blades in a razor loses all the points for grooming and hygiene. Further no distinction is made between maximum physical assistance and supervision for safety reasons. According to Mahoney and Barthel, this lack of distinction may interfere with the sensitivity of the evaluation in measuring problems over time. It seems more reasonable to divide the scale into more detailed items and score them separately. The scoring of ADL items on ADL instruments used in rehabilitation preferably should distinguish between the need for heavy nursing as opposed to minimal supervision, because such information is crucial when it comes to placement of patients after the rehabilitation period. The distribution of scores across categories seems questionable. The instrument was obviously not developed by an occupational therapist.

The Katz Index of ADL, according to Gresham et al., is an ordinal scale on which the six functions of "bathing, dressing, going to toilet, transferring, continence, and feeding" (p. 357) are scored. Independence in these activities is assumed to be obtained in a sequential order in this evaluation. The patients are ranked from A as most independent to G as most dependent. According to Avlund (1988), the scoring spans three levels: performs independently, performs with help, or unable to perform. Like the Barthel Index, the Katz Index of ADL keeps no record of how an activity is performed. Avlund reports that the index has high reliability and validity, and that it is informative in terms of the amount of assistance needed for performance and thus in determining placement of patients. The Katz Index was based on observations of patients with multiple sclerosis, hip fractures, and strokes, according to Gresham et al.

The Kenny Self-Care Evaluation is a numerical scale on which six functional categories containing a total of 17 items are scored, including "bed, transfer, locomotion, dressing, personal hygiene, and feeding activities" (p. 357), according to Gresham et al. The scores in each major category range from 0 as dependent, to 4 as independent. The total score of the combined categories thus ranges from 0 as totally dependent, to 24 as independent. Nursing care was considered to be reversely related to functional independence when the scale was developed.

Avlund (1988), in her review of ADL instruments, states that the Kenny Self-Care Evaluation was developed to measure effects of treatment of the hospitalized elderly. She reports that hemiplegic patients with scores of 5 to 14 out of the possible 24 at the time of admission to a hospital have been shown to have the most use for rehabilitation. For scoring, the different levels of assistance are termed *minimal, moderate,* and *severe,* but the exact distinction does not seem to be provided, calling for a subjective judgment. Further, the scores of the six groups are added up to a total score, as in the Barthel Index, but they are not necessarily additive. Avlund points out that validity studies have indicated that an equal time is needed to assist patients in each of the six activity groups on the Kenny Self-Care Evaluation.

Avlund compares the three instruments just described, and states that the *Katz Index* is the only one that reveals information about which functions are deficient. The others rely on total scores. Further, the Kenny Self-Care Evaluation is the most sensitive to functional progress over 1 month's time. Total scores may be informative for placement, but it seems evident that they lose much important information, especially in terms of treatment considerations.

The computed differences between the three ADL indexes obtained by using a z-test were not found by Gresham et al. to be statistically significant. The Spearman rank-order coefficient and the kappa coefficient of agreement *(k)* were used for statistical comparisons. A high degree of agreement was reported between the derived scores of the Barthel Index and the Katz Index of ADL $(k = .774)$. The agreement between the Barthel Index and the Kenny Self-Care Evaluation was reported to be lower $(k = .420)$, but statistically significant. These authors also reported that all the indexes classified stroke survivors adequately as independent or dependent. However, they concluded that the Barthel Index appeared to possess "certain advantages which include completeness, sensitivity to change, amenability to statistical manipulation, and greater familiarity due to more widespread use" (p. 355); thus, they disagreed with Avlund (1988) regarding sensitivity to change.

All of these ADL indexes are concerned with measuring functional independence. The ADL categories are very superficial, from an informatory point of view, including only one item each. Dressing, for example, revealed no information as to which areas of the dressing were completed, and where the difficulties lay. These evaluations did not look specifically at neurobehavioral impairments, nor did they identify specific problems resulting in a lack of independence. Thus, they revealed nothing about the causes of dysfunctions, and therefore no conclusions regarding suitable treatment aims or approaches for treatment can be drawn. A new scale that considers these factors should be developed to make specific predictions about neurobehavioral dysfunctions that can be formulated from ADL observation. This information is necessary for choosing the most efficient treatment to improve functional performance in daily activities.

The Klein-Bell Activities of Daily Living Scale (Klein and Bell, 1979) was developed to meet the need identified by the authors for a unique, valid, and reliable ADL scale. According to their conclusions after a literature review, the existing ADL scales include items that are too global, presenting such categories as dressing by a single score, rather than recognizing the complexity of this function. When a patient fails an item on a test, the score does not specify what the specific problem is. Further, global items are not very sensitive to changes in functional performance. These authors also criticized the fact that existing scales do not lead to treatment plans for patients according to the assessment results. This agrees with my own findings, reported earlier in this section.

Some of the scales reviewed by Klein and Bell are often applicable to certain types of patients only, according to them, and when a patient makes progress, different scales may be needed. This, of course, makes measures of progress over time very cumbersome and subject to errors. Additionally, some scales include items that are not pertinent to all patient categories. According to these authors, despite scales having been developed for one patient category (such as the Katz Index for elderly patients with hip fractures), they are used by therapists to evaluate other groups of patients.

The authors of the Klein-Bell ADL Scale (1979) also reported that it has been difficult to determine the specific level of assistance needed by patients, because arbitrary point-values have been used for levels of assistance and then added up, resulting in disparities in interpretation. Further, the scoring of level of assistance is often subjective without specific guidelines to differentiate, for example, between minimum and maximum levels.

Klein and Bell criticized the fact that when scores are assigned, the interval between the categories is often uneven. They also addressed the issue of timing ADL activities, which is not a realistic measure for functional activities performed by patients, according to them. In addition, for those who require physical assistance, such a measure reflects the attendant's efficiency and skill, and should therefore not be confused with the true measures of the patient's performance, according to these authors. They also criticized assigning different values to walking as compared to wheeling a wheelchair, these behaviors claimed to be "essentially the same."

According to the authors of the Klein-Bell ADL Scale, it addresses only basic ADL skills, which I call primary ADL skills. It was designed so that the wording of items would apply to all persons, regardless of the methods used to achieve the skills (such as bathing position during bathing). The scale consists of 170 behavioral items, all of which are considered either as achieved or failed, indicating the need for verbal or physical assistance. A point-value was determined for each item by opinions from 10 experts in the fields of occupational therapy, nursing, and physical therapy. The scores only reveal whether a patient is independent or not, not the type or amount of assistance needed. The scores within each ADL category are summed to yield an overall independence score for purposes of team communication. In addition to raw scores, percentage scores are calculated for communication purposes. Scores can also be plotted on a graph to display progress. Interrater reliability was obtained from six pairs of occupational therapists and nurses on 20 patients, with agreement reported to be 92%. A validity study revealed a significant correlation between ADL scores at discharge and the number of hours of assistance received by 14 patients, obtained by a structured phone interview several months later.

Through the Klein-Bell ADL Scale, the authors certainly reached some of their aims with regard to developing a uniform scale: it can be applied to different patient diagnoses, it is detailed enough to detect changes, and it facilitates communication with team members and the patient's family. However, I feel that the scale is not suitable for detecting neurobehavioral deficits or providing ideas for specific treatment considerations for such conditions. Although it would be possible to incorporate my analysis and methodology for detecting neurobehavioral deficits into other evaluations, such as the Klein-Bell ADL Scale, this is not considered suitable for several reasons. First, it would make the Klein-Bell ADL Scale, which already contains 170 items, so long that therapists would be unlikely to use it. Second, it would not be clinically suitable to use a scale that covers all diagnostic categories. It is more pertinent to have scales that are sensitive to the dysfunctions of a particular patient group, which can provide specific information for planning treatment. To create such an informative and treatment-oriented scale that would cover all diagnoses, one would have pages and pages of irrelevant items or considerations.

This was a factor in formatting the A-ONE for patients with neurobehavioral dysfunctions. This scale breaks down ADL domains into different items to a greater extent than, for example, the Barthel Index, but not in the same amount of detail as the Klein-Bell ADL Scale. On the other hand, it provides information regarding the specific problems of this patient population, which I believe is more valuable for planning treatment than are more details regarding functional items. These details are meant to be written in the comment section of the A-ONE, if needed (see Chapter 10).

The sensitivity to progress of the Klein-Bell ADL Scale is reflected in the number of items. In the A-ONE, sensitivity to progress is related to scoring, according to the type of stimulus information needed to evoke the neuronal processing necessary for the required activity components to occur, and according to the independence and assistance levels needed for each item. Thus, I would argue that evaluations should not be too cumbersome and that items do not need to be broken down into their smallest details because the comment sections are supposed to cover the details needed. However, a certain degree of complexity is needed if the scale is to be effective in providing important treatment information. Further, CNS localization of the origin of the dysfunctions that cause the neurobehavioral deficits that interfere with independence is introduced in the A-ONE instead of expanding the functional and physical details that can be included in the comments columns.

Items that are important to primary ADL functions are omitted from the Klein-Bell ADL Scale. An example of this is the category of "emergency communication." Only emergency telephone communication is covered. This includes one item related to language and verbalization. The other five items in the category of communication all refer to the patient's physical ability to approach the phone. General communication, such as comprehension and speech, is never considered. This overemphasis on physical detail in certain areas of the evaluation is not desirable for a "generalized" OT-ADL evaluation in my view. The imbalance between physical and organic mental aspects of function makes the assessment insufficient for evaluating patients with neurobehavioral impairments. The reader is referred to the previous section on cognitive and perceptual tests, where the majority of studies reviewed identified cognitive-perceptual abilities as important components of self-care independence in brain-damaged patients.

In addtion to the differences just described in the purposes of the Klein-Bell ADL Scale and the A-ONE, the Klein Bell ADL Scale is designed to be accessible for different team members, as well as for the family. The A-ONE evaluation, on the other hand, is designed to complement the expertise of occupational therapists. It is intended for use by occupational therapists in evaluation and the formation of treatment plans. The therapist is then responsible for reporting this information in a meaningful way to other team members and the families of patients, which should be easy once the assessment has been completed.

Before leaving the subject of occupational therapy evaluations, a few points from the head-injury literature should be considered. Sbordone (1987) comments on the need for qualitative dimensions in addition to the quantitative ones in the scoring of many standardized tests. According to him, the lack of qualitative information on quantitative tests may be misleading because factors such as motivation may contribute to the outcome. Thus, the process of obtaining a score needs to be considered, "not just the level of performance" (p. 16). He recommends that all the factors that influence behavior during a task be examined, as well as "the type of errors made by the patient" (p. 16). Further, a note should be taken of emotional signs, motivation, responses to errors, and cues affecting the patient's performance. However,

Sbordone points out that qualitative observations are subjective and may require training and an experienced examiner. Sbordone also stresses that scores from standardized test batteries are not necessarily of much value when it comes to planning treatment for cognitive rehabilitation. Benton (1987) supports the need for inclusion and consideration of emotional factors, affective disturbances, and cognitive processes, such as attention, concentration, communication skills, and memory, when interpreting tests of cognitive performance. Similarly, Diller and Ben-Yishay (1987) support the idea of "more comprehensive and precise" (p. 150) tests for evaluating the characteristics of head-injured individuals that are relevant for rehabilitation. To name some of the characteristic examples, level of attention; awareness of disability; "problem-solving abilities"; planning, organizing, and sequencing; and execution of behavior should be considered. Further, activity performance, as well as regulation of affect and emotion should be kept in mind. However, these authors identify the lack of specific and valid instruments to evaluate these factors.

The approach of the A-ONE supports the importance of including "qualitative" variables in the evaluation of neurobehavior; an attempt was made to include these considerations in the instrument. It is recognized that the observations are not specific or detailed for each variable and that for a comprehensive evaluation of memory, for example, different procedures are needed. However, the A-ONE has a different purpose. It is intended to provide an overview of how independence levels in primary activities of daily living are affected by neurobehavioral impairments. As such it might serve as a screening instrument to determine the need for more comprehensive evaluations in specific areas.

Diller and Ben-Yishay point out that the level of assistance needed for activity performance with the aim of decreasing dependency in ADL is an important indicator, and that it should be used as a scoring parameter on assessments of patients with neuropsychological problems. Such a scoring parameter is, according to them, both practical and of scientific interest. These authors further point out that "functional assessment measures" in rehabilitation medicine usually "sample the content of training programs" (p. 151). This certainly applies to ADL assessment, as well as other measures. Even cognitive retraining programs, including the practice of block building, overlap with some constructional tests. This is an important factor that should be kept in mind, as it produces a possible "practice effect" on a test that is administered after a treatment program, or a potential development of a "splinter skill" which has been drilled in. Thus, it is recommended that the same methodology as administered in the A-ONE be standardized for some secondary activities of daily living as well, for those who reach acceptable levels (or the ceiling) of the A-ONE. These secondary skills require more of the patient; they are not as basic as the primary skills. However, they may provide some indication of whether there are some residual impairments that interfere with performance, or if improvement in impairments identified on the A-ONE carries over to other situations.

Berk (1979) states that "the reliability index, in general, reflects the effectiveness of observer training and the degree of objectivity with which the target behavior can be measured" (p. 460). I consider that the training of therapists in the use of an assessment to ensure efficacy in skill use is a necessary goal to ensure better results. This method of training therapists is used for the new Sensory Integration and Praxis Tests, developed by Ayres (1989). The tests, which evolved from occupational therapy theory, are the most validated of all occupational therapy instruments.

In conclusion, the evaluation methods reviewed, which are used by occupational therapists to evaluate patients with neurobehavioral dysfunctions, fall into two categories. One is evaluation of the neurobehavioral impairment by using assessments similar to those used in neuropsychology. These tests are not based on occupational therapy theory, but appear to be "borrowed" from the discipline of neuropsychology. Further, these tests are not as reliable or standardized as those used within the field of neuropsychology. The authors categorized neurobehavioral deficits and then tested each one by a separate test or tests. This is different from the approach proposed by the A-ONE, in which skill performance in a daily activity is observed and many different deficits may be detected and scored during the observation of one activity. Many of the authors reviewed in this section agreed that validity and reliability are needed for instruments used in occupational therapy, and some of them have started processes of validation and the establishment of reliability for their instruments. However, it can not be overemphasized that occupational therapists need instruments based on occupational therapy theory. None of the authors reviewed identified this need.

The other assessment category used by occupational therapists is an ADL functional evaluation. Here, the same problem of lack of validity and reliability is present. Further, the evaluations are not sensitive to the specific problems that interfere with the independence of the patients assessed, and they do not address neurobehavioral deficits. Therefore, they are not suitable for suggesting accurate treatment approaches for diminishing patients' impairments. The use of two separate scales requires two assessments and then comparative studies so that the neurobehavioral deficit score can be used to predict function—a procedure that is too cumbersome in my view. A new ADL instrument was needed, an instrument that would address both functional performance in life skills and the neurobehavioral dysfunctions that interfere with skill performance. Such an evaluation would retain all the traditional requirements of an ADL evaluation, adding to the information gathered by identifying impaired performance components and thereby explaining the results, thus providing clinical considerations regarding treatment approaches without replacing the focus of a functional outcome.

All the authors reviewed recognized the use of either ADL evaluation or cognitive-perceptual assessments within the discipline of occupational

therapy for patients with neurobehavioral dysfunctions. Most of them also supported the existence of a perceptual component of ADL. The development of an evaluation that combines these two evaluation methods seemed to be a logical solution; the A-ONE provides an evaluation that identifies the origin of the neurobehavioral impairments interfering with functional independence. Needless to say, I propose that ADL evaluation instruments be used before other cognitive-perceptual tests to obtain information regarding neurobehavioral function for the purpose of establishing rehabilitation goals and selecting the type of treatment to reach these goals. ADL is the primary level of function, much more basic than block constructions and writing, and easily verifiable by looking at human developmental sequences. Thus, the patients will be ready earlier for an ADL evaluation than they are for a traditional cognitive-perceptual evaluation. Such tests can then be used as follow-up evaluations, where necessary.

Scores from some of the tests reviewed are presented in a point form. This makes it difficult to realize what the real problem is, and how it is related to a patient's function, especially for other team members. Further, adding of scores across different ADL domains may be of value for specific purposes related to studies of outcomes. However, such additions are questionable and not informative regarding the exact problem area. The results from a combined ADL-neurobehavioral assessment should be more informative regarding problem areas and treatment aims. The scoring and the conclusion should therefore be in more descriptive terms than information from many of the cognitive-perceptual evaluations is presently. Such a combined assessment should also reveal information regarding brain function and information processing that should contribute to the expansion of knowledge regarding the CNS.

Neuropsychological tests

Neuropsychological tests are commonly used to evaluate neurobehavioral deficits in an objective and quantified way. These tests, according to Strub and Black (1985), provide important information about behavior and its association with brain function. According to them, such tests are more comprehensive and more detailed than the mental-status examination performed by a neurologist for screening such deficits. Further, the tests have usually been standardized with samples of normal individuals, thus enabling comparison of test results from patients with brain dysfunction. As mentioned in the earlier section on occupational therapy evaluations, many authors have pointed out the limitations of neuropsychological evaluations in terms of their completeness regarding the holistic consideration of an individual and his performance in a realistic environment. Thus, many of the impairments are evaluated in situations that are not realistic from the point of view of everyday life.

Lezak (1983) supports this view in stating that "naturalistic observations can provide extremely useful information about how the patient functions outside the formalized, usually highly structured, and possibly intimidating examination setting" (p. 129). However, according to him, neuropsychologists rarely evaluate patients during performance of daily activities.

The importance of "how" an individual performs, as compared to only "what" the results are, has been stressed, as well as the impact of historical facts from the patient's life and factors affecting test performance, such as motivation and emotion, which contribute to test results. Lezak (1983) supports the importance of "how" patients solve problems, as compared to "what" score they obtain. He indicates that failure as such is not informative by itself. In his extensive publication on neuropsychological assessment, he mentions the contrasting roots of neuropsychology. These include what he terms the *clinical-theoretical approach* pioneered by Luria, a Russian neurologist and psychoanalyst, and approaches stressing statistical and operational importance in accordance with American psychology. The clinical approach develops from intensive case studies analyzing the qualitative nature of behavior. The psychological approach stresses the quantitive aspect of outcomes from standardized

tests, which (in its extremes) may not necessitate contact between the patient and the neuropsychologist. Lezak states that "in the strictest applications of this approach, the diagnostic possibilities are generated by a computer" (p. 3). Further, he suggests that a continuum can be established between the two approaches, with one extreme being based on pure quantification and the other on qualitative observations, which do not include objective standardization. Lezak recommends an approach drawn from the middle of this continuum. Although he supports the use of standard test conditions, he acknowledges the need for "a little more flexibility and looseness in interpreting the standard procedures" (p. 121), if the examiner is to be able to "make the most of the test and elicit the patient's best performance" (p. 121). Lewis et al. (1979) also support this view. They state that "a marriage between flexibility and standardization appears desirable" (p. 1004) as a basis for a neuropsychological battery. According to them, this calls for refinements of neuropsychological batteries, and they state that such refinement can be found in the Luria-Nebraska Neuropsychological Battery. The A-ONE was developed with these thoughts in mind. It uses detailed, holistic, clinical observations in an attempt to objectively systematize the information gathered. It is recognized that with such information, complete objectivity and standardization will not be reached without sacrificing a lot of information. Thus, for the time being, test administration and interpretation of the resulting clinical information will only be standardized to a level where important clinical information can be retained.

A wealth of psychological evaluation tools is reported in the literature, some of which are comprehensive, while others deal with restricted areas of testing. Lewis et al. consider comprehensive test batteries, as compared to the single tests necessary for distinguishing brain-injured patients from patients with other disorders, and for localizing brain damage. Lezak (1983) does not agree with Lewis et al. on the role of what he calls "ready-made batteries" (p. 110). Their popularity stems, according to him, partially from "a general lack of knowledge about how to do it" (p. 110). Further, such batteries may require more testing than a particular patient needs, and they will not necessarily provide specific enough information regarding his or her needs. According to Lezak, such batteries "can provide a good starting place for some newcomers to the field, who may then expand their test repertory and introduce variations into their administration procedures as they gain experience and develop their own point of view" (p. 110). The purpose of the A-ONE was to attempt to provide structured guidelines for clinical observations of patients in daily life situations, which reveal how neurobehavioral impairments interfere with normal function, especially for the less-experienced therapists and to provide a systematic format for research purposes.

For the purpose of this book, only three comprehensive neurologic batteries and one clinical test manual for neuropsychological assessment will be reviewed. The reader is referred to comprehensive texts on neuropsychological assessment for further review (Lezak, 1983).

The Halstead-Reitan Battery includes a series of neuropsychological tests that, according to Strub and Black (1985), have been well standardized. According to Lezak (1983) its most commonly used subtests include the Category Test for abstracting ability, the Finger Oscillation Test for manual dexterity, the Rhythm Test for nonverbal auditory perception, the Speech Sounds Perception Test for sound discrimination, and the Tactual Performance Test, a tactile memory test. Test results provide an Impairment Index that is intended to make diagnostic discriminations. Further, age-graded norms are available for the battery, but according to Lezak, the educational level of those being tested may affect the test performance significantly. There are other tests that belong to this battery, including the Trail Making Test of visual-conceptual areas and visuomotor tracking; different modifications of the Aphasia Screening Test; tests for finger agnosia, graphesthesia, tactile, auditory, and visual sensory extinction; a dynamometer mea-

sure for grip strength; and the Minnesota Multiphasic Personality Inventory (MMPI), an objective personality test, which, according to Lezak, "has only questionable usefulness in the evaluation of personality components of a neuropsychological complaint or disability" (p. 607). Lezak further states that administration of the complete battery takes between 6 and 8 hours.

The major limitation of the Halstead-Reitan Battery, according to Strub and Black (1985), "include its length, the minimal emphasis on important areas such as memory and language, and a lack of descriptive data" (p. 181) regarding test results so that they can be understood by the nonpsychologist. Otherwise, Strub and Black consider this battery to be "one of the best standardized methods of identifying patients with brain damage" (p. 181) available.

Luria's Neuropsychological Investigation is another well-known test battery. According to Lezak (1983), it is "Christensen's collection of Luria's material" (p. 566), which she has organized into 10 functional scales. The battery includes techniques that assess arithmetic skills, acoustico-motor organization, expressive and receptive language, higher cutaneous and kinesthetic functions, higher visual functions, intellectual processes, memory, motor functions, reading, and writing (Lezak, 1983; Strub and Black, 1985). According to Strub and Black, "interpretation of some items" is restricted "to a very well-trained and highly experienced examiner" (p. 181), because the tests lack normative data. However, these authors felt that the Luria Neuropsychological Investigation could be readily adapted "to meet the needs of each individual case" (p. 181).

According to Lezak (1983), the drawbacks of the evaluation are the lack of normative data for many of the test items and incompleteness related to omission of factors such as attention, concentration, and mental tracking, as well as limitations in the evaluation of nonverbal memory and concept formation. Lezak points out that many examiners use some of the subtests of the battery selectively. However, because of the test's incompleteness, he feels that "supplemental testing will be needed for most patients" (p. 568).

The Luria-Nebraska Neuropsychological Battery was developed as an attempt by Golden and his colleagues to standardize selected items taken from the Luria Neuropsychological Investigation, according to Lezak's (1983) comprehensive review on neuropsychological assessment. Thus it has the same drawbacks regarding limitations of content. Lezak considers that by timing the item performance, additional problems have been introduced—problems that disregard the quality of slow performance. The Luria-Nebraska Neuropsychological Battery has been criticized concerning its ability to differentiate patients with brain damage from both normal and psychiatric patients (Adams, 1980; Lezak, 1983; Strub and Black, 1985). Adams, for example, criticized the methodology used in the validation of the battery and argued that the test has lost its flexibility, that is, the potential of changing the assessment conditions according to the clinical patient's needs. Golden (1980), on the other hand, claimed that there were errors in Adams's criticism.

The controversy over having a test that can be adapted to each individual's needs and one that requires a more skilled examiner and loss of flexibility in order to get more standardized and valid data was found to be of interest when considering the constitution of the A-ONE. Preferably, as previously stated, such an evaluation should be closer to Luria's original ideas of flexibility because each patient is different. One of the goals in occupational therapy is for a therapist to be adaptive and able to use critical thinking skills, which certainly allows for and requires flexibility. It is hoped that the A-ONE, with the theoretical background provided earlier in this part of the book and its Manual in Part II, will succeed in providing the necessary basic information for therapists to be able to master these clinical skills, with practice. The comments on flexibility, the previously mentioned components of reliability, as well as Geschwind's (1985) comment that it seemed to be more difficult for doctors to become skilled in the evaluation of peo-

ple with neurobehavioral deficits, pointed to the necessity of *training* therapists for this kind of evaluation, rather than just handing out a manual, if the results were to be reliable. Such training, including case examples, should provide therapists with the necessary skills to use this kind of an assessment.

The *Clinical Manual* by Benton, et al. (1983) consists of 12 tests used to evaluate patients with brain damage. There are three tests of orientation and learning, and nine perceptual-motor tests. The tests for orientation and learning include tests of right-left orientation, serial digit learning, and temporal orientation. The perceptual and motor tests include tests for facial recognition, finger localization, judgment of line orientation, motor impersistence, pantomime recognition, phoneme discrimination, tactile form-perception, three-dimensional block construction, and visual form-discrimination. The manual includes directions on administration and scoring, as well as normative observations for all the tests. Many of these tests include normative data obtained from normal adults, others from children. Information regarding the performances of patients with brain diseases is also included for many of these tests.

On the test of temporal orientation, three items are scored: date, weekday, and time. One error point is given for each day and weekday counted away from correct answers, and one error point for each incorrect 30 minutes in time. Five error points are given for each month removed from the correct one, and 10 for each year. A normative study revealed that a score of more than three error points can be considered defective, according to Benton et al. (1982). The is valuable information when administering the A-ONE. Right-left orientation is evaluated on a 20-item test, scored by 20 points. Patients are asked to show specific body parts, to point to body parts both in crossed and uncrossed fashion, and to point to the examiner's body parts. In the normative group, 96% scored between 17 and 20. In the A-ONE, only one question is systematically used to address this dysfunction. Because of the test's flexibility, however, it is always possible to add further questions if needed. On the basis of the information provided by Benton's normative study, any incorrect response should be considered suspicious and checked further.

The purpose of the neuropsychological review was not to include comprehensive information regarding such tests. There are other extensive sources for such information. Rather, it was to bring up from that literature some general points about which considerations would be of value in instrument development within the field of neurobehavior, since the fields are obviously related. Further, rather than reviewing specific tests, the emphasis was on providing some idea of testing areas that neuropsychologists engage in, and pointing out what may be lacking in those tests as a result of the limitations of neuropsychological evaluations, which, on the other hand, may be found in occupational therapy evaluations concerned with daily living performance.

The neuropsychological tests seem to use methods similar to those used in formal occupational therapy cognitive-perceptual evaluations, except that the neuropsychological tests are usually standardized and validated better than the occupational therapy evaluation instruments. The neuropsychological tests are used to observe neurobehavioral dysfunction and then to hypothesize with regard to the cortical lesion. However, these tests do not reveal direct, comprehensive, and descriptive information regarding the patient's functional ability in real-life situations, as do the ADL evaluation instruments; they usually assess dysfunction in a test situation that is outside the context of daily reality. Therefore, if ADL evaluations can be structured so that they reveal reliable information regarding neurobehavior, they will be a more natural assessment method for the patient, and will reveal more practical information for other team members than do the neuropsychological tests.

In conclusion, I feel that the ADL assessments currently used by occupational therapists could be designed to be sensitive to neurobehavioral dysfunction. Similarly, these tests could be used to predict localization and processing defects in order to aid therapists in their treatment speculations. Such assessments would make valuable clinical contributions to deficit identification and treatment recommendation. Further, such assessment tools would be very practical because they would identify the exact problems that interfere with functional independence. The A-ONE was designed with these ideas in mind. The role of occupational therapists is not limited to evaluation and treatment recommendation. They are also responsible for the treatment and for evaluating the outcome of the treatment they provide, as well as the quality of their evaluation and treatment. No one is in a better position than occupational therapists to evaluate the everyday functions of patients with neurobehavioral dysfunction and how these functions are affected by neurobehavioral impairments, and, in turn, to formulate and evaluate the most suitable treatment methods.

TECHNOLOGICAL INVESTIGATION METHODS

Brain damage or disorders of brain function can sometimes be related to the structure, or architecture, of the brain. They can also be a result of, or result in dysfunction of, electrical and chemical processes of the brain (Kety, 1979). There has been a rapid development in technological investigation methods during the last years. Consequences of brain damage vary, and different methods are used to detect them. The availability of technological investigation methods also varies greatly in different hospital settings and in different countries. However, some methods have become almost clinically traditional, such as the use of CT scans; others are rare and are used by institutions that emphasize research heavily, as well as clinical aspects. Most of these methods are used primarily for diagnostic purposes; however, some of them may be used at times for research purposes to gather information regarding the function of the CNS. The aim of this section is to provide a brief overview of some of the techniques used to assess the CNS. Information from such investigations is of interest for all team members when they are making decisions regarding the treatment and prognosis of particular patients. In addition, I stress the importance of combinative studies of the association between results from clinical behavioral observations and the more direct measures of structural abnormalities and cerebral dysfunctions.

Abnormal function of the cerebral cortex can be detected by clinical observations, some of which were discussed in the section on neurobehavioral assessment methods. The following chapter on neurobehavioral deficits will also refer to behavioral manifestation of impairments. Structural changes can be detected by CT scanning. Angiography also sometimes provides information related to structural changes. Impaired electrogenesis can be detected by EEG or EP measurements. Altered metabolism can be detected by cerebral blood-flow measurements (Jennett and Teasdale, 1981). Further, MRI is used to examine both cerebral structure and function on the basis of magnetic information. Only methods that relate directly to structural or functional changes in regard to neurobehavioral dysfunctions, as previously defined, are reviewed here. The aim is to provide a superficial methodological review of evaluation techniques that can aid in the study of the CNS and in gathering comprehensive data about patients. There are several factors that should be kept in mind when considering the use of such methods for research purposes. These include the availability of the technology, the cost of the tests, and the risks or inconvenience for the patients.

Computerized tomography (CT) scanning

CT scanning is an X-ray technique that combines information obtained from different angles to produce a three-dimensional image of internal structures (Kety, 1979). X-ray beams are emitted from an X-ray tube that is rotated 180° around the skull. The X-rays go through the person's head, where brain tissue absorbs the radiation, according to the density of the different components. Consequently the X-rays are picked up by sensitive crystal detectors at the site opposite to their emission. A computer processes the information obtained and subsequently produces the images. The images represent 8 to 10 consecutive sections, or slices, of brain tissue, which are 5 to 10 mm thick. Scanning time ranges from 20 to 60 minutes.

The technique reconstructs an image, or density map, based on the degree of absorption of the X-rays by different tissues. The density, measured in Hounsfield units, is measured by a scale that spans from 500 + representing bone, which appears white on the image, to 500 − for air. Water has a density of 0, which appears black on the image. Clotted blood appears close to white, as it is denser than the normal brain, whereas edema and infarcted tissue are less dense than normal brain, and thus appear darker (Bradshaw, 1985; Jennett and Teasdale, 1981). According to Bradshaw, the slices are produced in a transverse plane, sequenced from the base of the brain upward. However, new machines are able to recalculate the data into sagittal or coronal planes. Further, the anatomical features and details that appear depend on the thickness of the section, head position during the scanning, and the quality of the scanner.

Discrimination between normal and abnormal brain tissue on a CT scan can be enhanced by intravenous injection of iodine-contrast compounds. By this process additional features, such as blood vessels, also become evident. The contrast agent does not cross the blood-brain barrier, unless there is a lesion that disrupts the barrier (Netter, 1983). Some abnormal CT scan appearances include displacement of ventricles, suggesting a mass lesion, or abnormally large ventricles, suggesting hydrocephalus or brain atrophy. Areas of increased density may suggest bleeding. Areas of reduced density may suggest edema or infarcted brain tissue (Jennett and Teasdale, 1981). See Fig. 6-1 for an illustration of a CT scan.

One must keep in mind, however, that it may take time for some changes to develop before they can be detected by a CT scan. Thus, a recent infarction may not appear on the scan, and contusions are more marked several days after injury (Caplan and Stein, 1986; Cummings and Benson, 1983; Jennett and Teasdale, 1981).

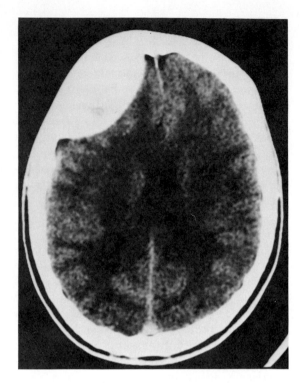

FIG. 6-1 CT scan from a man who was struck by a baseball bat on the right forehead. The CT scan shows a lenticular (lens-shaped) white mass frontally to the right, indicating an epidural hemorrhage as consequence of the injury. There is also displacement across the midline of the anterior portion of the falx cerebri. The right ventricle (the darkest areas in the middle indicate the ventricles) is also displaced towards the left side. Note that the white matter appears darker than the gray matter on a CT scan. (From Novelline, R.A., and Squire, L.F.: *Living Anatomy.* Philadelphia: Hanley & Belfus, Inc., 1987, with permission.)

Computerized tomography is a simple and comparatively safe method (Cummings and Benson, 1983) of assessing structural abnormalities of the cerebral cortex. Therefore, it can be used to provide diagnostic information, as well as to indicate changes occurring over time, such as evolution and resolution of lesions, by using repeated scans.

Restak (1984) stated that the CT scan has provided "a tremendous advance in terms of visualization of brain structure" (p. 82). However,

according to him, because it does not provide "information regarding brain function" (p. 82), he considered it to reveal a static as opposed to a dynamic image. As mentioned previously, static measures that reveal structural or anatomical defects are only one of the technological approaches used to examine the nervous system. A "normal" structural appearance does not necessarily mean normal functioning or processing in the neurons forming the structures. Therefore, other measures may be needed in order to detect function or physiological processing of the CNS.

In conclusion, CT scans reveal information on structural changes and their localization. The procedure is reported to be a simple and comparatively safe method.

Magnetic resonance imaging (MRI)

MRI is a recently developed diagnostic brain-imaging technique. According to Oldendorf (1985), it uses magnetic fields as a probe which is introduced into body tissues, in order to measure and localize different chemical characteristics of these tissues. The technique measures radio frequency signals emitted from hydrogen atoms within the brain tissue when affected by a magnetic field. These signals are then converted into multiplanar colored images of the brain by computer processing (Norman and Brant-Zawadzki, 1985; Restak 1984).

According to Oldendorf (1985), during the MRI scan the "patient is placed in a strong magnetic field" (p. 247) that corresponds to the earth's gravitational field. The hydrogen nuclei, which have an odd number of protons, are "driven into a higher energy state by the exciting radio-frequency pulse" (p. 251). The activated hydrogen nuclei act as small magnets. They move in order to align either parallel or antiparallel with "the direction of an externally imposed magnetic field" (p. 259), according to Norman and Brant-Zawadzki (1985).

Further, the nuclei that are aligned parallel to a magnetic field "have a lower energy state than those aligned antiparallel to the field" (p. 259). Protons have a tendency "to be in the lower energy state" (p. 259). The radio-frequency pulse causes a rapid "flipping," or "resonance," of protons between the two energy states (Norman and Brant-Zawadzki). The nuclei release energy at their resonance frequency as their kinetic energy decays. According to Oldendorf this energy can be picked up by a receiver. Further, the decay is important because the nuclei cannot be energized again until after the decay, and the slow decay results in long scan times. The imaging results from applying a sequence of energizing radio-frequency pulses and then "analyzing frequency versus amplitude versus time of the reradiated energy" (p. 251), according to Oldendorf. Further, after the radio-frequency pulse that drives the hydrogen nuclei into a higher energy state is turned off, "the hydrogens in tissue water reradiate that energy as a shortwave radio signal" (p. 251).

According to Martin and Brust (1985), it is fortunate that hydrogen is a strong resonator, as 75% of the human body is water (water molecules being composed of two hydrogen nuclei). Because body tissues vary in their water content (bone, for example, contains little water), they allow tissue differentiation on the images. According to these authors, as well as Norman and Brant-Zawadzki, the gray cortex contains 10% to 15% more water than does the white subcortical matter. However, it contains considerably less lipid than does the white matter. Differences in water and lipid content thus account for the contrast differences. Further, the water content of abnormal brain tissue (for example, in small brain tumors and infarctions) varies from that of normal brain tissue, allowing discrimination between the two. See Fig. 6-2 for an illustration of MRI.

Many authors, including Martin and Brust, Metter (1986), Norman and Brant-Zawadzki, and Restak consider MRI superior to CT scans because it can depict anatomical detail and because ionizing radiation or intravenous contrast agents are not required in order to differentiate pathologic from normal tissue. As stated by Norman and Brant-Zawadzki, MRI has proved to be more sensitive than CT scans in detecting tumors, demyelination changes, and infarcts. Further, it is at least as effective in detecting hemorrhage as the CT scan is. These authors predicted that MRI will replace "CT scanning as the primary screening modality" (p. 268) for those CNS patients who need imaging techniques. However, Caplan and Stein state that despite the apparently better "anatomical definition" (p. 57) of MRI as compared to CT scans, it "does not separate brain hemorrhage, tumor and infarction as well as CT" (p. 57) does. Further, Martin and Brust state that MRI has a better resolution than the PET scan, which will be reviewed later in this section.

Angiography

Angiography, a technique that uses an arterial catheter to inject an iodinated contrast agent into the cerebral circulation, in combination with serial X-rays, has been used for several years to provide visualization of the injected cerebral artery and its branches, according to Netter (1983). Femoral angiography, in which a catheter is entered through the femoral artery and maneuvered into the cerebral arteries, is becoming more common than direct puncture of the common carotid artery, according to Jennett and Teasdale, which creates a risk for the patient (Cummings and Benson, 1983; Jennett and Teasdale, 1981; Netter, 1983). Although this risk has been reduced with femoral angiography, the use of angiography is still controversial and requires a skilled angiographer. It is an important technique in locating a bleeding aneurysm, or source of intracerebral bleeding, as well as in providing information regarding occlusive lesions, according to Caplan and Stein (1986), and Cummings and Benson (1983). It is used for precise diagnosis in head-injured individuals, according to Jennett and Teasdale. Some of the abnormal findings indicated by an angiogram are, according to Jennett and Teasdale, a lateral arterial shift, indicating a mass lesion in a hemisphere; a marked slowing of the flow of the contrast agent, indicating a reduced blood flow caused by elevated intracranial pressure; a systemic hypotension; leaking of the contrast agent, indicating bleeding; and occlusion of an artery, indicated by little or no flow. Further, irregular

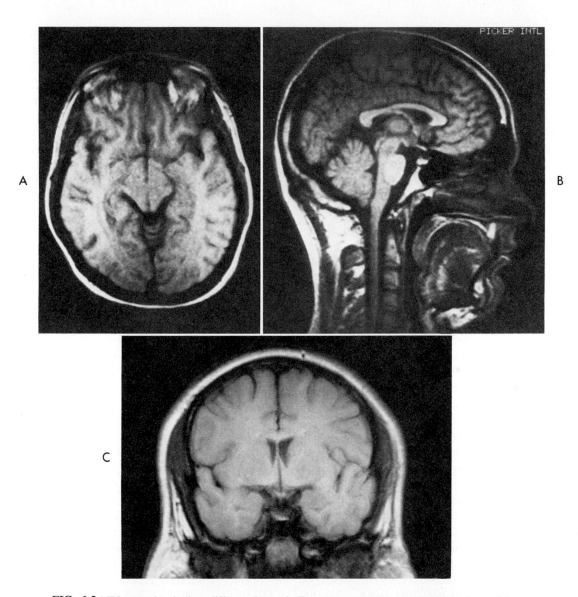

FIG. 6-2 MRI scan taken in three different planes. **A,** Transverse or axial image taken at the level of the midbrain illustrating the tops of the orbits, cerebellar vermis, and the bases of the frontal, temporal, and occipital lobes. **B,** Midline sagittal image at the level of the interhemispheric fissure. The cerebellum, brain stem, and corpus callosum are clearly illustrated, as well as the cerebral cortex. **C,** Coronal image taken at a level anterior to the central sulcus separating the frontal and the parietal lobes. The interhemispheric and lateral fissures are evident as well as the ventricles, insula, temporal, and frontal lobes. On these scans, intense signals appear white, whereas low or absent ones appear black. Thus fat appears white, whereas air and bone appear black. Blood vessels also appear black because of the constant movement of blood, which hinders the formation of strong signals. White matter, containing more lipid than gray matter, appears lighter than the gray matter. (From Novelline, R.A., and Squire, L.F.: *Living Anatomy.* Philadelphia: Hanley & Belfus, Inc., 1987, with permission.)

maneuvering of arterial segments can point to arterial spasms, which accompany subarachnoid bleeding.

In summary, angiography reveals information regarding the vascular system. This information may suggest structural abnormalities of the brain, or the effects of a defective blood supply on brain tissue and function. It has a potential risk to the patient.

Measurement of regional cerebral blood flow (rCBF)

The rCBF procedure is based on the chemical processes of brain function, according to Kety. It examines how the cerebral cortex utilizes energy by measuring the blood flow to the cortex and the consumption of oxygen or glucose. Lassen et al. (1978) have used a method based on these principles to observe functional localization within the cerebral cortex directly. According to them, the theory behind the technique is that "the flow of blood through the tissues of the body varies with the level of metabolism and functional activity in those tissues" (p. 62). Thus, during tasks that involve specific cortical functions, local changes in neuronal activity are required, which call for increased oxygen consumption and metabolic rate. This, in turn, calls for increased blood flow to the active area, indicating localization of function within the brain (Lassen et al).

The methods used by Lassen et al. involved the use of xenon 133, a radioactive isotope of the inert gas xenon. A small volume of this gas was injected via arterial catheters into the main arteries of the brain. The radioactivity from many cortical areas on the lateral surfaces is followed by a camera with 254 external detectors, each detector scanning approximately 1 cm^2 of brain surface. In this way both arrival and washout of radioactivity are examined. A digital computer processes the information from the detectors and produces graphic images on a color television monitor. According to these authors, the superficial cortex is responsible for the radiation.

Roland (1985) states that the rCBF measure-

ments with xenon 133 have "been useful for functional mapping" (p. 103) and what he calls "functional dissection of the cerebral cortex" (p. 103) in human beings. Some of the studies used for functional mapping were reviewed in the chapters on processing in this book. These studies have, according to Roland, used four different kinds of cortical activation; "language production, voluntary movements, focusing of sensory attention, and somatosensory discrimination" (p. 90). He further claims that the results showed that behavioral manipulations can be used to dissect different "sensory and motor functions . . . into anatomical and informational subcomponents" (p. 103). Further, according to Roland, these studies have shown that cortical fields are activated prior to the actual performance of a specific activity. They thus manifest brain work in awake individuals, including planning of voluntary movement, processing of sensory information, work of a cognitive nature, and memory retrieval. Lassen et al. state that rCBF studies of complex tasks such as reading support the view that several cortical areas are required for performance (see Fig. 6-3, p. 114).

Roland et al. (1980) pointed out the limitations of the rCBF method; with rCBF "the time relations between the different cortical activations" (p. 129), cannot be studied, and because rCBF measurement takes 45 seconds, "it is likely that cortical regions with only brief activation may be missed" (p. 129). Further, because rCBF represents "the total oxidative metabolism regionally" (p. 129), including both neuronal and glial metabolism, rCBF increases cannot be assumed to result exclusively from increased neuronal activity. Further, there is a "lack of control of mental activity during the reference state" (p. 129), that is, the rest condition. One can control somatosensory input, but not prevent subjects from thinking. It is also possible that marked blood-flow changes of deeper structures that are close to the brain surface (such as the basal ganglia) get recorded where the overlying cortex is "relatively inactive" (p. 131). In addition, Lassen (1985) pointed out that with this technique only one side of the brain can be studied at a time and that it potentially produces a trauma to patients. Lassen et al. mentioned that because xenon is usually injected into the carotid arterial system, structures supplied by the vertebro-basilar system, such as the primary visual cortex, do not show up on these two-dimensional blood-flow images. Jennett and Teasdale comment regarding the lack of knowledge of the partition coefficient for xenon in the abnormal brain, stating that this "limits the value of any comparisons" (p. 133) for abnormal brains.

According to Jennett and Teasdale, Lassen et al., and Lassen, the limitations of the technique are also related to the fact that it reflects events in the superficial layers only, and omits deeper structures. These authors noted that instruments that measure distribution in three dimensions, allowing analysis of deeper parts, have recently been developed, and Lassen stated that it is time for this two-dimensional imaging method to be replaced by the three-dimensional PET scan. Roland agreed with this view. He stated that "in a single folded structure like the cerebral cortex, single photon detection cannot distinguish between activation of the more deeply located cortex and the superficially located cortex" (p. 88). According to him, one would have to "move the detectors relative to the cortex" (p. 88) in order to overcome this problem. Thus, Roland concluded that the PET scan provides a solution for the problem.

Two-dimensional blood-flow measurements were never widely available, and are now being replaced by more advanced methods. They seemed to be used mainly for research purposes to investigate functional localization within the brain, rather than for diagnostic purposes and clinical evaluation of dysfunction. They have thus, with other imaging techniques, contributed to a paradigm shift in the evolution of knowledge and understanding of the CNS.

Positron emission tomography (PET)

PET is a technique based on some of the same principles as the previously reviewed rCBF, that is, the relation between blood flow and functional activity, according to Kety. Similarly, the method allows imaging of the brain and its neuronal activity during fuction (Kety, 1979; Mazziotta et al., 1985; Restak, 1984). According to Martin and Brust (1985), emission tomography images are based on the tissue distribution of a positron-emitting isotope that has been either injected into the blood stream or inhaled. The technique utilizes radioisotopes of natural elements, including ^{11}C, ^{13}N, ^{15}O or ^{18}F, which have short half-lives. The isotopes are bound with compounds such as water, glucose, or transmitter molecules, and the cortical distribution of these can subsequently be mapped (Martin and Brust, 1985; Phelps and Mazziotta, 1985; Sokoloff, 1985). After the isotope has entered the circulation, it can cross the blood-brain barrier over to the brain. Its decay takes place by positron emission. The positrons combine with electrons, resulting in the formation of gamma rays. The rays penetrate the head and are detected by specific detectors located inside the tomograph, which surrounds the patient's head. This information is used to form a colored tomographic image representing brain activity by a technique similar to computerized tomography (Phelps and Mazziotta, 1985; Restak, 1984).

The two most commonly used isotopes are ^{15}O, which is inhaled and enters the pulmonary capillaries as H_2O, and ^{18}F, which is used with glucose metabolism, according to Leenders et al. (1984). They further state that ^{18}F is injected and that sampling of arterial plasma is required after the injection.

PET scans have been used to study cortical responses to stimuli of different complexity in normal individuals. They have revealed which cortical areas are involved in hearing, memory, movement, sensation, thinking, and vision (Lenzi and Pantano, 1984; Mazziotta and Phelps, 1985; Phelps and Mazziotta, 1985; Restak, 1984). According to Phelps and Mazziotta, such studies have revealed on one hand a relation between stimulus content, stimulus size, and the strategy used to solve tasks, and on the other, flow magnitude in auditory and visual cortexes during auditory and visual stimu-

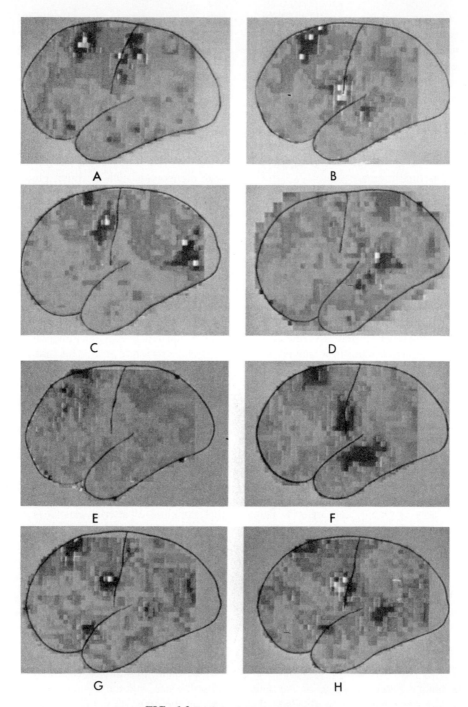

FIG. 6-3 For legend see opposite page.

FIG. 6-3 Two-dimentional measure of regional cerebral blood flow (rCBF) by xenon 133 during performance of different tasks. The figures show changes in flow as compared to a previously established resting state, which indicated relatively active frontal lobes bilaterally during rest, described as departure from the "hyperfrontal resting pattern." The shades indicate increased flow, but the areas of activation have "shrunken" in this black-and-white preparation, as compared to the inital colored scale. The posterior cerebral circulation (occipital lobe) does not appear as the injection of xenon only included the internal carotid artery. All the illustrations have the same orientation as illustrations from studies of the right hemisphere have been reversed. **A,** Cortical activation during movement of fingers on the contralateral body site. The hand areas in the primary sensory and motor cortices are active, as well as the supplementary motor and premotor areas. **B,** Cortical activation during speech. The subject counted to 20 repeatedly. The primary sensory and motor mouth areas are active, as well as the premotor and supplementary motor areas and Wernicke's area. Wernicke's area comes into play as the person comprehends the counting. **C,** Cortical activation as a result of sensory processing while a subject visually follows a moving object. The visual association cortex, frontal eye field, and supplementary motor area are active. **D,** Cortical activation as a result of sensory processing while a subject listens to spoken words. The primary auditory cortex in the temporal lobe and Wernicke's area are active. The next two figures show different flow patterns during internal speech and speaking aloud. **E,** Cortical activation during "internal speech;" a person imagines counting from 1 to 20. The premotor and supplementary motor areas are activated. **F,** Cortical activation while speaking aloud. Broca's area and Wernicke's area, as well as the auditory cortex and the mouth area of the somatosensory cortex, are active in addition to the areas mentioned in *E.* The next two figures show different flow patterns in the left hemisphere during different types of reading. Similar activation has been reported in the right hemisphere during reading. **G,** Cortical activation during silent reading. The visual association area, the frontal eye field, the supplementary motor area, and Broca's area are active. **H,** Cortical activation during reading aloud. Increased flow is demonstrated in the sensory motor mouth area, the auditory cortex, and Wernicke's area as compared to flow levels during silent reading. (From Lassen, N.A., Ingvar, D. H., and Skinhoj, E.: Sci. Am. 239(4):62-71, 1978.)

lation. They have also shown increased lateralized flow and glucose utilization during presentation of both verbal and nonverbal stimuli, which supports localization of verbal functions in the left hemisphere and nonverbal in the right, according to the same authors. Mazziotta and Phelps consider it important to establish and define the relation between biochemical and physiologic processes in numerous normal individuals, and to determine their range of variability. Subsequently, examination of these processes can be performed in diseased states. However, Phelps and Mazziotta support a progressive formation of paradigm complexity in order to study "higher-order" human processes such as language. See Fig. 6-4 for PET scans.

According to Restak, PET scans have been used for diagnostic purposes in psychiatry, for example, to evaluate patients with schizophrenia and manic-depressive disorders. PET scans have been used to examine the extent of metabolic reduction in relation to the extent of impairment in ischemic

disorders, epilepsy, tumors, and dementias of different severity, and to normal aging (Lenzi and Pantano, 1984). Further, Reivich et al. (1985) used PET scans to study various visual-field defects of vascular origin. They concluded, on the basis of a small sample, that a PET scan might detect altered cerebral function that was not detected by a CT scan, emphasizing the importance of examining the nervous system from more than one viewpoint.

Martin and Brust, as well as Ziporyn (1985) state that use of specific radioactive neurotransmitter tracers for PET scanning will enable the study of transmitter distribution. This may provide a biological approach to brain function and anatomy at a cellular level, which may lead to revisions of present knowledge, including clinical abnormalities.

There are several major drawbacks to PET scanning. These include the short half-lives of the tracers, which require close access to the cyclotron that produces them (Duara, 1985; Leenders et al.,

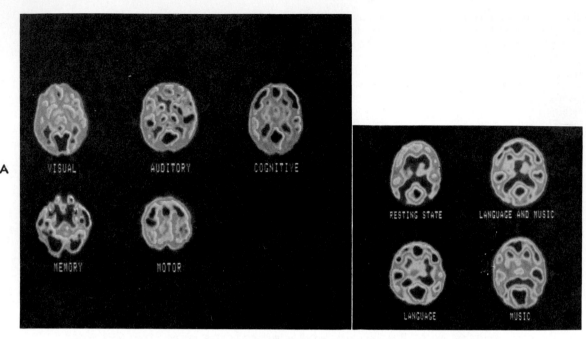

FIG. 6-4 PET scan. **A,** Illustration of different patterns of glucose utilization (increased utilization being indicated by arrows), depending on task requirements. These include visual stimulation activating the primary visual cortex, located at the medial side of the occipital lobes; auditory stimulation activating the transverse temporal cortex asymmetrically according to anatomical assymmetry of the area; activation of the frontal cortex during a cognitive task based on auditory input; bilateral temporal activation of hippocampus and parahippocampus in the temporal lobe during a memory task based on a verbal auditory stimulus and activation of the left primary motor cortex and supplementary motor area during sequential finger movement of the right hand. Note that anterior is toward the top of the figure. **B,** Different cortical activation as indicated by level of glucose metabolism during rest (ears plugged and eyes open); verbal auditory stimulation with predominant left cerebral involvement and nonverbal musical stimuli with predominant right cortical involvement in right-handed subjects. When presented simultaneously language and musical stimuli resulted in bilateral activation. Note that indications of highly increased and decreased glucose consumption both appear dark in this figure. (From "Positron Emission Tomography: Human Brain Function and Biochemistry," by Michael E. Phelps and J.C. Mazziotta, 1985, *Science Magazine,* 228, p.799. Copyright 1985 by the AAAS. Reprinted by permission of the author and *Science Magazine.*)

1984; Ziporyn, 1985), and the long stimulation time, requiring repeated stimulus presentation (Mazziotta and Phelps, 1985; Roland, 1985). The excessive cost of the method limits its use to a few research centers (Duara, 1985; Leenders et al., 1984). There are also error-producing factors that are hard to control, such as head movement during the scanning and cognitive activity, which cannot be controlled in the same way as visual stimuli and speech (Duara, 1985; Lenzi and Pantano, 1984). Duara concluded his discussion by identifying the

additional problems of "analyzing the images in a coherent way, given the enormous quantities of data available at the end of each successful study" (p. 343). Leenders et al. also pointed out the present underdevelopment of "evaluation and validation of the theoretical models describing the fate of various tracers in the body" (p. 33).

According to Phelps and Mazziotta there is a "need to develop a better understanding of the structure, organization, and chemical basis of normal cerebral function" (p. 799). Better understanding of normal CNS processes is also needed for identification and treatment of its diseases. They considered that the PET was a method of combining "basic and clinical research to achieve these goals" (p. 799). However, when considering PET scans, one needs to keep in mind their limited availability and their cost, which restricts routine clinical use considerably, together with many other limitations. There is certainly an identified need to expand knowledge regarding the CNS. Therefore, the A-ONE was developed to provide a structured occupational therapy assessment to obtain clinical data that later might be compared to results from technological evaluations to contribute to better understanding of the nervous system, including mechanisms that contribute to improvement of neurobehavioral deficits as manifested through daily living task performance. This is important because at present no imaging techniques exist that can tackle such complex performance as daily activities, where there is little control of input stimuli, as compared to experimental stiuations, and the response requirements are complicated.

Electroencephalogram (EEG)

The EEG is a record of amplified electrical brain activity. The record consists of fluctuating lines on paper, which represent electrical activity generated by cortical cells (Martin, 1985; Tyner et al. 1983). Scalp electrodes detect the electrical activity, which has been "associated with the summed activity of the individual cells" located under the electrode, according to Martin (1985, p. 644), although, according to Tyner et al. (1983), the exact knowledge of how electrical potentials are responsible for the lines on the EEG is not yet complete. They state that simultaneous changes of potentials in the neurons beneath the electrode, in an orderly sequence, are responsible for various rhythms. Further, the synchrony and the resulting rhythms may be affected by cortical neurons at distant locations.

For EEG recordings, an active electrode is placed over the recording area where activity is supposed to take place, and an indifferent electrode is located away from this site, according to Martin (1985). Numerous active electrodes are used for the recording. Usually these are positioned on the scalp according to the 10–20 International System, in which each electrode is placed 10% to 20% away from adjacent electrodes (Fig. 6-5, *A*). The electrodes on the left side are identified by odd numbers, those on the right by even numbers, those near the midline by small numbers, and the ones located more laterally have larger numbers. The name of each electrode is also identified by the first letter of the cortical area (central, frontal, parietal, temporal, and occipital) where the electrode is attached. The indifferent, or inactive, electrode is located away from the scalp at the ear, nose, or chin (Hughes, 1982).

The recordings always measure the difference between two electrodes. Electrodes may be connected in two ways: monopolar, where the difference between an active and an indifferent, or inactive, electrode is measured; or bipolar, where the difference between two active scalp electrodes is measured (Hughes, 1982; Martin, 1985). The electrical activity picked up by the electrodes is amplified and filtered on its way to the writer units where the electrical rhythms are recorded on paper, usually moving at 30 mm/s (Hughes, 1982).

The rhythms, or waves, of the electrical activity from the brain are named according to their frequency and amplitude, measured in cycles per second (c/s) or Hertz (Hz). There are four main rhythms: delta refers to rhythms that are less than 4 Hz; theta waves are between 4 and 8 Hz, alpha waves are between 8 and 13 Hz; and beta waves are greater than 13 Hz. The waves are shown in Fig. 6-5, *B* (Hughes, 1982).

Normal background rhythm is, according to Hughes, the dominant frequency observed in the record. It is "a general indication of the exitability of the central nervous system" (p. 18). These background rhythms vary with age and wakefulness or sleep. For example, the normal background rhythms seen in awake adults are 8 to 10 Hz (alpha), whereas the background rhythm seen in light sleep is 5 to 6 Hz (theta) and in deep sleep 2 to 3 Hz (delta). Beta waves are normally seen under three conditions, according to Hughes, usually in frontal and central areas: (1) suddenly appearing

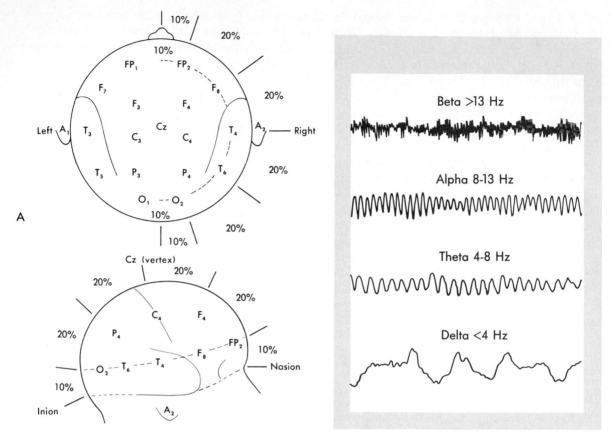

FIG. 6-5 A, Placement of electrodes on the scalp according to the 10-20 International Placement System for EEG recording. Electrodes A1 and A2 are termed inactive electrodes. **B,** The four basic EEG frequencies. (**A** adapted from *Medical Neurobiology,* p. 445, by W.D. Willis and R.G. Grossman, 3rd ed., 1981, St. Louis: Mosby. Copyright 1981 by C.V. Mosby. Reprinted by permission. **B** adapted from *Medical Neurosciences,* p.150, by J.R. Daube and B.A. Sandok, 1978, Boston: Little, Brown. Copyright 1978 by Little, Brown.)

beta waves in light sleep, (2) in anxious people, and (3) in patients on drugs that depress cortical action.

The normal alpha rhythms are "usually maximal on the occipital areas, but at times higher on the parietal areas" (p. 57), according to Hughes. Further, in general, decreased alpha rhythm on the right side can be considered suspicious, whereas slight decreases on the left are usually normal. According to Tyner et al. decreased voltage of alpha rhythms will occur during activity engagement, such as solution of an arithmetic problem.

Abnormal patterns of electrical activity are seen in either slow waves and sharp waves, or spikes, according to Hughes. Depression of normal rhythms may also indicate abnormality. Slow waves, such as delta and theta, should not appear in the adult waking record, as they indicate neuronal damage. Sharp, or spike, waves are seen in patients with seizures, and often signify an epileptogenic brain region. Focal slow waves can reflect disturbance in any part of the brain, whereas diffuse slow waves point to a generalized brain abnormality.

According to Cummings and Benson, the major role of EEG is in demonstrating epilepsy.

They stated that the most commonly seen EEG activity in patients with tumors, hematomas, abscesses, or other space-occupying lesions are focal slow waves. In dementia, they reported a diffuse slow-wave activity. Jennett and Teasdale reported a slowing of EEG activity in head-injured individuals that correlates with the severity of the injury. However, according to them, artifactual abnormalities are very possible. Further, it is "difficult to obtain reliable records in the restless patients" (p. 137), this necessitating considerable experience of the interpreter.

Regan (1979) felt that EEG recordings of the combined electrical activity of neurons did not reveal much about perception, "because they are not usually correlated with specific perceptual stimuli" (p. 139). However, just as the PET scan has superseded the rCBF, and the MRI is by some authors considered to be ready to replace the CT scans, computerized mapping of EEG and evoked potential (EP) measures may soon compensate for some of the limitations of EEG technology by providing, for example, specific perceptual information in addition to measurement of CNS electrical activity. As will be evident later, computerized mapping is used to enhance the EEG, not as a substitute for it.

In conclusion, the EEG reveals information regarding brain electrical activity that is too general for specific behavioral considerations. More precise methods regarding brain function are needed. Development of such methods, based on the EEG technology, has been attempted, as will be evident later in this section. Therefore, understanding the most fundamental EEG mechanisms, as reviewed here, is a necessary background.

Evoked potential measures (EP)

Evoked potentials are defined by Spehlmann (1985) as "computer averaged electric responses of the nervous system to sensory stimulation" (p. 6). The potentials are elicited by sensory stimulation during the performance of specific tasks. The electrical activity is recorded as the potentials pass from the periphery to the cortex at subcortical levels, and at the reception areas in the cerebral cortex by surface electrodes located on the skin and the scalp. The recordings are in waveform, characterized by upward and downward deflections or peaks (Jennett and Teasdale, 1981; Restak, 1984; Spehlman, 1985). According to Martin (1985), the computer averaging program allows the EPs to be detected from the background EEG. According to Spehlman, evoked potentials are used clinically to test conduction of sensory information in order to detect lesions. Abnormalities may be detected anywhere in the pathway from the periphery to the cortex. However, the obtained information does not indicate what is causing the problem.

There are three major types of electical potentials, which are differentiated by the stimulus modality used. These are (1) visual evoked potentials (VEPs), (2) auditory evoked potentials (AEPs), and (3) somatosensory evoked potentials (SEPs) (Jennett and Teasdale, 1981; Spehlmann, 1985; Springer and Deutsch, 1981). The VEPs can be subdivided according to the method of stimulation, such as checkerboard patterns or flashes, according to Spehlmann (1985). Further, AEPs evoked by a click or a tone can be subdivided by latency, and SEPs are divided according to stimulus location. The median nerve at the wrist is usually chosen for the electrical stimulation in SEP (Jennett and Teasdale, 1981; Spehlmann, 1985). According to Jennett and Teasdale it is important to check which subcortical levels are intact when an abnormal response is obtained, before cortical dysfunction is inferred.

According to Chiappa (1983), EP wave forms can be identified by numbering the components in sequence by polarity, for example, N1, N2, N3, and P1, where N stands for a negative and P for a positive wave. However, different nomenclatures are being used with EPs; another common way of identification is the use of polarity and latency information, resulting in labels such as P100 and N20 (Fig. 6-6).

In addition to visual, auditory, and somatosensory potentials, which are evoked by peripheral sensory stimulation, there are also event-related potentials (ERPs). These potentials are, according to Spehlman, a result of cognitive processes, either

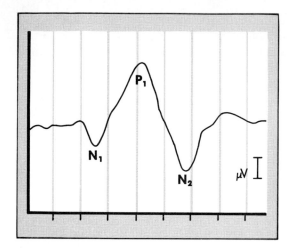

FIG. 6-6 General characteristics of evoked potentials. The letters refer to polarity, *P* indicating a positive wave, *N* a negative wave. The numbers refer to appearance in time.

as a result of sensory reception, or as a preparation for a response, such as movement. According to Stuss and Benson (1986), these potentials "vary more with the psychological significance of the stimulus" (p. 71) than do the evoked potentials. One of these ERPs is the contingent negative variation (CNV), which, according to Stuss and Benson, is useful for assessing frontal lobe function. Further, the N2, which is a component of the ERP, has been related to attention and functions of the frontal lobe. In addition, the same authors reported that the N400 potentially reflects "a more generalized function, perhaps the initiation and supervision of higher levels of perceptual processing controlled by the frontal lobes" (p. 71). According to Ragot et al. (1982), the P300 has been associated with cognitive information processing.

According to Jennett and Teasdale, there are practical limitations to the use of evoked potentials. One is that a comprehensive study requires at least 2 hours, during which time the patient must be cooperative and a skilled operator must be present. Further, according to them, it has to be determined whether evoked potentials provide information that is different from available clinical methods, and if so, in which cases specifically. Springer and Deutsch (1981) comment on the limitations of

evoked potential studies in studying cerebral asymmetry. According to them, "attempts to replicate findings have frequently met with failure, and studies that do obtain asymmetries sometimes fail to agree on which aspect of the electrical recording shows the asymmetry" (p. 93). When looking at electrical recording techniques, one should further consider the limited number of data points obtained from the head, that is, usually no more than 32 electrodes.

In conclusion, the EP measures that have grown out of the EEG technique reveal information about the conduction of sensory information from the receptor organs to receptive cortical areas, where they can be "dissected" from the background EEG noise. Such measurements usually reveal conductance and cortical reception, but some information-processing components have also been studied. The technique is used clinically for diagnostic purposes, although its superiority over clinical measurements has been questioned. The method is also commonly used for research purposes to study the CNS.

Computerized mapping of electrical activity (CMEEG)

According to Nuwer (1988a), the EEG technique has changed little during the past 50 years, despite many new discoveries that have contributed to the development of neuroimaging techniques. Recently, however, with the advancement in microcomputers, this has changed (Nuwer, 1988b). Color-coded topographic maps are now being used as a method "of quickly conveying EEG data to persons who are untrained in traditional EEG" (p. 2), although they do not carry much different information from the traditional methods. Computerized mappings are used to condense and summarize the available traditional information obtained about electrical activity of cortical neurons by means of scalp electrodes (Nuwer, 1988a). This condensing is important because of the wealth of information produced by an EEG (Duffy et al. 1979; Nuwer, 1988a). According to Nuwer (1988a), there are many possibilities of quantitative analysis of an EEG. These include, for example,

Frontal lobes

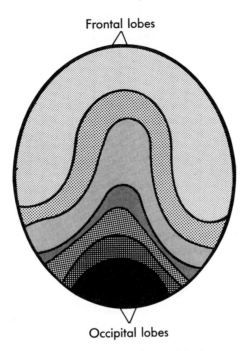

Occipital lobes

FIG. 6-7 Adaptation from a colored CMEEG printout of mean alpha frequency from several frames. This is a symmetrical, normal map indicating maximum alpha activity in the occipital lobes, as indicated by the darkest shade. Similarly, maps can be obtained from the other frequency bands. An asymmetry between the two hemispheres would indicate abnormal electrical activity, as would abnormally increased or decreased appearance of waves in different frequency bands from the usual distribution. An example of this would be no alpha activity in this figure.

"frequency analysis," "topographic mapping," and "compressed spectral arrays," as well as "significance probability mapping" (p. 2). Such quantification can be performed on either EEG or EP data, usually with recordings from 16 to 32 electrodes. Recordings can be obtained at rest or during specific sensory stimulation, or even during paradigms designed to measure higher mental functions (Duffy, 1985; Nuwer, 1988a). These include, according to Nuwer (1988a), so-called "free-running behavior such as reading" (p. 4). However, only a small movement can be incorporated into the recordings.

The voltages that are reflected in the lines of the EEG record can, according to Nuwer (1988a), be transferred over to color on "head format displays" by using topographic mappings. Here positive potentials are represented by the color red,

and negative activity by the color blue, with yellow and green shades representing voltage in between the two extremes. According to Nuwer, topographical mapping of neuronal electrical information can be represented in three domains. They can be represented over time in the time domain; as bands of the power spectrum (alpha, beta, delta, and theta) in the frequency domain; and in the significance domain, allowing subsequent statistical testing of potentials and power spectra, such as the z statistic for examining deviation from norms, or by a t-test for group comparison. Results from such analysis can subsequently be displayed on the head format, according to Nuwer (1988a) (Fig. 6-7). This methodology was used by Duffy as the procedure of significance-probability mapping (SPM) during brain electrical activity mapping (BEAM), which statistically delineates abnormal regions (Duffy,

1981, 1982; Duffy et al. 1981; Lombroso and Duffy, 1980; Nuwer, 1988a; Restak, 1984). The grid-sector analysis is used to quantify the degree of overall and focal abnormalities in BEAM images, according to Duffy (1982).

Nuwer (1988a) considers the head format convenient for representing electrical information, because it resembles the representations from other imaging methods, such as CT scans and MRI. However, he points out that they only represent 12 to 32 real data points, and thus 99% of the display consists of interpolations between the real data points. This is different from, for example, CT scans, which present 100% real data.

According to Nuwer (1988a), quantitative topographical analysis has both advantages and disadvantages. It reduces and compares considerable amounts of available data automatically. However, identification of artifacts, which may lead to errors in interpretation, is a problem. Some abnormalities may be blurred or overlooked. Norms must contain information on age, gender, and alertness state, and they must consider effects of medication and environmental artifacts. Further, the test may be misleading in exaggerating some difference that, in reality, may be neither clinically nor statistically significant. Thus, according to Nuwer, the statistical analysis of EEG data necessitates cautious interpretation.

In Nuwer's reviews of quantitative EEG, he states that "the clinical use of quantitative EEG still seems to be in its infancy" (p. 78). He concludes that these tests should be used as an adjunct to traditional EEG analysis and not a replacement.

According to Nuwer (1988b), many clinical reports of quantitative EEG have methodological problems in areas such as the sensitivity of the test, specificity, and lack of reproducibility, to name a few. The clinical importance of quantitative EEG seems most apparent in detection of abnormalities of cerebrovascular disorders, where it can detect dysfunction where symptoms are too weak to be noticed, or when it is too early for abnormalities to show up on a CT scan. Further, in this patient population, Nuwer states that it can measure

changes during progress, but in terms of localization it will probably never be able to obtain comparable results to CT or MRI. In terms of dementia, the computerized mappings are approaching clinical usefulness. Further, mass lesions do not have sufficient research background yet for clinical use, and very few studies have been attempted with the head-injured population. In terms of dyslexia, schizophrenia, and depression, the use of the method is still investigational. Thus, to some degree Jennett and Teasdale's statement regarding "sophisticated methods of analysis" offering "little advantage over standard EEG recordings" (p. 137) may still hold.

According to Nuwer et al. (1987), the principal advantages of electrophysiologic neuroimaging techniques are as follows. Firstly, they measure functions of physiology as opposed to structure. They do not involve a risk to the patient. The cost of equipment and cost of each test are relatively low, and finally changes over time can be monitored with a temporal resolution of seconds. These authors stated that neuroimaging of EEG is superior to CT scanning, in patients with fluctuating symptoms, marginal ischemia, or during the first days after deficit onset. However, as stated earlier, Nuwer (1988b) has pointed out that these measures will never equal either CT or MRI in their ability to localize lesions.

It is interesting to note that Nuwer (1988b) is much more critical in his evaluation of the present clinical usefulness of the technique than are some of the previous reporters (Duffy, 1982). He further sets a useful criteria for evaluating clinical usefulness, which should be reconsidered with different patient populations.

In conclusion, the computerized analysis of electrical data recorded from the CNS offers information on the dynamic functional electrical activity of the cortex. The technique, although not yet clinically sound across different patient populations, could possibly (with further validation), complement the information provided by the static measures of structural abnormalities, such as CT scans. Although use of the technique during behavioral activities sounds fascinating, as described by, for example, Duffy, Albert, and McAnulty (1984); Duffy, Albert, McAnulty, and Garvey (1984); and Duffy et al. (1980), such methods are not used extensively, let alone in real-life behavioral performances, which produce movements that would result in EEG artifacts. Such behavioral examinations have not been validated, nor has their reliability been established.

Bergland (1985) criticizes the view held by many scientists that the brain is "driven" by electricity. According to him, "the committment that science made to the understanding of brain electricity did not help patient care" (p. 3). He states that "knowing about brain electricity has given scientists knowledge of the shape of the brain, of its inner circuits, but it has provided physicians who care for patients with brain illnesses very few tools for therapy" (p. 3). Unfortunately, this is also true for some other testing methods, such as clinical observations of cognitive-perceptual dysfunction. Clinical evaluations must be more focused towards treatment goals and the functional performance of patients in daily activities.

SUMMARY

In summary, several technological evaluation methods of the CNS have been reviewed. These include both static measures, which evaluate structural aspects, and dynamic measures, which evaluate function, both by chemical and electrical measurements. The CT scan provides information regarding structural changes. It is widely available and used currently as an evaluation method, with minimal risks to patients. MRI has some reported advantages over the CT scan in terms of structural information as well as patient safety, but this method is not yet as widely available as are the well-established CT scans.

Availability of two-dimensional blood-flow measures has been limited, and the technique is now being rapidly replaced by the PET technology, which is more appropriate for use as a diagnostic tool in hospitals. PET scans are reported to have been used both to map the normal brain function and as a source for diagnostic information regarding functional CNS abnormalities, providing information regarding the chemical dynamics that take place in the brain during behavior. They can be used only in certain specially equipped facilities, they are expensive, and they are not used routinely. They also include factors that may produce errors, such as the length of time needed for the information processing by the tomograph.

According to the literature review, the EEG is not suitable for use in correlations with sensory stimuli and information processing, because the information it provides is too generalized. The EPs with auditory, visual, and somatosensory conduction responses similarly seemed to reveal more information in regard to sensory conduction and reception than of perception and sensory processing within the brain. However, some cognitive information or event-related potentials are also being studied by this method. Both the EEG and the EPs are noninvasive methods of no risk to the patient and are reasonably common. Computerized analysis of EEG and EP data, which gives a dynamic representation of neurophysiological cortical activity in a summarized form, has been developed; however, it is not considered a replacement for the other methods. It has so far mainly been used for research purposes, and it still has a considerable way to go to be useful for general clinical purposes.

To conclude, the literature on technological evaluation methods including both static and dynamic imaging measures of CNS structure and function were reviewed. It would be interesting to combine the results from such neuroimaging methods with results from clinical observations. Further, those techniques that do not produce risks to patients could be used in comparative studies of clinical change.

CHAPTER
7
Neurobehavioral Deficits Related to Cortical Dysfunction

Neurobehavioral deficits related to cortical dysfunction depend on the localization and the extent of the lesion (Cummings and Benson, 1983; Daube and Sandok, 1978; Jennett and Teasdale, 1981). Thus as stated in Chapter 4, localization of cerebral function where a match is made between anatomy and function is one perspective for considering neurological dysfunction resulting from brain lesions. It is also the foundation for the evolution of the concept of parallel processing, where complex functions are reported to depend on the combined activity performed by different cerebral regions. Thus, to understand more complex processing dysfunctions, knowledge of localization as reviewed in this chapter is necessary. Perception of the processing dysfunctions reviewed in Chapter 8 requires a holistic perspective of the brain and its function, and this perspective is limited to the cerebral cortex in this text.

As indicated in Chapter 4, the performance of daily activities is composed of integrated functions of different cerebral areas. To some extent, it is possible to analyze requirements for task performance into subcomponents, such as planning complex movement patterns, or sequencing activity steps. These components can subsequently be related to specific cortical areas. Thus, although task performance can be considered a holistic activity based on integrated functions of many cerebral areas, deficits that manifest in a function

may, to a certain extent, be analyzed into components that can be related to specific cortical areas. The A-ONE attempts to analyze manifestations of behavioral defects as neurobehavioral impairments, which can subsequently be related to cortical areas.

Kandel (1985c) states that only elementary operations or subfunctions that are required for more complex functions are localizable to specific cortical areas. More elaborated functions, he believes, depend on the interconnections of different cortical areas. Kandel postulates that the interconnections on which elaborate function is based are like the links of a chain. A break in a single link in a subchain will affect function in one of the "parallel" subchains; however, such a break will not necessarily interfere with the function of the whole system, at least not permanently. This analogy emphasizes that neurobehavioral deficits have subcomponents that originate from different cerebral areas. It further refers to the concept of brain plasticity. Individual differences could, as mentioned in Chapter 2, possibly be a result of defects taken care of by neuronal plasticity during early development. One needs to keep in mind that localization is not absolute, but it does apply to many patients and can be of help in their evaluation.

For the purpose of this presentation, neurobehavioral signs of impairment are associated with different lobes for localization purposes, but because of the extensive connections within the cerebral cortex and the nature of neuronal processing, it is hardly possible to isolate signs to just one location, except for the receptive areas. Rather, they are a result of disrupted processing or communication between several areas. Signs of neurobehavioral impairment can be associated with each other, as the same location can contribute to different functions, and they can be composed of more than one factor. For example, as stated by Benton (1985b), the phenomenon of right-left discrimination has three components: verbal, sensory, and visuospatial. Thus a sign of impairment may be a result of several different factors. For nonaphasic patients with right-hemisphere lesions, visuospatial disability seems to be the underlying cause for impaired right-left discrimination, whereas a deficit in language processing seems to be the cause of this impairment in aphasics.

Heilman (1983) concurred with Hughling Jackson's point of view, which stated that behavioral manifestations of neurobehavioral deficits caused by brain lesions are not "a result of the missing or damaged tissue but rather of how the remainder of the brain acts in the absence of that tissue" (p. 2). According to this view, lesions may change behavior in two ways: they may interrupt a critical system, and they may also affect other areas that may be either inhibited or facilitated physiologically by the area in which the lesion lies. This is in agreement with Kaupfermann (1985a), who states that "no part of the nervous system functions in the same way alone as it does in concert with other parts" (p. 686). This view is very important when assessing brain damage and synthesizing treatment models. It is not enough to consider how the lesioned area can be affected through treatment modalities; we must also consider how those areas affected by the lesion can be influenced.

A review of neurobehavioral deficits is necessary at this point, because it is very important for therapists to recognize them as they appear in an assessment, and to be able to relate this information to a dysfunction within the cerebral cortex. This information is essential for making a complete evaluation of a patient's functional status and subsequently choosing the most effective treatment. The outcome from such a review, which includes information on CNS localization and functional disorders, was used to develop a valid, theoretically based ADL evaluation of neurobehavioral deficits. Examples from the evaluation will be used throughout the chapter in order to form a link between signs of neurobehavioral impairment, their cortical location, and functional performance in daily activities. It should be emphasized that the purpose of this review is to gather clinical information. Readers are referred to classical texts in neurology and neuropsychology for further details and studies in specific areas as well as historical facts (Geschwind and Galaburda, 1987; Heilman and Valenstein, 1985; Luria, 1980; Walsh, 1987).

DYSFUNCTION OF THE FRONTAL LOBES

As stated in Chapter 3, the frontal lobes are the most recent structures of the cerebral cortex. They are the least differentiated areas of the brain, and thus their individual areas are the ones most capable of replacing one another. Therefore, according to Luria (1973), disturbances of the frontal lobes are most clearly manifested in the case of massive bilateral lesions. However, Stuss and Benson (1986) maintained that a moderately severe frontal lobe impairment is readily recognized by clinicians. Walsh (1987) pointed out that some patients with frontal lobe dysfunction might appear normal before undergoing tests that are specifically sensitive to such dysfunction.

Lesions of the frontal lobes cause motor and neurobehavioral deficits, including personality changes, emotional changes, and memory defects (Damasio, 1985; Daube and Sandok, 1978; Luria, 1980; Strub and Black, 1985; Stuss and Benson, 1986). These impairments will be dealt with on the basis of their assignment to cortical locations within the primary motor, premotor, and prefrontal areas.

Primary motor cortex

Limited lesion of the primary motor area will result in flaccid, hyporeflexive paralysis or muscle weakness, depending on the severity and extent of the lesion (see Fig. 3-1 for topographical distribution within the primary motor cortex). On the other hand, when there is a lesion in the premotor area in conjunction with a lesion of the primary motor area, the result is a spastic, hyperreflexive paralysis. The spasticity will result in increased muscle tone, which is manifested in adduction of upper limb, elbow flexion, forearm pronation and flexion at fingers and wrist. In the lower limbs, spasticity is manifested by increased muscle tone in hip adductors and extensors, knee extensors and ankle plantar flexors. Severity of spasticity varies with extent of the lesion (Daube and Sandok, 1978).

Premotor cortex

As stated in Chapter 3, the premotor cortex programs skilled motor activity. Dysfunction of this area results in apraxia and motor perseveration. Disturbances of speech and eye movement can also result from lesion of this or adjacent cortical areas.

Apraxia

Isolated destruction of the premotor area will result in motor apraxia, according to Daube and Sandok. Apraxia can be defined as a disorder of skilled, purposeful movement that is neither caused by deficits in primary motor execution nor comprehension problems (Heilman and Rothi, 1985). Apraxia has been subdivided into many different groups by many authors. Unfortunately there is much inconsistency in the classification and the nomenclature, as is true for many other neurobehavioral dysfunctions.

Motor apraxia. Motor apraxia was defined by Siev et al. (1986) as loss of kinesthetic memory patterns so that purposeful movement cannot be achieved, even though the idea and purpose of the task are understood. Ayres (1985) differentiates between ideomotor and ideational apraxia. She defines ideomotor apraxia as a breakdown of planning and programming of action. Luria (1980) differentiates between kinetic and kinesthetic apraxia. Kinetic apraxia results from a premotor dysfunction that disturbs the organization and timing of motor acts that are components of skilled, complex movements. This affects speed, smoothness, and automaticity of movements. Components of activities such as typing, piano playing, and handwriting that were previously performed automatically by the patient now require separated effort for each step. Kinesthetic apraxia, on the other hand, refers to sensory disturbances due to a lesion located in the parietal lobe. It is discussed under Dysfunction of the Parietal Lobes later in this chapter.

Limb-kinetic apraxia is related to the premotor areas as well as to the parietal lobe in Stuss and Benson's review of "The Frontal Lobes" (1986). Heilman and Rothi (1985) also indicate possibilities for premotor involvement in this deficit. They state that manifestation of the dysfunction is particularly prominent during rapid finger movements, such as tapping. Examination of rapid alternate movements can also be used to test for such dysfunction, as well as premotor perseveration. This functional description of limb-kinetic apraxia undeniably sounds similar to Luria's (1980) explanation of the manifestation of kinetic apraxia. Heilman and Rothi state that limb-kinetic apraxia can be seen during pantomiming, imitations of gestures, or actual object use. Stuss and Benson (1986) describe four different groups of limb-kinetic apraxia. The "proper" type of this group is described as an executive deficit when performing complex serial acts, resulting in sequencing and timing abnormalities. Their explanation is consistent with Heilman and Rothi's description of the impairment. Stuss and Benson classify apraxia of gait as limb-kinetic apraxia. Damasio (1985) describes the presence of abnormal gait and posture due to frontal lobe lesions, such as use of short steps, loss of balance, or gait apraxia.

Heilman and Rothi define ideomotor apraxia as impairment of the selection, sequencing, and spatial orientation of movements when gesturing or pantomiming, for example, patients may have problems with pretending to use an object. Imitation may improve performance, and so may actual object use. However, performance often remains defective. As stated earlier, Ayres (1985) describes ideomotor apraxia as a breakdown in planning and programming where ideation is intact. The idea of the movement, or of how to use the object, is present, and the person may be able to verbally describe the plan but will not be able to execute it. Ideomotor apraxia can be manifested either unilaterally in the left extremities or bilaterally. Heilman and Rothi describe a model of the processing pathway involved in motor praxis. This pathway involves the parietal as well as the frontal lobes, as was outlined in Chapter 4. Both premotor and primary motor areas of the frontal lobes are involved in their model, and the exact lesion site along this pathway plays a role in the type and extent of the impairment, as will become evident in Chapter 8.

Ideational apraxia. As mentioned earlier, Ayres (1985) listed ideational apraxia as another form of defective praxis. According to her, "ideational apraxia is a breakdown in *knowing* what is to be done." Further, "the mental representation or neuronal model of what is to be done is lost" (p. 9). In ideational apraxia there are problems with object use, due to the inability to sequence the necessary actions or to sequence the use of several objects in relation to each other, although the objects themselves can be recognized according to Ayres. Thus, both spatial and temporal factors play roles in the sequencing of action components.

Heilman and Rothi commented on the immense confusion regarding the term *ideational apraxia* in the literature. They describe it as causing difficulties in sequencing the steps involved in an activity. It can even involve the lack of knowledge of the use of a present object, indicating some kind of conceptual disorder. These authors state that although this disorder has commonly been associated with profound conceptual disorders, focal lesions of the corpus callosum have also resulted in such impairments.

According to Ayres (1985) there have been different views regarding the two forms of apraxia.

Some authors claim that different neuronal pathways are responsible for ideomotor and ideational apraxia; others claim that they are different levels of processing. Observations, according to the different levels of processing, suggest that ideational apraxia occurs with ideomotor apraxia but that ideomotor apraxia can occur independently. Some authors have connected ideational apraxia with both the frontal and parietal lobes just as for ideomotor apraxia, but they link ideational apraxia to the prefrontal areas rather than the premotor area. However, different blood-flow studies during ideation or imagination of movement support the involvement of both the supplementary motor area and the orbitofrontal cortex during ideation, as mentioned in Chapter 4 (Ingvar and Philipson, 1977; Roland et al., 1980).

According to Siev et al. (1986), tests for the two different types of apraxia are very similar and are only differentiated by the quality of the response. They include demonstrations of object use, with or without the object in sight. They also include actual object use. The objects used for testing are, for example, a hammer, a glass, and a toothbrush. Meaningful movements, such as saluting or lighting a candle, are commonly used, as well as nonmeaningful movements, such as imitation of hand postures (Fig. 7-1).

The A-ONE simplifies and combines the different apraxia categories with the purpose of a functional evaluation in mind. Pretended object use and imitation of nonmeaningful movements, for example, do not serve a functional purpose in real-life situations unless the person has expressive aphasia. The three-step classification of praxis described by Ayres (1985) that is: ideation, planning, and motor execution is used in the A-ONE. The motor execution is the end result of the process performed by the primary motor areas, and will not be discussed further at this point. Ideational apraxia will be understood to refer to lack of knowing what to do, and how to perform, using correct objects. Ideomotor apraxia will be divided into its ideational and motor components due to deficits in motor planning. The term *motor apraxia* will be

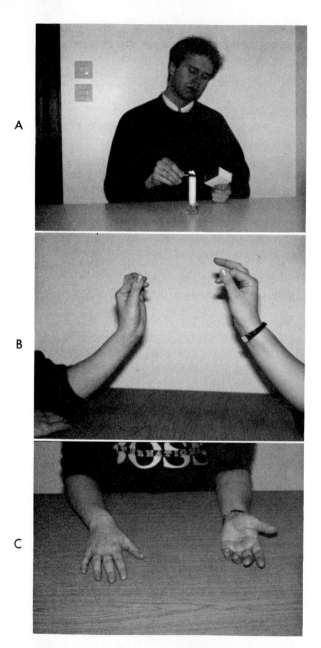

A

B

C

FIG. 7-1 Testing for apraxia. **A,** Testing by demonstration of object use with the actual objects. **B,** Testing by having the patient imitate different hand positions. **C,** Testing for motor apraxia and premotor perseveration by having the patient perform rapid alternate movements.

used for what has been described in the previous pages as *ideomotor* and *limb-kinetic* apraxia. It refers to "clumsiness," where planning and execution of motor programs are defective due to the dysfunction of the premotor cortical areas, or the parietal lobes, where motor engrams (kinesthetic or visual) for such planning are stored. The deficit refers solely to "clumsiness" in object manipulation and lack of knowing how to plan a movement correctly, but not to the lack of an idea of object use. *Ideational apraxia* will be used to refer to the lack of an idea. Examples of its functional manifestation will be covered later on under dysfunction of the prefrontal areas.

Following are a few examples that demonstrate motor apraxia as it appears during performance of functional ADL activities. In dressing, a person with motor apraxia may grab a shirt or a sock, but has trouble planning and executing movements in order to adjust the grasp according to the requirements of subsequent steps in the process. Clumsy hand movements may also interfere with buttoning a shirt, where the person cannot plan (or has difficulties with planning) the necessary sequencing of finger movements in order to complete the task. Note that tactile agnosia (covered in the section on parietal lobe dysfunctions) can also result in difficulties with buttoning, but this deficit manifests a little differently and would have been termed *kinesthetic apraxia* by Luria (1980). Thus, for motor apraxia, one should rule out tactile agnosia if in doubt.

During grooming and hygiene, a patient with motor apraxia may be unable to change an awkward grasp when holding a washcloth. These patients sometimes fragment the activity steps, in order to complete a task and might, for example, release the cloth and try to pick it up differently, when unable to program the finger and hand movements to alter the grasp without releasing the cloth (Fig. 7-2). One of the most obvious indications of motor apraxia appears when a person with this deficit attempts to comb the hair. After grasping the comb, the person is unable to change (or has difficulties with changing) the grasp to a more func-

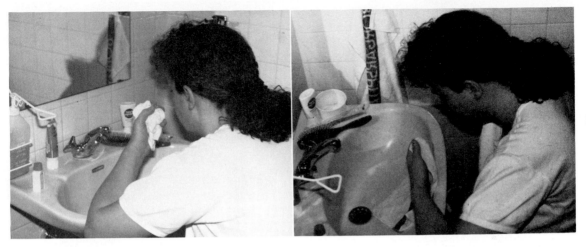

FIG. 7-2 Manifestation of motor apraxia during washing. **A,** The patient with a flaccid right arm grasps the washcloth and is unable to plan and sequence the hand movements of the left hand to straighten the cloth out. **B,** The patient has to let go of the washcloth and straighten it out on the sink before grasping one corner so that the cloth will fall straight over the hand. The right hand is paralyzed, and if it were not completely paralyzed, one would expect motor apraxia there too as a result of bilateral motor apraxia when the left hemisphere is impaired.

tional one. The person may be able to comb the hair on one side of the head, but reaching to the other side with the same hand requires that the person be able to plan adjustments of movement sequences if the comb is to follow the shape of the scalp (Fig. 7-3). Inability to adjust these movements very often reveals the deficit. Similarly, it may be manifested when the patient moves from one side of the face to another with an electric razor, without being able to adjust the grasp according to the different requirements of the activity. Observation of brushing the teeth can also reveal motor apraxia, because the person has to adjust movements when turning the toothbrush up and down, as well as moving it to the right and the left sides.

Motor apraxia can be manifested during performance of transfer activities and mobility. As mentioned earlier, apraxia of gait can lead to short, wide base steps. In addition, a person with this deficit may have difficulty programming movements in order to orient the body in terms of spatial directions according to the intended activity. In this case there may be an overlap with the deficit of spatial relations described in the section on parietal lobe dysfunction, as the memory engrams for movement are stored in the inferior part of the parietal lobe, a part which also integrates spatial information from visual and tactile-kinesthetic sensory modalities.

During feeding, people with motor apraxia may use clumsy, inflexible movements that lack goal-directed sequencing to hold a cup, a fork, or a spoon. Further, they may spill food because of inability to adjust movements (Fig. 7-4). The direction of the spoon, for example, must be adjusted by very fine hand movements on its way from a soup dish, in order to remain level as it reaches the mouth, without spilling.

Premotor perseveration

Another common sign of a lesion in the premotor area of the frontal lobe is motor perseveration. In this case, patients have difficulty in shifting from one pattern of response to another (Damasio, 1985; Luria, 1973; Strub and Black, 1985). Luria (1980)

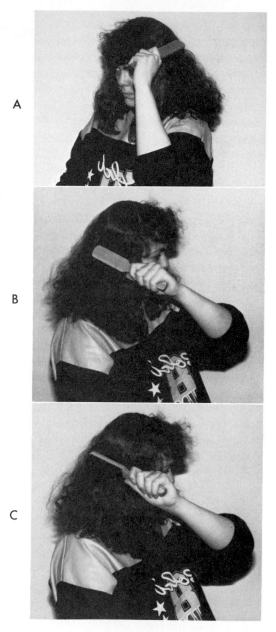

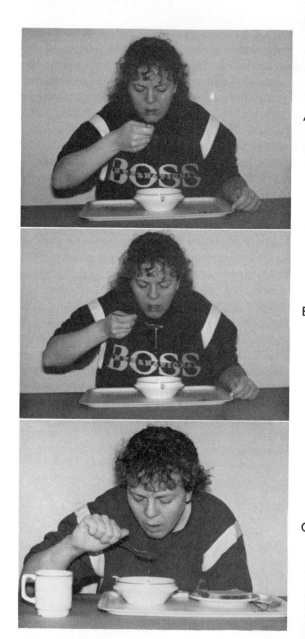

FIG. 7-3 Manifestation of motor apraxia during combing. A, The left apraxic hand may hold a brush and have no observable problem with brushing the hair on the left side of the scalp. B, Under normal circumstances, when the hand is moved to brush the right side, adjustments of hand position are automatically made by sequences of organized hand movements directed towards the goal of changing the position of the brush. C, The patient with motor apraxia is unable to perform and sequence the required movements when the hand is moved over to the right side, resulting in an awkward grasp when considering the task requirements.

FIG. 7-4 Manifestation of motor apraxia during feeding. A, During normal performance, the patient adjusts the movements of the wrist and forearm when approaching the mouth with the spoon. B, A patient with motor apraxia may be able to hold the spoon correctly but unable to adjust the movements when approaching the mouth, resulting in spilling from the spoon. C, The patient holds the spoon with a very "clumsy" and inflexible grasp. She is totally unable to adjust her grasp when approaching the mouth, again resulting in spilling of the soup from the spoon.

Stimulus illustration   Response

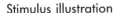

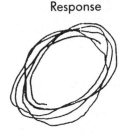

FIG. 7-5 Premotor perseveration during drawing. The person draws a circle according to instructions but is unable to stop the movements involved in the task, resulting in many circles being drawn on top of each other. The figure on the left indicates the stimulus illustration; the figure on the right, the patient's response.

describes two kinds of motor perseveration that can both be related to a particular location within the frontal lobe. One is inertia of the "effector components" of action, resulting in compulsive repetition of the same movement once initiated, due to a lesion in the premotor area. The patient is unable to shift to another action. The other is inertia of the scheme of action, resulting in repetition of a whole action program or a whole activity after having engaged in a particular task. The latter form of perseveration is due to a lesion in the prefrontal cortex, and will be discussed in more detail later.

Premotor perseveration has often been tested by use of paper-and-pencil activities in patients who are able to engage in such activities. Fig. 7-5 is an example of premotor perseveration of the action of drawing a circle. An ADL example of this deficit would be the repetition of movements or acts when, for example, attempting to put on a shirt without any progress. Here the patient may start pulling the front end of a long sleeve up the arm and get stuck in these motions, continuing to pull long after the initial intention of getting the sleeve over the hand to wrist level has been accomplished. The person may match many button holes with the same button, or persist in manipulating the toe end of a sock in order to find the hole. This person may also be unable to stop the movements of washing the face once they are initiated. The person will be stuck at the same spot repeating the same movement components compulsively, and it may be necessary for the therapist to stop the movements physically and direct the patient's movements to another body part (Fig. 7-6). Although the A-ONE does not currently differentiate between prefrontal and premotor perseverations, it should be of interest for therapists to be able to differentiate between the two.

Speech and language dysfunction

Several types of speech disturbances are related to frontal lobe functions. These include Broca's aphasia, oral apraxia, speech perseverations, mutism, and dysarthria.

Broca's aphasia. Dysfunction of Broca's motor speech area results in a loss of speech production: speech becomes nonfluent, dysarthric, and effortful (Daube and Sandok, 1978; Geschwind, 1979; Strub and Black, 1985). An isolated lesion of this area leaves comprehension relatively intact. Transcortical motor aphasia results from a disconnection of Broca's area from the other language areas, according to Stuss and Benson (1986). Benson (1985) differentiates between three subtypes of transcortical aphasia: motor, sensory, and motor and sensory combined. Transcortical motor aphasia results, according to him, from a lesion superior to or anterior to Broca's area. These patients have nonfluent speech but excellent ability to repeat words and echo. Comprehension is relatively intact. Transcortical sensory aphasia, characterized by fluent output, frequent echoing, and limited comprehension of spoken language, as well as impaired reading and writing abilities, is reported to be rarely diagnosed. The suggested lesion site is the posterior left hemisphere at the parieto-occipital junction. Echolalia, which according to Benson refers to an "almost mandatory tendency to repeat what has just been said" (p. 35), is also a dominant characteristic of mixed transcortical aphasia. Patients with this subtype of transcortical aphasia are reported to be nonfluent in speech, noncomprehending, anomic, alexic, and agraphic. In the watershed area, lesions due to insufficient blood flow

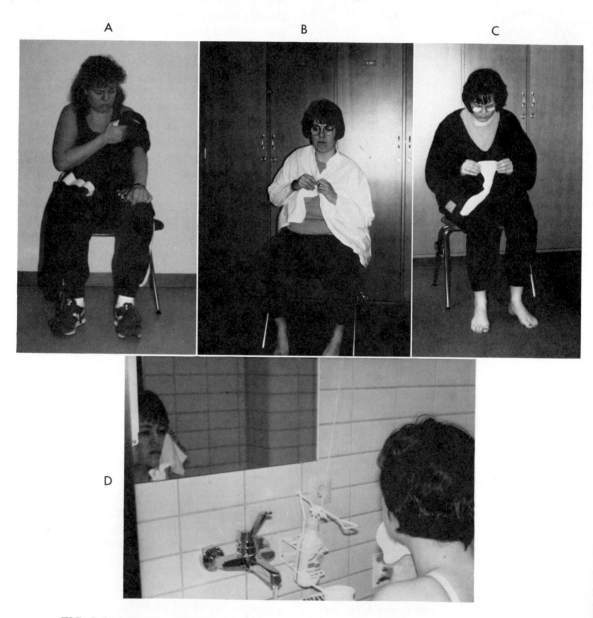

FIG. 7-6 Manifestation of premotor perseveration during ADL. **A,** During dressing, the patient repeats the movements of pulling up the sleeve long after the sleeve has cleared the hand, as was the initial intention. **B,** During dressing, the patient gets stuck when buttoning and attempts to button many buttonholes on the same button. **C,** During dressing, the patient persists in looking for the hole of the sock at the toe end. **D,** During washing, the patient repeats the movements of washing the same part of the face numerous times without moving on to other areas or stopping the motions.

of the distal branches of the middle cerebral artery have been reported. Daube and Sandok reported that 95% of all patients with a disturbance of language function in the cerebral hemispheres have a disease in the left hemisphere. According to them, 99% of those who are right-handed and have a language disorder, have left cerebral dysfunction. Further, 70% of left-handed individuals with language disorders have left-hemisphere dysfunction.

Oral apraxia. Ayres (1985), as well as Stuss and Benson (1986), report inconsistencies in the operational definitions of oral apraxia and verbal apraxia. According to them, some researchers group the two as a single deficit; others keep them separate. According to Ayre's review (1985), oral apraxia has been defined as difficulty with planning movements of the tongue, the cheeks, the lips, and the jaws on command. Verbal apraxia, on the other hand, manifests in omitting consonants and syllables, as well as in difficulty with phonological sequences. According to Ayres, oral apraxia has been localized in the left cerebral hemisphere. Perseveration of certain sounds or words due to an inability to overcome fixed stereotypes or pathological inertia can be associated with oral apraxia, according to Luria (1980).

Mutism. Mutism has been associated with lesions of the supplementary motor area of either hemisphere and the cingulate gyrus on the medial side according to Damasio (1985). Mutism refers to a dysfunction of speech, where a patient makes no effort to communicate. The communication defect refers to both verbal communication and gestures. Damasio further states that in addition to being silent these patients may also be motionless. Mutism is usually associated with bradykinesia and akinesia. Eye blinking, however, is preserved. Damasio claims that when verbal output is provided, it is well-articulated, thus supporting the view that mutism is a nonlinguistic deficit.

Disturbed eye movements

Other impairments related to motor performance of the frontal lobes may occur. There may be changes in the control of eye movement due to a lesion in the frontal eye field, which is responsible for control of conjugate gaze. In the case of such a lesion, the eyes will deviate to the side of the lesion, because the activity of the frontal eye field in the opposite hemisphere is unbalanced (Daube and Sandok, 1978). The patient will not be able to voluntarily move the eyes when attempting to follow a moving object across the visual field (Barr and Kiernan, 1983). According to Damasio (1985), impairment of head and eye movement toward new stimuli in the frontal-lobe-damaged patient is possibly associated with an impairment of orienting responses.

Prefrontal cortex

The prefrontal cortex is a functional extension of the premotor cortex concerned with cognitive aspects. Some deficits in this area can be localized to the dorsolateral areas, others to the orbitofrontal areas, and still others are common to lesions of either location, according to the literature.

Dorsolateral prefrontal cortex

The dorsolateral prefrontal cortex is concerned with executing goal-directed activities, according to Luria (1980). He states that a lack of intention to perform a motor task, as well as attention to the command and regulation of complex actions may be caused by a prefrontal lesion. Further problems in planning, organizing, and sequencing steps in a motor program that is composed of several steps may become apparent. The organization problems affect not only motor functions but also mental activity. In addition, disability in noting errors may be manifested, because the person is unable to compare the performance with the initial intention. Inadequate and irrelevant stereotypic actions will not be inhibited, and will replace selective goal-directed actions corresponding to specific tasks. The deficits related to these changes include perseveration and inertia, both of initiation and determination of activity performance, as well as impulsiveness related to elementary orienting reflex or field-dependent behavior, according to Luria. They also include ideational apraxia associated with the lack of an idea for performance; impairment of organization and the sequencing of activity steps; general slowness in response during performance, or bradykinesia; rigidity, which is manifested in lack of flexibility in approach to situations; and diminished ability to shift from one concept to another. A prefrontal lesion will also prevent performance of more than one motor program simultaneously. Some of the preceding impairments, such as perseveration, ideation, and field-dependency also apply to lesions of the orbitofrontal areas (Luria, 1980).

Cognition, concrete thoughts, and diminished problem-solving ability. According to Walsh (1987), intellectual deficits, as measured by intelligence tests, more often result from dorsolateral lesions than orbitofrontal ones. He bases his view on reports from case studies of patients who have undergone brain surgery. Loss of abstraction, or decreased flexibility of conceptual behavior, resulting in the use of more concrete thoughts and problem solving, has been attributed to frontal lobe function (Walsh, 1987). Damasio (1985), however, relates disturbances of abstract reasoning to the orbitofrontal rather than the dorsolateral areas. Walsh points out that patients may perform poorly on tests of abstraction for different reasons, because abstraction has many subcomponents. These include the abilities to detach oneself from external and internal experiences; to "assume a mental-set"; to verbalize or utilize internal speech; to shift mentally back and forth from one situation to another and yet be able to keep the various aspects in mind simultaneously; to grasp the general idea of a whole and be able to analyze its components and synthesize them; to classify concepts and form hierarchies of concepts; to plan ahead by the use of ideation, and realize the consequences of an action; and to use symbolics in thinking or performance. From this it is evident that abstraction and ideation as described by Ayres (1985) and explained previously in relation to apraxias are related to each other and seem to have common components. The problem solving and foreseeing the consequences of one's actions are common to both of these functions.

Luria (1980), states that the problems that patients with prefrontal lobe damage may have in terms of abstraction may be related more to an inability to inhibit irrelevant connections than to the disintegration of the meaning of the abstract ideas. This may become evident on categorical tests or when retelling stories. Similarly, simplification of arithmetical operations, omission of task components, or perseverance of operations may lead to calculation mistakes. According to Walsh (1987), the patient lacks a total plan for two- or three-step operations. He works with a fragment of the necessary operations, and on impulses. During hygiene and grooming, this person may fragment the body and wash and dry only one fragment at a time, such as the face, the left arm, or the right arm, without a total plan for the activity.

According to Luria (1980), patients with frontal lobe impairments have problems with proverbs, amongst other things. These difficulties are related to an inability to inhibit irrelevant alternatives that may be related to the concrete words.

Concreteness or inflexibility of thinking may manifest during ADL activities in a patient's inability to generalize from one situation to another. A patient may ask what time of day it is while eating breakfast. When asked how to wet a dried-out roll-on deodorant, the patient will put it under running water instead of turning it upside down (Fig. 7-7). Thus she is not able to think of simple solutions that require some thought. The patient will wash the body with ice-cold water without liking cold water, rather than turning on the hot water, too.

Ideational apraxia, organization, and sequencing problems. In ideational apraxia there is a breakdown in knowledge of what is to be done in order to perform, according to Ayres (1985). This is often tested by tasks such as lighting a candle, as mentioned previously. Luria (1980) explains that during such tasks, patients with prefrontal lesions may often only perform a fragment of the task or completely replace the act by another, simpler one. According to him, a patient may thus light the match and then immediately put it out (Fig. 7-8).

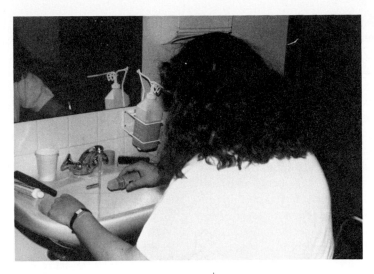

FIG. 7-7 Manifestation of concrete thinking during grooming. The patient attempts to wet a dry roll-on deodorant by putting it under running water. The concrete concepts of dry and water allow for no flexibility in thinking, in this case.

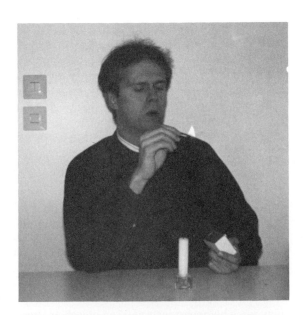

FIG. 7-8 Testing for ideational apraxia. Simplification of an action as a result of an ideational problem. The patient who is instructed to light a candle lights the match and blows it out instead of continuing with subsequent steps in the process.

According to Luria (1980), prefrontal disturbances are particularly pronounced in patients with lesions of the left dominant frontal lobe, which is closely connected with the cerebral organization of speech. According to him, voluntary, goal-directed movements and actions seem to be based on regulatory programs controlled by speech. Disturbance of internal speech interferes with the formation of such programs. This results in a lack of inhibition of irrelevant stimuli, and stereotypic repetitions of previous behavior.

Several examples follow of how ideational apraxia is manifested during primary ADL tasks. As mentioned earlier, organization and sequencing-of-activity tasks are related to ideation, and so is bradykinesia, or slowness during performance. (Bradykinesia is termed *performance latency* in the A-ONE.) Thus examples of organization and sequencing problems will precede examples of the more severe forms of ideational apraxia. It should be kept in mind that organization and sequencing problems can manifest as mild forms of ideational problems. These can also manifest as residuals of ideational apraxia after impairments have improved.

During dressing activities, a patient may have problems in sequencing the activity steps. An unaffected arm may, for example, be dressed before the affected or paralyzed arm, so that the person runs into problems with dressing the affected arm. Here the patient is aware of the affected arm and intends to dress it, as opposed to body neglect, where the patient "forgets" the affected arm completely. The patient with organization and sequencing problems may also leave out steps in an activity. Fastenings, such as buttons, zippers, and laces, may, for example, not be completed according to the functional nature of the activity; sequence may be out of order, so that the person puts shoes on before pants. Further the patient may stop the activity after each step and need to be "programmed" by the therapist to continue.

During grooming and hygiene activities, the patient may not turn off water after washing, or turn off an electric shaver. He may not wring out the washcloth after washing, or even during the washing, so that water drips from the washcloth all over the patient. One activity may not be completed before another one is started. A patient may, for example, stop in the middle of washing when she sees uncombed hair in the mirror. Subsequently, she will reach for the comb and start combing. This example relates to field-dependent behavior, an attention deficit that will be described later. In such cases, an irrelevant stimulus will interfere with activity performance and take over voluntary, goal-directed activity.

Further examples of organization and sequencing disorders during grooming and hygiene are that a patient does not take off his glasses to wash his face, or does not wet his hands before applying handsoap when washing his hands. It is also possible that a patient may fragment the activity, washing first the face only, then one shoulder only, followed by one arm only, before proceeding to the other shoulder or neck. Each fragment will be finished before the next is started, including washing and drying off. A person who performs this way is likely to have somatoagnosia, as well as a problem with organization and sequencing.

Similar impairments during the performance of transfer and mobility tasks are evident in a patient who does not put breaks on a wheelchair before transferring, or does not place her feet correctly on the floor before standing up. It should be kept in mind that during functional activities, there are great possibilities of overlapping deficits. In the last example, a recent memory problem may, for example, interfere with learning new organization and sequencing procedures according to altered abilities. The inability to make use of corrected actions was mentioned previously as an example of inertia, along with the inability to shift from one system to another. The inability to learn and use new sequences thus may have many related components, and all of these should be considered during the therapist's decision making regarding the impairments. Lack of judgment may also contribute to performance defects, and so may neglect of or inattention to body sites.

During feeding, a person with organization and sequencing problems may attempt to eat food without cutting it or asking for it to be cut. This person may also keep stuffing food into the mouth without swallowing in between. The last example may also relate to premotor perseveration of movement or lack of judgment.

Bradykinesia refers to a slow performance of tasks, (Damasio, 1979), slowness in responding to the therapist's instructions, and taking an abnormally long time to perform ADL tasks. This is sometimes referred to as a latency period for performance. Bradykinesia relates to slowness rather than problems with the initiation of an activity.

As mentioned earlier, ideation may also refer to an inability to carry out activities automatically, or on command. In more severe ideational apraxia, the patient may no longer understand the concept of the act (Siev et al., 1986). The patient may not have any idea of what to do with ADL items, and may therefore misuse them. Further, the patient may use a body part instead of an object. In dressing, the patient may, for example, not know what to do with a shirt, a pair of pants, or socks. He may thus just sit without performing. When asked what to do with the clothes, he will not be able to answer the question, although he is able to name the items. This lack of a verbal plan for action in patients who are able to speak, can aid in differentiating between difficulty with ideation and other deficits, in this case from lack of initiation. A patient lacking initiative can often describe the intended activity.

During grooming and hygiene activities, a patient with ideational apraxia may not understand what to do with a washcloth or a bar of soap. The patient may hold a washcloth and reach for the toothpaste, thus lacking the proper idea for object use. The patient may be unable to figure out what to use to turn on the water. She may grab the side of the water faucet automatically, instead of using the handle. Thus, she may pull or attempt to turn in the wrong places. A washcloth may be placed where the water should be running to wet it, although the water is not running, indicating a simplification of the activity (leaving out one step, as previously mentioned). The patient may use a washcloth to wash the sink instead of the face. Tools may be used inappropriately. A toothbrush, for example, may be used for combing the hair, the hair or the eyebrows may be shaved with a razor, or toothpaste may be smeared over the face. In severe cases, a patient may get confused if she grabs an incorrect object, such as a glass instead of a toothbrush, resulting in attempts to squeeze the toothpaste into the glass or stirring the toothpaste in the glass. A patient with ideational apraxia may bite on a toothbrush as it is placed in his mouth, or grab the therapist's hand and put it towards his mouth when the therapist attempts to point to the patient's mouth to get him to take out his dentures. Further, the patient may use her own hand as an object, attempting to wash the face with the hand, without a washcloth.

An automatic performance may interfere with an activity where ideation is lacking. A right-handed patient may, for example, place a washcloth into the dominant paralyzed hand and attempt to use the unparalyzed arm to move the paralyzed one to complete the activity of washing. When a patient combs her hair with the unaffected left hand, the affected hand may move as well. Fig. 7-9 illustrates several examples of ideational apraxia during grooming and hygiene tasks.

During the performance of transfer and mobility tasks, ideational apraxia may become apparent, because the patient may not have an idea of what to do in order to move. She may, for example, get trapped in the sheets without knowing why, or what to do in order to release herself. A patient with an organization and sequencing problem may get trapped in the sheets because the step of removing blankets when sitting up in bed was omitted. Further, a patient may attempt to get into bed by turning sideways, having no idea of how to sequence activity steps to perform the activity (Fig. 7-10). This particular example may also be a sign of a spatial relation problem, which brings up the previously mentioned fact that ideational apraxia is not solely a result of dysfunction in the frontal lobes, but can also result from a dysfunction of the parietal lobes, where engrams for motor movements based on visual and kinesthetic components are stored. Thus, where common factors contribute to different deficits, their overlapping should not take anybody by surprise. A patient with ideational apraxia may also be unaware of how to use a stool to climb into a high bed, although his extremities are motorically intact. Further, attempts may be made to wheel a "one-hand-drive" wheelchair by automatically grabbing and pushing down on the armrest (on the intact side) without the patient's noticing the mistake (Fig. 7-11).

During feeding activities, ideational apraxia may manifest in misuse of utensils. A patient may, for example, use a knife instead of a fork to get food to the mouth. A patient may take a long time, because of a delay in conceptualization about what to do. The patient may not have an idea of what to do with food or utensils. She may, for example, attempt to eat an egg with a knife, or the bread with a spoon. This patient may also use her own body parts as objects and eat, for example, with the fingers instead of a fork or use her hand to butter bread (Fig. 7-12).

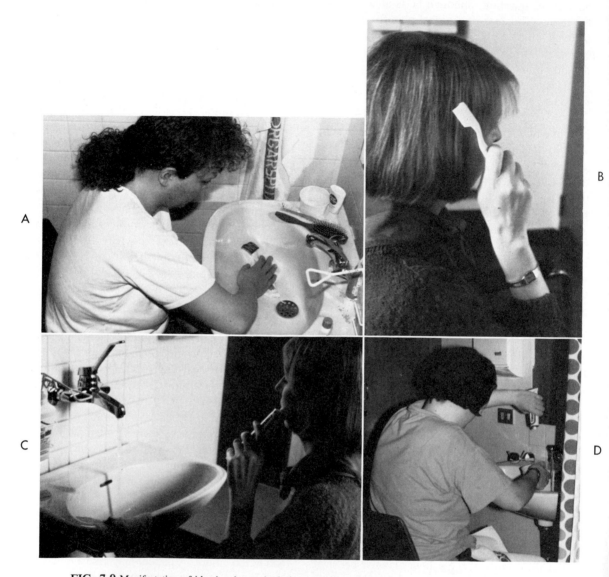

FIG. 7-9 Manifestation of ideational apraxia during grooming and hygiene. **A,** A patient with ideational problems may use a washcloth to wash the sink instead of the face. **B,** The patient who lacks ideas regarding correct object use uses a toothbrush to comb the hair instead of a brush. **C,** The patient, not having an idea of what the toothpaste is intended for, attempts to smear it over the face. **D,** The patient's plan of action is completely disrupted by grasping an incorrect object, a cup, instead of a toothbrush when reaching for a toothbrush. As a result of that, the patient tries to get the toothpaste to go into the cup, again without having an idea of how to go about it.

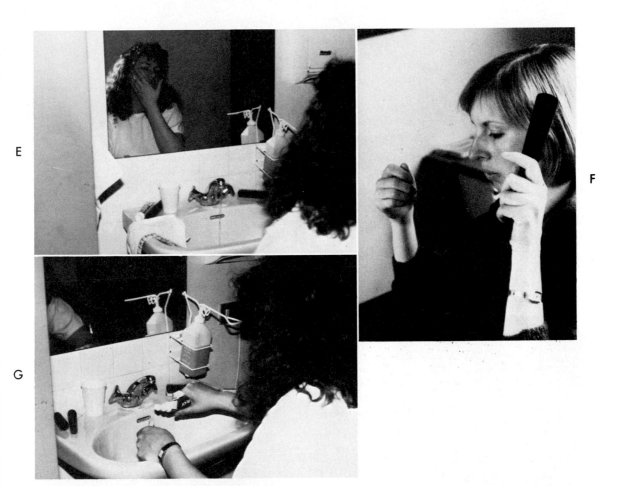

FIG. 7-9, cont'd E, The patient simplifies the activity of washing the face by wetting the hand and using it as an object, in this case, as a washcloth. **F,** The patient who is unable to use the right "dominant" hand because of a severe motor apraxia uses the left hand to comb. However, the right hand moves simultaneously, automatically, as if it were participating in the combing activity. **G,** Organization problem manifested by a patient who leaves out one step: removing the toothpaste tube from the box.

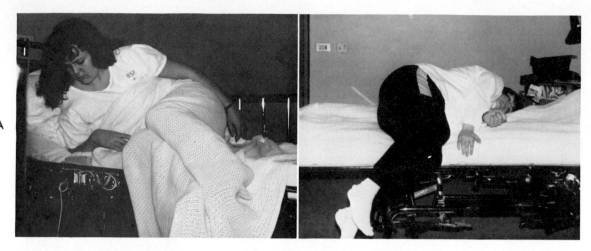

A   B

FIG. 7-10 Manifestation of ideational apraxia and problems with organization and sequencing manifested during transfers. **A,** The patient who is ready to get out of bed omits the step of taking off the sheets before sitting up. **B,** The patient has no idea of how to get over to the bed. After managing to get in the bed sideways, she does not realize what is wrong, or that anything is wrong.

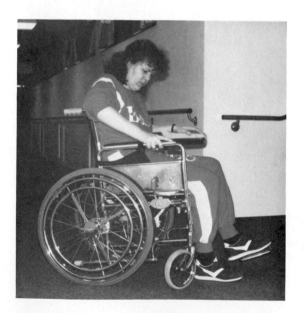

FIG. 7-11 Ideational apraxia during wheelchair mobility. The patient attempts to push down on the armrest on the intact side to propel the chair, instead of using the wheel.

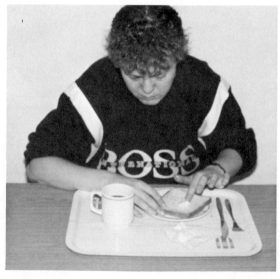

FIG. 7-12 Ideational apraxia during feeding. The patient uses the hand as an object to butter the bread.

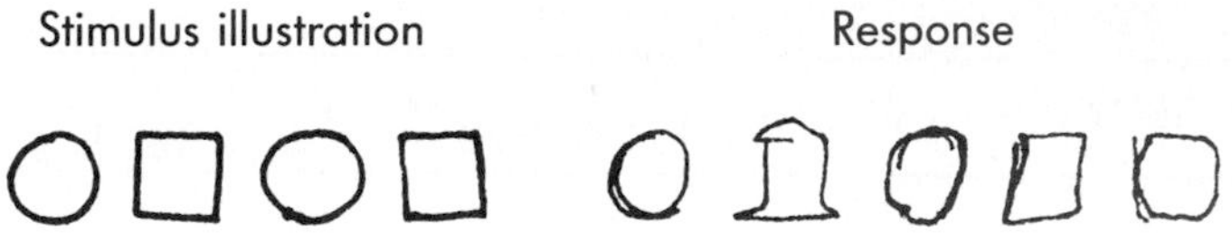

Stimulus illustration   Response

FIG. 7-13 Prefrontal perseveration during drawing. The patient perseverates a component of a previous figure when asked to draw a circle, a square and a circle again. The second circle has kept some components of the action of drawing a square. The figures at the left indicate the stimulus illustration, the figures at the right, the patient's response.

Prefrontal perseveration. Prefrontal perseveration is manifested, as stated earlier, in inertia of a particular program and the inability to change over to other tasks (Walsh, 1987). The following testing methods indicating the presence of this dysfunction have been described by Luria (1980). A patient may be able to draw a simple figure, but when asked to draw a different figure, he will repeat the previous one. He may even draw the same figure numerous times. He may also be able to draw the new figure requested but may include some component of the previous design in the latter figure (Fig. 7-13). When asked to change the system of action and, for example, write a word after drawing a figure, the patient may not succeed in going back to figure drawing on command; rather he will write out the word for the requested figure.

One characteristic of these patients is that they are unaware of their mistakes. When mistakes are pointed out to them, they are unable to learn from the corrections and carry the information over to subsequent activities, which indicates a dissociation between thought and action (Luria, 1980). Such perseveration of systems or problem solving strategies also becomes evident during card sorting tasks, according to Walsh. Here the patient is unable to sort by colors after sorting by forms. Performance of rapid alternate movement sequences with the hands has also been used to test for this deficit.

Prefrontal perseveration can show up during ADL activities. A patient may be able to complete the activity of washing the face, including the actions of wetting the washcloth, moving it over the face, and rinsing off the soap, without repetitions

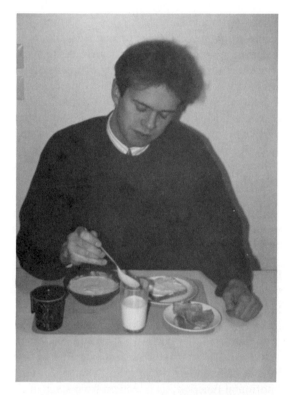

FIG. 7-14 Prefrontal perseveration manifested during feeding. The patient is eating porridge with a spoon. When intending to have a drink of milk, instead of releasing the spoon, the patient reaches with the spoon over to the glass and keeps "eating or drinking" with the spoon.

of action components, such as being "glued to" washing the face, as previously described for premotor perseveration. However after completing the entire activity once, instead of going to the next activity, the person will start washing the face a

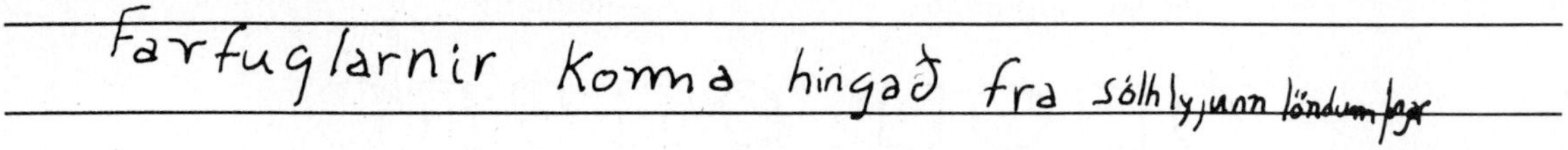

Farfuglarnir komma hingað frá sólhlyjunn löndumfax

FIG. 7-15 Prefrontal perseveration of spatial orientation. The patient "gets stuck" at the end of the line perseverating with writing, attempting to solve the problem by writing with smaller letters toward the end of the line, in order to continue the task. The pencil is not moved independently to the next line, and the patient may need verbal or physical clues for doing so.

second time, and then possibly a third time. The person might also go over to another activity and then start to wash the face over again. An example of prefrontal perseveration during eating would be a person who has used a spoon to eat porridge and will then reach with the spoon for a glass instead of taking a drink from it (Fig. 7-14). Perseveration of spatial orientation may also become evident (Fig. 7-15). In this case a patient who needed to switch lines during a writing task, was unable to move to the far left of the page. A difficulty in shifting lines was also noted, as at times the patient would attempt to proceed, although he was at the end of the line, by reducing letters and writing over previous letters.

Orbitofrontal cortex

The orbitofrontal cortex has close connections to limbic structures. Thus, lesions of this area cause disturbed emotions, personality, consciousness, cognition or higher cognitive functions, and memory (Luria, 1980). In some instances it has been hard to differentiate dorsolateral function from orbitofrontal function, as is evident from some of the impairments mentioned previously.

Emotional impairments and affective disorders. Emotional impairments, or affective disorders, that are seen with orbitofrontal lesions include aggression, apathy, euphoria, frustrations, irritability, pseudodepression, and restlessness. These impairments may be related to altered cortical tone or a lack of inhibitions necessary for behavioral regulation, due to prefrontal dysfunction. There are fluctuations in mood that are not consistent with changes in external stimuli nor with the intensity

of the emotional changes. Euphoria refers to inappropriate gaiety. Apathy refers to a shallow affect, blunted emotional responses, and indifference towards environmental stimuli such as pleasure or pain. It is accompanied by slow performance and inaction. Depression with sad affect or expression may be evident, and yet the depression does not seem to be profound. Lability, where there are mood-swings out of proportion with external stimuli, resulting in inappropriate cries or laughs, may also be displayed. Patients with orbitofrontal lesions may reveal psychopathic-like behavior, and yet they lack the necessary goal-directed organization for the behavior to be effective, according to Damasio (1985). He further states that there is a marked disturbance of behaviors associated with rewards, and that both sexual drive and exploratory drives are impaired. Anxiety will be diminished, and so will judgment.

Lack of regulatory mechanisms, impaired modulation of sensory information, and disturbances in the orienting response may also result in restlessness, frustrations, irritability, or aggressions. These behaviors may manifest in emotional changes, verbal responses of patients, or physical actions, which are usually related to external stimuli.

Heilman et al. (1983), in their review of the association of affective disorders with hemispheric disease, suggested that patients with brain damage in the right hemisphere have difficulty with interpreting or expressing emotions. The studies used to research this area included auditory and visual processing examinations. These patients were also found to have decreased arousal, as determined by psychophysiological measurements, thus supporting the hypothesis of right-hemisphere emotional dominance. These findings of Heilman et al. are in keeping with the observations of other authors (described in Chapter 8) of depression occurring in patients with left-hemisphere damage as opposed to the indifference, or emotional flattening, observed in patients with right-hemisphere lesions.

Damasio and Van Hoesen (1983) reported that electrical stimulation of the cingulate gyrus in humans suggests its role in heightening attention and changes in affect, including anguish, euphoria, fear, or sadness. According to these authors, this suggests that the cingulate gyrus is associated with both the experience and the expression of affect. They reported that the cingulate projects to the supplementary motor area of the cortex, and that electrical stimulation of that area has been shown to interrupt ongoing voluntary activity, be it movement or speech. This is in keeping with the previously mentioned importance of the supplementary motor cortex for intention of movement.

Damasio and Van Hoesen also related bilateral orbitofrontal lesions to emotional disturbances, including bluntness of affect, euphoria, facetiousness, impaired social judgment, intolerance, irritability, and sudden depression. They reported that these changes are not a permanent feature and that the type of emotion displayed varies with time and place. Similar changes were noted with unilateral orbitofrontal lesions, according to these authors, although the intensity was less severe in these cases. Orbitofrontal lesions were also reported by these authors to have been associated with memory deficits in both remote and recent memories. Recent memory deficits may appear as aggression, distractability, frustration, and restlessness (Damasio, 1985; Luria, 1973). According to Luria (1973), the memory process of recall and the reproduction of material are impaired.

Geschwind (1979a and b) discriminated between types of emotional reactions, depending on which hemisphere has been affected by the lesion. According to him, lesions on the left side are accompanied by feelings of loss, in which the patient is disturbed by the disability, and may be depressed. Lesions in the right hemisphere, on the other hand, result in inappropriate emotional responses regarding the patient's own condition, as well as impaired recognition of emotion in others. Kaupfermann (1985c) reports similarly that tests involving sodium amylate injection support the idea that left-hemisphere dysfunction produces depression, whereas right-hemisphere dysfunction produces euphoria.

Behavior revealing emotional and affective disorders may be manifested in daily activities. Restlessness may be evident when a patient has trouble staying in one place during an activity without being short of time. He may also be impatient and unable to wait for the therapist to arrive before starting the activities, although requested to wait. Frustrations may become evident when a patient gets emotionally excited or intolerant when trying to perform, or when he is unable to perform. The frustrations indicate a lowered threshold when considering the stimulus that evoked them. Water of unexpected temperature or a sandwich ending upside down on a plate may result in verbal explosions. Similarly any unexpected touching of the patient (tactile stimuli) or an unexpected movement of a wheelchair (vestibular stimuli) may produce irritation and an outburst of annoyance and possibly physical aggression. Thus irritability or annoyance may be verbally expressed as a dislike, and in people with frontal lobe damage this may be out of proportion to the stimuli that provoked the emotion. The aggressive patient may show hostility or aggression toward an activity or people. Things may be thrown at the therapist, for example, when the latter attempts to motivate the former to perform a task (Fig. 7-16). According to Luria (1980), these patients show a diminished concern for their failure and a lack of critical judgment. Damasio (1985) states that emotional disturbances are more related to right or bilateral damage as compared to left-hemisphere damage.

Arousal deficits. Prefrontal impairments related to alterations in cortical tone, arousal, and consciousness may manifest as decreased alertness, de-

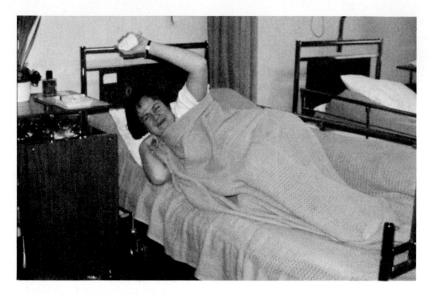

FIG. 7-16 Aggressions manifested during ADL.

creased attention, distractability, field-dependent behavior, decreased orienting response, decreased initiative, decreased motivation, slowness in responding, and absentmindedness. Such patients may have difficulties in dealing with incoming information, sorting out relevant stimuli and inhibiting other stimuli. Sometimes relevant stimuli may not be taken into account, whereas irrelevant stimuli will distract the person's attention and interfere with or interrupt an ongoing activity. The person may not be able to carry out the details of an activity because of lack of attention to either his own body or to the external environment. A patient holding a bottle of after-shave in the affected hand may forget the bottle in his hand when looking into the mirror, resulting in the fluid's spilling from the bottle (Fig. 7-17).

An activity may also be interrupted when a patient hears or sees a person walk into the room, or she may join in on a conversation in the next room or make remarks about it. This is sometimes termed *orienting reflex* (Luria, 1980). The alertness deficit may momentarily become so profound that the patient forgets what she is doing and must be instructed to go back to the prior activity. (Atten-

tion defects are discussed later with unilateral neglect and parietal lobe dysfunctions, as well as processing dysfunctions.) Brief periods of absentmindedness may also become evident. The patient may sit for a few moments without being aware of the environment. This may occur between activity steps, during activity steps, or after the entire performance. A patient who has finished dressing and grooming activities may just sit and look "disconnected" from the environment. He may then begin to move away from the sink area spontaneously or after reminding. He may state that he "got lost." Patients with more severe attention deficits may not blink when a hand is moved in front of their eyes. This may be related to epileptical episodes in the temporal lobe. Inertia of the gaze is also related to an attention deficit, when a person cannot follow a moving object, according to Luria (1980).

Patients with attention deficits may act on irrelevant impulses. They may, for example, discontinue an activity when they see a light switch on the wall. They may fixate on the switch, during, for example, a grooming activity and feel compelled to push it. When perseveration is predominant, or inertia of an activity termination, the per-

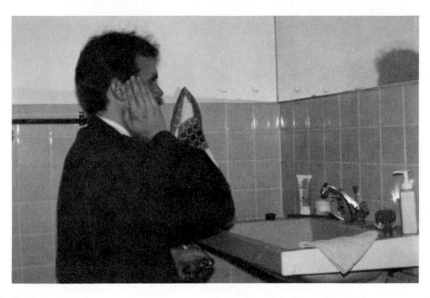

FIG. 7-17 Manifestation of unilateral body inattention during ADL. The patient holding an open after-shave bottle in the left hand, forgets it in the hand that drops down. Thus the liquid spills as the patient looks in the mirror while applying the after-shave to the face with the right hand.

son may turn the light off and on numerous times before stopping. This would be classified as distraction, field-dependent behavior, and premotor perseveration, depending on the performance (Fig. 7-18). A patient who is eating breakfast may also be distracted by orienting his attention on a small breadcrumb that fell down on his napkin. This behavior will take up all the available attention, and the patient will focus on the breadcrumb, perseverating while trying to grasp it and forgetting that he was in the middle of eating a meal. During this activity, verbal comments from the therapist often do not reach the patient's attention. Attention decrease may also be evident when a patient does not become aware of his own mistakes. When these are brought to his attention, he may not be able to correct them. This problem relates to judgment and lack of self-criticism.

There may also be a loss of interest in activities, or of motivation to perform (Fig. 7-19). Patients may want to stay in bed and refuse to get up in the morning. They may be very hard to motivate in terms of any functional activity. Lack of initia-

tive may also be present. A patient may sit by a sink for a long time without performing any of the grooming activities. Such patients may have an idea of what to do and be able to state the action plan, but be unable to start performing. This deficit has been related to inertia of starting actions (Luria, 1980).

Impaired judgment. In prefrontal damage there may be a lack of judgment, a lack of identification of one's own errors and of self-criticism, as well as diminished awareness of social rules. These patients are not able to make use of feedback from their own errors (Damasio, 1985; Luria, 1980; Walsh, 1987). Lack of judgment may be shown in the performance of self-care activities, where a patient does not turn off the water faucets after washing and does not realize that the brakes need to be applied on a wheelchair before he transfers either to it, or from it. A patient with this dysfunction may also go to the dining room without dressing or combing the hair. He may not pay attention to clothes that are inside out or only pulled halfway down at the sides. Such a patient may even walk

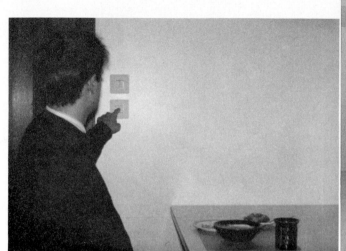

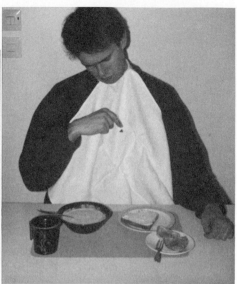

A

B

FIG. 7-18 Impaired attention and premotor perseveration manifested during feeding. **A,** The patient's attention is shifted from the food he is eating over to a light switch on the wall because of field-dependent behavior. He has to touch it and keeps perseverating pushing it back and forth until he is stopped by the therapist. **B,** The patient's attention is shifted from the food over to a small bread crumb that has fallen on the napkin. The patient's attention is devoted completely to the bread crumb, even for a matter of minutes, and then he may have problems orienting to his previous activity (field-dependent behavior).

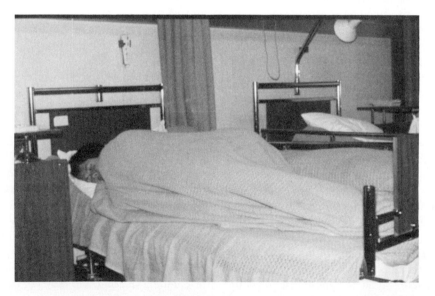

FIG. 7-19 Lack of motivation.

into the hospital hallway without putting his clothes on and not realize that it is not the proper way to perform, or that it disturbs other people. This person may be incontinent and unaware of being wet, and he may not care whether he is wet or not, even though he notices it. The patient may also urinate in a corner of the hospital's hallway rather than going to a toilet.

Lack of insight. Patients with prefrontal lobe dysfunction may lack insight into the disease or disability. They may make unrealistic comments regarding their disease or disability, such as being able to go back to work tomorrow, or in a week, despite recent extensive paralysis. They may further make unrealistic statements regarding future plans.

Impaired memory. Patients with orbitofrontal lesions may have severe short-term memory defects. Luria (1980) relates this deficit to generalized loss of cortical tone. Learning from mistakes and learning new strategies may be difficult, due to a lack of recent memory and memory-storage problems. A patient may comment on a bandage on her arm, not remembering a blood test she had 15 minutes earlier, or may be unable to remember instructions throughout an ADL evaluation. A patient may deny having eaten as soon as a food tray has been removed. The question, "What do you want me to do next?" may be asked frequently during hygiene and grooming tasks, even though the activity sequence was outlined in the beginning. There may also be manifestations of disorientation with respect to hospital stay or time in patients who do not present language problems. The patient may experience difficulty in providing the therapist with his personal history and may also have difficulty in following what time of the day it is and whether it is morning or night.

Confabulations, where patients make up stories or excuses to fill in memory gaps and "cover up," are not uncommon. Patients may respond to an external stimulus from an open question such as, "How was your weekend?" by replying, "Fine, I went to a movie and had a good time," in spite of severe physical handicap and an intravenous needle that should provide orienting information if judgment was unimpaired. Confabulations may be so severe that they do not consider the rules of reality and thus are easily identified. However, confabulations may also be within the limits of reality rules and verification of such information may require more detailed personal knowledge related to the case. There is not necessarily any consistency in confabulations. The story may change from one extreme to another in just a few minutes.

When the patient does not remember an answer to a question he will attempt to guess. If the guess is wrong, he may attempt to deny the error and rationalize to support his answer. He may sooner claim that the therapist is wrong than admit to his own failure. When, for example, a patient is asked whether he had had any visitors that day, he may claim that he didn't even if he did. When shown photos brought by a visitor that day, he will claim the particular visitor had been there the previous day. Sometimes, however, the patient may give in to the person he is talking to, depending on the level of his perseverance. On other occasions the patient may become aggressive without giving in to logic.

• • •

Certain types of intellectual disturbances become evident in patients with prefrontal damage. According to Luria (1980), these patients may display impairments in constructional praxis, arithmetic, and abstractions. He further states that this may, for example, be indicated by tests of proverbs, classifications, and generalizations.

The constructional difficulties are not related to spatial-relation problems in patients with frontal lobe damage, but to the patient's ability to form a whole plan for an operation, according to Luria (1980). She may start on a particular aspect of the pattern and continue from there, without ever forming a gestalt plan. These difficulties may also relate to an attentional deficit to details or space, or spatial perseveration when, after starting to write or perform in one place, the person will limit the activity to that particular area. Perseverations of movement and concepts, where a person who has picked up a black block perseverates in lining up the blocks with the black side up throughout the activity, may be present, or there may be a perseveration of a particular part of a pattern. Further, after making an error, this person will not notice it. Even though the patient does recognize the errors, or is told what is wrong, she may not be able to correct it. According to Walsh, these patients may need a program for the constructional performance. Sometimes the staff members who present cognitive tests have been reported to function as such a program.

Prefrontal speech deficits

Some speech defects may also be attributed to dysfunction of the prefrontal lobes. These include echolalia, anomia, and paraphasia.

Echolalia. According to Luria (1980), echolalia refers to the repetitions of words occurring in the environment. A patient may, for example, repeat words after the therapist. Thus, a patient may not remember that he has just finished eating breakfast, and when the therapist states, "You have to believe me, you just finished eating," the patient may state, "You have to believe me, I have not eaten." A less severe form of this deficit occurs when a patient takes up some verbal stimuli from the environment and adds it into his verbal output and elaborates on it. These impairments reveal the difficulties that patients with frontal lobe dysfunctions face when they are required to form their own schemes of expression, which is necessary for spontaneous speech (Luria, 1980). (See also Premotor Cortex, Speech and Language Dysfunction.) Frontal mutism also was discussed with the premotor frontal dysfunctions, as was perseveration of speech.

Anomia. Benson (1985) states that anomia refers to difficulties in recalling the names of objects or people. This deficit in word-finding has also been described in relation to verbs or action words (Luria, 1980). According to Benson (1985), word-finding problems, or anomia, are very hard to localize within the cerebral cortex. He states that

dysfunction in almost any aspect of the language processing path of the dominant hemisphere can result in such difficulties, and even lesions in the nondominant hemisphere can do so.

Paraphasia. Paraphasia is an expressive speech deficit characterized by misuse or replacement of words during active speech. The word that is used for replacement is from a conceptually related sphere, according to Luria (1980).

Prefrontal motor disturbances

Abnormal reflexes such as the grasp reflex may appear as an indication of the release of primitive forms of a reflex response that is normally kept inhibited by the function of the dorsolateral aspect of the frontal lobe. Fluctuating rigidity may also be present. Changes in sphincter control can be associated with orbitofrontal lesions and are probably due to a loss of inhibitory action over the spinal detrusor reflex. Incontinence may also result from lessened awareness and lack of social judgment.

Impaired motivation and drives

Listlessness and diminished sexual drives may be manifested in patients with prefrontal lobe lesions, especially at the orbitofrontal side (Damasio, 1985). Lack of inhibition regarding eating may also manifest. These changes may be related to altered motivation, drives, and control mechanisms. The reader is referred to Chapter 4 regarding processing of attention. Pleasure and motivational factors, such as food, may drop to more primitive and concrete levels. Connections of the frontal lobe, for example, via the medial forebrain bundle to the hypothalamus, and hormonal control mechanisms play a role in these impairments.

To summarize, dysfunctions specific to behavioral manifestations as a result of faulty programming and verification, other than motor problems, are associated with prefrontal lobe lesions (Damasio, 1985; Luria, 1973). These include changes in alertness and attention, affect, and regulation of emotional responses. Appropriate control of regulatory behaviors may be decreased, and creativity may be lacking. Thinking may become concrete. However, intelligence is relatively preserved. The capacity to learn diminishes. Planning becomes disturbed, and strategies for problem solving become less effective (Damasio, 1985; Luria, 1980).

In conclusion, frontal lobe deficits include personality changes; motor changes (paralysis, apraxia, bradykinesia, perseverations, and loss of speech production); changes in alertness, attention, intention, affect, and emotional responses; memory deficits; impaired problem-solving ability, ideation, judgment, behavioral organization and sequencing, and perseveration of actions. See Table 7-1 for an overview of frontal lobe deficits.

DYSFUNCTION OF THE PARIETAL LOBES

The parietal lobes have three functional areas: primary, secondary, and tertiary. The tertiary area in the inferior parietal lobes overlap the temporal and occipital association cortices.

Primary sensory cortex

Damage to the primary somatosensory cortex located in the postcentral gyrus on one side results in sensory deficits on the body side that is contralateral (opposite) to the lesioned hemisphere (Daube and Sandok, 1978; Werner, 1980). These deficits include lack of light-touch sensation and conscious proprioception. Proprioception refers, in this case, to the conscious awareness of information from joints, muscles, tendons, and ligaments. According to Ayres (1985), the primary somesthetic area also receives vestibular input, but so does the rest of the parietal lobe, as well as all the other cortical lobes. To test for light touch, a patient is touched, for example, with a cotton ball and required to indicate verbally each time he or she is touched. Two aspects of proprioception are tested: position sense and kinesthesia. For evaluation of position sense, different joints and body parts on one side are moved while the patient is blindfolded. The patient is asked to imitate the movements with the other side, or verbally explain

the positions. Kinesthesia is tested similarly, but it does not refer to the position of joints but to the movement of body parts around joints and the direction of the movement (Scott, 1983).

Superior parietal lobule

A lesion in the secondary parietal area, which is the somesthetic association cortex located in the superior parietal lobule, can result in loss of discriminative tactile and proprioceptive sensation, including localization of touch, two-point discrimination, sharp-dull discrimination, graphesthesia, and stereognosis. Tactile localization is tested by touching different locations of the skin of the hands and arms while the patient is blindfolded. The patient is subsequently asked to point to or name the area touched. Graphesthesia refers to the ability to recognize figures, such as letters or forms, traced on the subject's hand while vision is occluded. A pencil may be used for the tracing.

Stereognosis refers to the ability to recognize objects and forms by touch only. For this recognition, a person needs to be able to discriminate between shape, texture, size, and weight with vision occluded. Astereognosis, sometimes referred to as *tactile agnosia,* is a failure of tactile recognition based on this kind of discrimination, although tactile sensation is intact. It has both tactile and proprioceptive components, which are necessary for object recognition by object manipulation when vision is occluded. Astereognosis is usually tested by having the patient manipulate objects in one hand at a time, with vision occluded, and verbally identify the objects by name, shape, size, and texture (Fig. 7-20). Ayres (1985) reported an apparent superiority of the right cerebral hemisphere for somesthetic processing.

An example of how this neurological deficit can interfere with functional performance during primary activities of daily living would be a patient who has trouble manipulating fastenings without any motor involvement. An indication of this deficit during ADL might be that the patient needs to observe the performance closely, for example, when buttoning a shirt, to complete the dressing

TABLE 7-1 Frontal Lobe Deficits

Cortical location of dysfunction	Deficit	Cortical location of dysfunction	Deficit
Primary motor cortex	Muscle weakness Flaccidity/(spasticity)		Speech deficits* 　Echolalia 　Mutism 　Speech perseveration of 　　thought 　Anomia 　Paraphasia
Premotor cortex	Apraxia 　Motor apraxia (kinetic) 　Ideomotor apraxia 　Ideational apraxia Impaired intention Planning and sequencing 　Problems related to move- 　　ments Perseveration 　Premotor: repetition of 　　movements Speech and language disor- 　ders 　Broca's aphasia 　Oral apraxia 　Mutism Disturbed eye movements 　Deviation of eyes to one 　　side	Orbitofrontal area	Emotional/affective disor- 　ders 　Aggression 　Apathy* 　Euphoria 　Pseudodepression* 　Frustration 　Irritability 　Restlessness Cognition* 　Lack of abstraction 　Arithmetic problems 　Lack of judgment 　Lack of insight Arousal deficits* 　Altered cortical tone 　Decreased alertness 　Field-dependent behavior 　Impaired orienting re- 　　sponse
Prefrontal cortex 　Dorsolateral 　　area	General arousal level 　Impaired intention to per- 　　form 　Altered attention to stim- 　　uli 　Impulsiveness related to 　　orienting response 　　(field-dependent behav- 　　ior) 　Slowness in performance 　　(bradykinesia) Intellectual deficits Loss of abstraction or de- 　creased conceptual flexi- 　bility Apraxia* 　Ideational apraxia 　Constructional apraxia Planning and sequencing 　Problems related to ac- 　　tions Perseveration 　Prefrontal: repetition of 　　action program, or 　　whole activity		Decreased initiation 　Decreased motivation 　Slowness in responding 　Absentmindedness Memory 　Short-term memory loss Impaired organization and 　sequencing of action* Personality changes 　Pseudopsychopathic per- 　　sonality Incontinence Diminished sexual drive Listlessness or abnormally 　increased appetite Abnormal reflexes and rigid- 　ity*

*Both orbitofrontal and dorsolateral prefrontal dysfunction may produce this deficit.

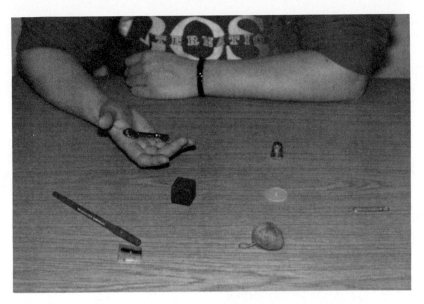

FIG. 7-20 Testing for astereognosis with vision occluded.

activity (Fig. 7-21). Thus the patient will not be able, for example, to talk to and look at the therapist when performing. A therapist who is in doubt regarding the actual presence of the deficit could bring small objects along and have the patient close his eyes and identify the objects placed in his hand. Another indication of tactile or astereognostic problems, which could also be related to unilateral body neglect or inattention, would be a patient who, while eating a piece of bread, shifts attention to other patients or things in the external environment, with the result that she drops the bread (Fig. 7-22). To differentiate this deficit from a unilateral attentional deficit (explained in the section on frontal lobe), it may be necessary to use the method of identifying small objects.

Motor impersistence is described by Carmon (1970, p. 1033) as the "inability of patients with cerebral disease to sustain simple motor activities which are initiated on command." She investigated the utilization of kinesthetic feedback in 60 patients, 20 with right-hemisphere lesions, 20 with left-hemisphere lesions, and 20 control subjects. They performed a simple manual motor-persistence task with the hand ipsilateral to the hemispheric lesion. She found that, in contrast to patients with

left-hemisphere lesions and to control subjects, patients with right-hemisphere lesions were "unable to utilize increasing amounts of kinesthetic feedback from the fingertip to improve their performance" (p. 1038). This feedback, according to the authors, "is normally used to regulate movements in relation to space" (p. 1037) in order to monitor the precision of limb and body-part movements. Thus it refers to using "spatial sensory information to control sustained movements" (p. 1038). Carmon's findings are in agreement with Ayres' (1985) report of an apparent superiority of the right cerebral hemisphere for somesthetic processing.

Carmon's study supported the view that the right hemisphere has a superior role in integrating kinesthetic feedback. Although a precise location of dysfunction within the right hemisphere in the case of motor impersistence is not indicated, it seems logical to suspect processing deficits of somesthetic sensory information in the sensory association cortex of the parietal lobe and in the premotor area of the frontal lobe. The deficit can be tested during an assessment by having the patient oppose the index finger and the thumb over a period of time. The ability to sustain this position would subsequently be noted by the examiner.

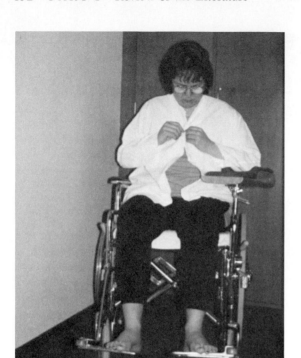

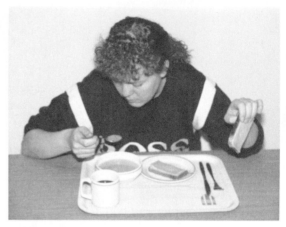

FIG. 7-22 Manifestation of tactile agnosia or unilateral inattention during feeding. Defective processing of tactile and proprioceptive information becomes evident when attention is shifted from the hand holding the bread. Unilateral inattention may manifest in the same way during this task. More specific tests for astereognosis may differentiate between the two deficits.

FIG. 7-21 Manifestation of astereognosis during dressing. The patient needs to observe her performance very closely in order to succeed, as tactile and proprioceptive processing are not sufficient to provide information regarding the activity performance.

Stuss and Benson (1986) suggested that motor impersistence is related to damage in the nondominant hemisphere, probably a lesion of the frontal lobe. However, they also stated that motor impersistence has been associated with apraxia as well as attention deficits and lack of initiation. Heilman et al. (1985) report that motor impersistence, in which patients are unable to sustain movements such as a protruded tongue with the eyes closed for a short period of time, often accompanies neglect and right hemisphere lesions.

Inferior parietal lobule

The neurobehavioral deficits related to dysfunction of the tertiary area in the inferior parietal lobe of the cerebral cortex can be divided into four main categories: apraxias, agnosias, body-scheme disorders, and spatial-relation disorders (Daube and Sandok, 1978; Matthews and Miller, 1975; Siev et al., 1986; Werner, 1980). A brief description of each of these categories follows, along with a list of subdeficits in each category related to the parietal lobes.

Apraxia

Apraxia has been defined as the inability, in the absence of paralysis, sensory loss, or disturbance of coordination, to voluntarily perform learned complex acts (Daube and Sandok, 1978; Liebman, 1979; Matthews and Miller, 1975; Siev et al., 1986). This inability can be related to three practic processes as proposed by Ayres (1985): ideation, or conceptualization; planning and choosing a strategy of action; and motor execution, as stated previously.

According to Ayres (1985), "Praxis is that neurological process by which cognition directs motor action; motor or action planning is that intermediary process which bridges ideation and motor execution to enable adaptive interaction with the physical world" (p. 23). Further, "praxis enables us to put together the components of the physical world and of our physical and intellectual selves in order *to do, to act,* to act purposefully *on* and *in* that world effectively" (p. 5). In addition, praxis includes both knowing what to do, and how to plan a strategy to achieve the goal. Knowing is a conceptual process, dependent on sensory integration and knowledge of the body's capabilities. It is not in itself sufficient for action; implementation of an action plan is also needed. Planning is also related to the cognitive process, as it requires thinking, according to Ayres. She states that if an individual has to think about actions, then he is probably planning his movements. If thinking is not required, the actions are probably automatic, not requiring motor planning. It is important to be aware of this difference when evaluating patients. Sometimes, for example during an ADL task, a person may be able to perform "on automatic." When this is suspected, it is possible to alter the task requirements slightly, in order to see whether problems will be encountered. A patient may, for example, be able to dress without obvious problems; however, if a sleeve is turned inside out, difficulties may arise.

Motor apraxia. Apraxias can be subdivided into four groups according to Heilman and Rothi: ideomotor apraxia, ideational apraxia, constructional apraxia, and dressing apraxia. Ideomotor apraxia, described in the section on premotor frontal dysfunction, and defined by Ayres (1985) as a breakdown of planning and programming of action (as mentioned previously), is reported to occur more frequently with damage in the dominant parietal lobe (Ayres, 1985; Heilman and Rothi, 1985; Siev et al., 1986). Ideomotor apraxia has also been reported as a result of a lesion in the left frontal lobe, as stated in the previous section, but it has been more often reported as a result of a lesion of the left parietal lobe (Ayres, 1985). Rothi and Heilman (1985) suggested two forms of ideomotor apraxia. One is due to destruction of motor engrams stored in the left parietal lobe, the other to disconnection

of the engrams from the motor areas in the frontal lobes. Neuronal processing deficits producing this deficit will be described in Chapter 8.

Basso et al. (1980) studied the relation of ideomotor apraxia to the CT scan locus of the lesion in 123 left-CVA patients. They considered the anterior-posterior dimension of the lesion location with respect to the lateral fissure, as well as lesion depth. The only difference found between patients with ideomotor apraxia and those without was that the nonapraxic patients had a higher frequency of deep lesions and small lesions. In the apraxic patients, the results supported the classical localization within the left hemisphere, including the anterior inferior parietal area. The researchers' conclusion is that apraxia is the outcome of widespread disruption in the left hemisphere, and of some callosal or even right-hemisphere lesions. This study, in agreement with other previously reviewed studies, supports the cortical localization pattern of apraxia and the processing model described previously. The authors emphasized that a CT scan location of a lesion was not as accurate as histological localization because it only occasionally gives sufficient information regarding the extent of the lesion in terms of the specific functional ability. This could be because the area of critical connections involved in the processing of ideomotor praxis is too diffuse. It could also be because the CT scans at the time were not suitable to demonstrate circumscribed lesions.

The study supported the view that ideomotor apraxia can result from lesions in either the frontal or parietal lobe, or from disrupted pathways between the two lobes. The authors concluded that the deficit occurred more frequently with left-side lesions. It also emphasized the limitations of CT scans when considering functional impairment. Neurobehavioral deficits due to disrupted neuronal processing can be expected during patient assessments, although the CT scan does not necessarily indicate the expectation of such deficits.

Kimura and Archibald (1974) studied the performance of manual activity in 30 patients with left- and 14 with right-hemisphere damage. Their findings indicated that the performance of patients with left-hemisphere damage was more impaired when engaging in complex motor sequences, whether they were meaningful or not. The impairments were reported to be bilateral and equal in both hands where hemiplegia was not present. The movement-copying defect in the left-hemisphere group was not significantly related to hemiplegia nor to verbal impairment, according to the authors. Further, it could not be explained in terms of perceptual deficits.

Kimura and Archibald suggested that the impairments were caused by a disorder of motor control, and that they were unrelated to representational content. They thus supported the idea that motor sequencing may be related to unique functions of the left hemisphere. They further provided support for the concept of task difficulty, suggesting that the performance of a movement in response to a verbal command would be the most difficult to perform, that imitating movements might be less difficult, and least difficult of all would be using actual objects, because an object would provide a certain reference point for manipulation.

The results of this study agree with those of previous studies—that apraxia related to movement-sequencing appears more frequently in left-side lesions, resulting in a bilateral apraxic affect, and that the left hemisphere has a unique function in sequencing movement. The sequencing function appears to be unrelated to language; the deficit depends on the severity of a lesion and can be manifested in task complexity; it may not show up in ordinary daily living, according to the authors, but it might in a more artificial situation. However, one needs to question the functional importance of artificial testing. The A-ONE does assume that the verbal perception of instruction is more complex than visual or tactile information, and this is reflected in the order of scores in the evaluation.

Kimura and Archibald further suggested that careful observation of object use within the normal environment might uncover mild impairments that would go unnoticed in the presence of gross and obvious difficulty in speech and locomotion. The A-ONE provides numerous ways in which motor apraxia can be detected, for example, during shaving or combing the hair (see Dysfunction of the Frontal Lobes).

Ayres (1985) discusses neuronal models as mental images. The neuronal models for body scheme are based on proprioceptive and kinesthetic information from the secondary somesthetic association cortex in the superior parietal lobe. These neuronal models also need visual spatial input from the secondary visual association cortex in the occipital lobe. Thus it seems logical that the necessary neuronal models or engrams for motor movement would be associated with the inferior parietal area, which is the area that integrates information from secondary visual and somesthetic cortices.

Luria (1980) describes kinesthetic apraxia, in which the patient's movements become clumsy as a result of disrupted kinesthetic schemes, which are necessary for the construction of motor movement. It leads to a disturbance of voluntary movements, as a result of lesions in the primary and secondary areas of the parietal lobe that affect kinesthetic information. The defect manifests as clumsiness in object use and imitation of, for example, hand movements. This deficit is not differentiated from other components of motor apraxia in the A-ONE. It may also overlap with tactile agnosia, or astereognosis (described above), which is based on tactile and proprioceptive perception.

All the authors reviewed agreed that ideomotor apraxia results most frequently from a lesion of the left hemisphere. Some of the authors have theories that are more developed than the speculations of others concerning the location of stored motor engrams in the left parietal lobe. Damage of this area, as well as disconnection of it from the motor areas in either frontal lobe, will result in ideomotor apraxia. None of the localization information above disagrees with this theory. Functional examples of the manifestation of ideomotor apraxia were given in the section on frontal lobe deficits, and will not be repeated here.

Ideational apraxia. Ideational apraxia, described in the previous section on frontal lobe dysfunction, is defined in Ayres' excellent literature review (1985) as a "breakdown in knowing what is to be done in order to perform" (p. 9). Thus, according to Ayres, the mental representation, or neuronal model, of what is to be done is lost. This cognitive deficit is usually associated with left-hemisphere cerebral lesions (Ayres, 1985). Others have associated ideational apraxia with lesions of the left parietal lobe or diffuse brain damage (Heilman and Rothi, 1985; Walsh, 1987). Frontal deficits, such as loss of abstraction, internal speech, decreased alertness or cortical tone, as well as defective sequencing and organization of behavior in general also seem to be important aspects in ideation, and the frontal lobes would thus contribute as a possible site of cortical disorders. Examples of the manifestation of ideational apraxia during functional activities were provided in the preceding review of frontal lobe dysfunction. It is timely at this point to quote Ayres (1985) and her view of evaluation related to neurobehavior: "By necessity, assessment creates an artificial environment. With the exception of construction or drawing, praxis is tested out of context. This is also the case with intelligence testing" (p. 6). This comment is in agreement with my own view and certainly supports the evaluation strategies used in constructing the A-ONE.

Constructional apraxia. Constructional apraxia, defined in the literature review by Siev et al. (1986) as "the inability to produce designs in two or three dimensions, by copying, drawing, or constructing, upon command or spontaneously" (p. 179), has been associated with lesions of the posterior parietal lobe, with a greater incidence in patients with right-side lesions.

Benton (1985a) describes constructional praxis as "any type of performance in which parts are put together or articulated to form a single entity or object" (p. 175). According to him, this refers to two dimensional drawings as well as block designs. Benton points out that the term *constructional apraxia* has been tested by use of different spatial-organization tasks, and that these tests evaluate visuoperceptual, visuospatial, as well as visuoconstructive disorders. He recommends the use of the term *visuoconstructive disability* to cap-

ture its original visuopractic or perceptual motor-executive qualities, as compared to the visuoperceptual emphasis included later. According to Benton's review, apraxia of the ideational type is closer to the original concept of constructional apraxia than is a spatio-agnostic constructional disability.

Benton (1985a) further points out that constructional tests are diverse and do not necessarily measure the same construct. He reports a low correlation between some tests that claim to be sensitive to constructional defects.

Geschwind (1975) reports that the term *apraxia* has often been misused. An example of this, according to him, is the tendency to label construction disorders as *constructional apraxia*.

The section on frontal lobe deficits has pointed out problems with the term *constructional apraxia* in testing situations. A test for constructional dysfunction can be sensitive to a number of other deficits as well, and careful analysis of performance, rather than an overly structured interpretation of passing or failing a test, is crucial if such tests are going to be of clinical value.

According to Ayres' literature review (1985), constructional apraxia has been identified with lesions in both hemispheres, but especially with those in the right cerebral hemisphere, due to the superior spatial ability of that side of the brain. She reported that the parietal lobes also have been most frequently identified as lesion sites in constructional apraxia. Ayres refers to *graphic praxis* as a separate term that applies to graphic designs or drawings. This term excludes agraphic errors due to language deficits.

Piercy et al. (1960) observed constructional apraxia to be more severe in lesions of the right hemisphere, and the lesions in that hemisphere to be more restricted. They also found that functional impairment could be bilateral.

Black and Strub (1976) studied the incidence and severity of constructional apraxia in 60 patients with missile wounds confined to one of four brain quadrants. They used psychological tests, the WAIS block designs, Object Assembly subtests, and the Bender Gestalt test for the evaluation of apraxia. They obtained a significant laterality effect on two of the three tests, with consistently lower performance from patients with right-hemisphere lesions. The caudality effect however, was found to be stronger than the laterality effect for all the test variables. The incidence of constructional apraxia varied in the four quadrants: the left anterior lesion sample showed little evidence of constructional apraxia, whereas patients with right posterior lesions showed a high incidence of such deficits.

Black and Strub, as well as Benton (1985), reported that constructional apraxia occurs more frequently and is more severe in patients with right-hemisphere lesions. They observed that posteriorly located lesions resulted in more severe constructional apraxia.

Black and Bernard (1984) studied the incidence and severity of constructional apraxia. They evaluated patients with penetrating missile wounds located in one of the four brain quadrants and found that patients with right posterior lesions tended to have the most impaired performance. Laterality of the lesion was found to be more important than caudality when considering the severity of apraxia, although neither analysis reached statistical significance. Lesion size correlated significantly with measures of impairment in the left posterior sample, but not in the other samples. According to the authors, the results supported "either a regional interpretation of the mass action theory or the possible role of deficient verbal mediation in the constructional performance of patients with left hemisphere lesions" (p. 119). Similarly Benton (1985) reported a study that revealed a high incidence of defect frequency on a three-dimensional block-building task in patients with receptive aphasia.

The authors reviewed were in agreement that constructional apraxia occurred most often in the right posterior cortex, or the parietal lobe. This area is important in terms of spatial relations, as will become evident later on. They also agreed that such lesions resulted in the most severe functional impairment and that a lesion in the left posterior hemisphere is also a possible cause for the deficit.

The frontal lobes were further considered a possible lesion site by many authors, especially on the right side. Their identification of the frontal lobes as possible locations of constructional difficulties agrees with the findings of Luria (1980) and Walsh (1987) reviewed in the previous discussion on frontal lobe deficits.

In occupational therapy, constructional apraxia is often evaluated as a single dysfunction. Constructional apraxia is not evaluated by the A-ONE. I do favor, however, breaking the constructional task and the constructional difficulties down into components according to their nature: spatial-relation difficulties, where the person aligns the cubes outside of the space required; perseveration of color or spatial fragments; unilateral spatial neglect, where the person leaves out blocks in a neglected visual field; a comprehension problem, where the person does not understand what she is expected to do; an ideational problem, where the person does not know what to do or know how to do it in order to perform; a motor-praxic problem, where the person does not have the necessary manipulation skills in order to perform; concrete thoughts, where the patient aligns the cubes on top of the stimulus figure instead of beside it; or an attention deficit (Fig. 7-23). The type of error analysis applied here to a constructional task is used to detect different neurobehavioral deficits as manifested during the performance of self-care skills in the A-ONE.

Following are a few examples of classical tests used to evaluate the presence of constructional apraxia. Paper-and-pencil tasks are commonly used to evaluate graphic praxis. These include the reproduction of geometric shapes, copying, and spontaneous drawing (Fig. 7-24). A reproduction of stick designs and two- and three-dimensional block constructions are also used to evaluate constructional praxis (Fig. 7-25). Unfortunately such tests often only include pass or fail evaluation of "constructional praxis," which is a very broad term, including many unrelated neurobehavioral deficits, as mentioned earlier. A scoring of 0–3, for example, does not solve this problem, where

Text continued on p. 161.

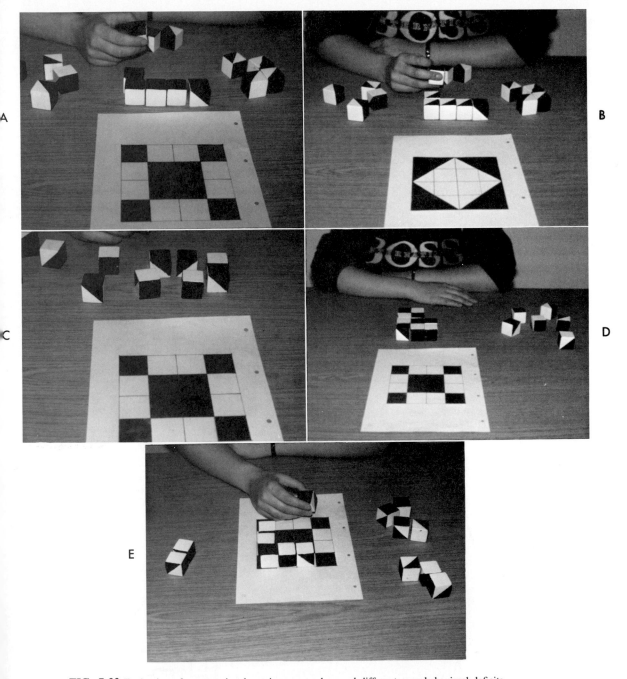

FIG. 7-23 Evaluation of constructional praxis can reveal several different neurobehavioral deficits.
A, Perseveration of color. The patient, after initiating with a black side up, continues to line up the black sides. **B,** Perseveration of shape. **C,** Spatial-relation difficulties. The patient has trouble relating the cubes to each other in an organized way according to the space provided by the design. So far she has picked up the correct blocks, but uses much more space than desired. **D,** Unilateral spatial neglect to the left side. The patient who has finished the task has left out the cubes that are located in the left visual field. **E,** Concrete thinking. The patient lines the blocks up on top of the design, lacking the flexibility needed for constructing beside the stimulus figure.

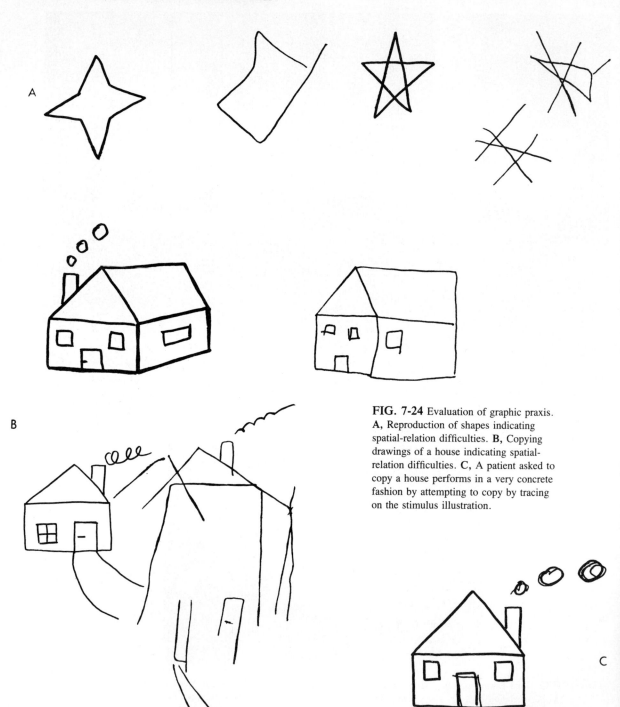

FIG. 7-24 Evaluation of graphic praxis. **A,** Reproduction of shapes indicating spatial-relation difficulties. **B,** Copying drawings of a house indicating spatial-relation difficulties. **C,** A patient asked to copy a house performs in a very concrete fashion by attempting to copy by tracing on the stimulus illustration.

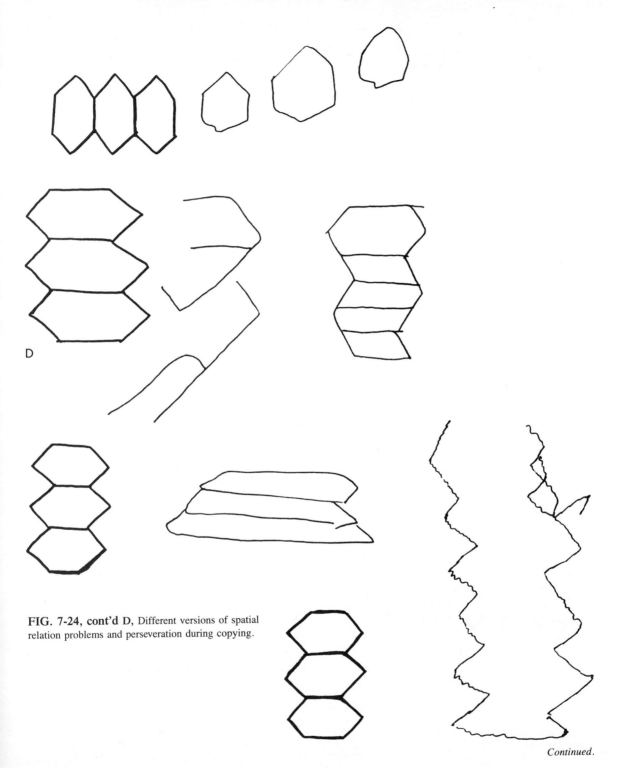

FIG. 7-24, cont'd D, Different versions of spatial relation problems and perseveration during copying.

Continued.

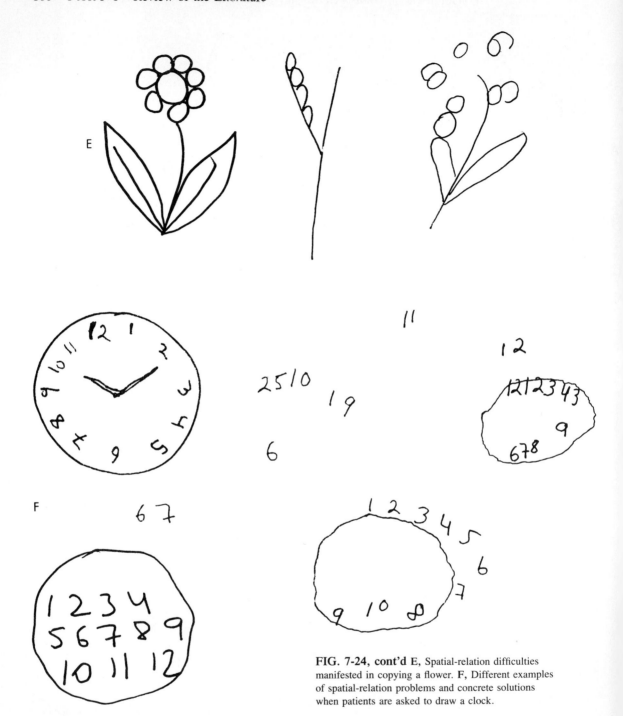

FIG. 7-24, cont'd **E,** Spatial-relation difficulties manifested in copying a flower. **F,** Different examples of spatial-relation problems and concrete solutions when patients are asked to draw a clock.

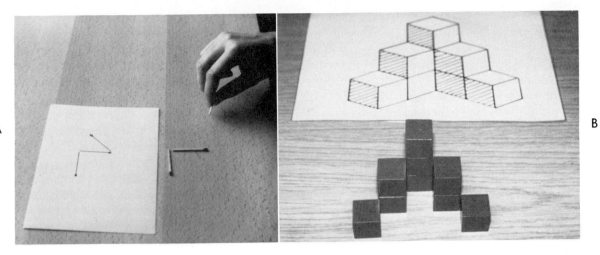

FIG. 7-25 Evaluation of constructional praxis. **A,** Construction of two-dimensional designs. **B,** Construction of a three-dimensional design. The patient is not able to cope with the oblique lines in the design.

the "failure" indicates a failure in other behavioral components than the visuomotor act—for example, failure due to perseveration problems.

Dressing apraxia. According to Matthews and Miller (1975), dressing apraxia, defined by Siev et al. as "the inability to dress oneself because of a disorder in body scheme or motor planning" (p. 179), is often seen in diffuse cerebral disease, and is probably due to parietal lobe damage. In accordance with what was stated in the discussion of constructional apraxia, I prefer looking at components of dressing apraxia as they are manifested through motor planning, ideation, spatial relations, or body-scheme disorders rather than grouping all these components together under the term of *dressing apraxia*. Therefore, this term is not used in the A-ONE.

Agnosia

Agnosia was defined by Daube and Sandok as the "inability to perceive the significance of sensory input" (p. 396) received by the primary cortical areas. Agnosias related to parietal lobe function include the previously described astereognosis. Other agnosias of the parietal lobe include apractognosia and visual-spatial agnosia.

Apractognosia. Apractognosia, which "consists of several different apraxic and agnostic syndromes," such as dressing apraxia, body-scheme disorders, constructional apraxia, unilateral spatial neglect, and visual coordination problems, all of which are derived from an impaired spatial perspective, according to Siev et al. (p. 178), was classified with agnosias by the same authors. According to them, the deficit is due to lesions in the parietal and occipital lobes of the nondominant hemisphere. Because this deficit is very diverse, spanning apraxias and agnosias, as well as spatial relations, and because I have preferred to break down deficits into their smallest components, it was not included in the A-ONE. Thus, in the A-ONE, *apractognosia* does not occur as a term, but was broken down into components such as spatial neglect or disorders of body scheme.

As stated earlier, agnosia refers to a disturbed recognition of stimuli presented through particular sensory channels: visual, auditory, or tactile. This recognition includes, for example, acknowledgment of all fragments of an object or a figure, and the ability to put these fragments together as a whole. In addition to this matching, it is necessary to link the information with previous experience through the function of the association cortex. According to Bauer and Rubens (1985), agnosia is usually modality-specific, which means that if, for example, a visually agnostic patient is allowed to use another type of sensory modality, such as the tactile sense, to investigate the object, it may lead to recognition. More complicated perception is based on these gnostic recognition processes. In general, Bauer and Rubens suggest three components that should be kept in mind during clinical evaluation: the ability to identify the stimulus, stimulus familiarity, and the adequacy of any kind of responses provoked by the stimulus.

Visual-spatial agnosia. Visual-spatial agnosia, according to Bauer and Rubens' literature review, refers to visual space-perception disorders and unilateral spatial agnosia. Thus it comprises several subcategories. Visual-spatial agnosia was defined by Siev et al. as a defective perception of spatial relationships between objects, or between objects and self, regardless of the presence of visual-object agnosia. Thus it is synonymous with spatial-relation impairment (discussed below). The reviewers agree with Bauer and Rubens that this term is a collective one, and that it has several subcategories, including spatial-relations syndrome, spatial-orientation deficit, topographical disorientation, and difficulties in judging distances and depth. These deficits will be covered in more detail later in this section.

Spatial-relations syndrome

The spatial-relations syndrome includes defects common to apraxias and agnosias, according to Siev et al. They related the following symptoms to parietal lobe dysfunction: trouble differentiating foreground from background; difficulties with form constancy, which (according to them) is the ability to attend to slight variations of forms; inability to interpret and deal with concepts related to spatial positioning of objects, which has been labeled *position in space;* difficulties with spatial relations; constructional apraxia; topographical disorientation; and perceptual deficits related to depth and distance. Walsh adds impaired memory for spatial location to this list.

Luria (1973) mentioned a tertiary zone of function in the posterior cortex, where the cortical areas for visual, auditory, vestibular, cutaneous, and proprioceptive sensations overlap. The center of this zone, according to him, is the inferior parietal region. He postulated that damage to this area was responsible for spatial-relations impairments, presenting varied problems in perceiving spatial relationships and distances between objects, or between self and objects.

Kinsbourne (1978) stated that the more elementary the space perception (not requiring conceptual or memory functions), the more it appeared to be confined to a focal area of the right hemisphere. Spatial orientation of a single element was exclusively performed by the right half of the brain in the posterior region. Semmes et al. (1963) reported that anterior lesions tended to impair personal but not extrapersonal orientation, whereas for right posterior lesions, the contrary was true.

Difficulties in differentiating foreground from background. Difficulties in differentiating foreground from background are related to spatial-relation problems by Siev et al., as well as to an attention deficit. This impairment is commonly tested by the use of superimposed figures (Fig. 7-26), where the patient has to identify the different components of such a figure. These authors give a functional ex-

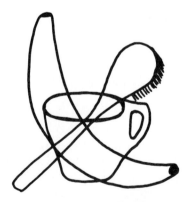

FIG. 7-26 An example of superimposed figures. The patient is required to identify the different figures, in this case a cup, a banana, and a brush.

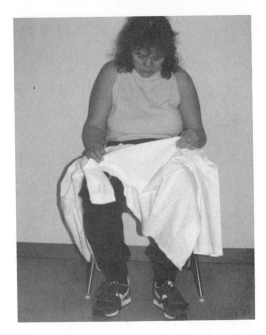

FIG. 7-27 Difficulties in differentiating foreground from background. The patient has trouble finding the sleeve of a unicolor shirt (visual-spatial agnosia).

ample of the impairment, where a patient is not able to locate a hairbrush in a cluttered drawer, or a sleeve of a unicolor shirt. Inability to find a sleeve of a solid color shirt is related to visual-spatial agnosia in the A-ONE (Fig. 7-27).

Spatial positioning. Spatial positioning concepts, such as beneath or above the sink, under the towel, and in the glass, require language comprehension, in addition to perception of spatial relations. This deficit is often tested by drawings: the patient is instructed, for example, to draw a circle beneath a box (Luria, 1980). It is also tested by asking a patient to rearrange objects, such as a cup, a saucer, and a spoon, or blocks (Fig. 7-28), or by having a patient identify whether different drawings are identical or different (Siev et al., 1986). In ADL, this impairment may become evident when the therapist instructs a patient, or gives verbal cues with prepositions that the patient is unable to comprehend. Luria (1980) describes receptive agrammatism, where patients have difficulties with genitive and prepositional instructions. He associates this difficulty particularly with spatial-relation situations. According to him, this is a parieto-occipital

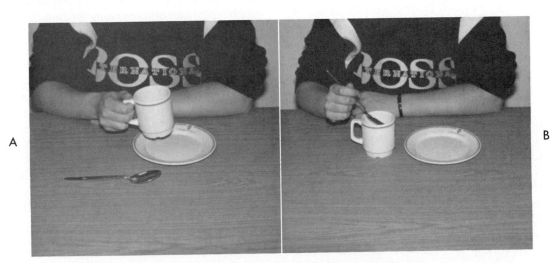

FIG. 7-28 Test for spatial positioning. **A,** The patient is asked to place the cup "on" the plate. **B,** The patient is asked to place the spoon "into" the cup.

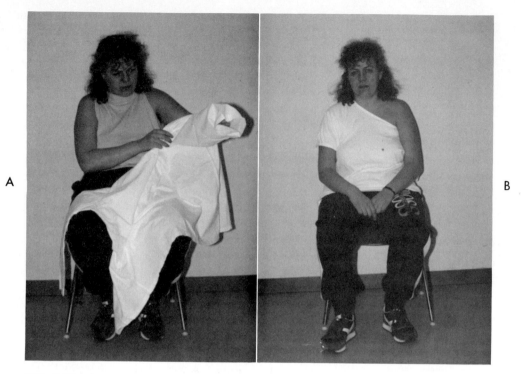

FIG. 7-29 Spatial-relation difficulties during dressing. **A,** The patient is unable to find the right armhole. **B,** The patient may start at the wrong hole, placing her arm through the neckhole instead of the left sleeve.

dysfunction involving defective simultaneous synthesis of, for example, two words related to each other by a preposition and spatial orientation. In the A-ONE, the spatial-positioning concepts are related to the impairment of spatial relations and comprehension deficits.

Spatial relations. Difficulties in relating objects to each other or to the self, termed *spatial-relation dysfunction,* has been evaluated by numerous tests. These include, for example, imitation of dot figures, or of the position of a cross on a paper, free drawings, or position form boards. Constructional praxis tests, including both two- and three-dimensional drawings and block constructions have been used to evaluate spatial-relations dysfunction. This impairment was dealt with earlier in this section.

Following are examples of how spatial-relation deficits can be identified through observation of a patient's performance during daily ac-

tivities. A patient with spatial-relation difficulties may have trouble differentiating the front from the back of clothes, or the inside from the outside during dressing. (This is not a person with an attention deficit who puts clothes on automatically without thinking.) This person may also be unable to find armholes, legholes, or the bottom of a shirt (Fig. 7-29). This could be related to problems of differentiating foreground from background. One should always keep in mind that deficits may (and will) overlap. If the therapist suspects ideational apraxia, for example, in the case where a person cannot find the hole she is looking for, the patient should be asked what she is looking for and what her intentions are. She could also be asked what the problem is.

A patient with spatial-relation difficulties may start to pull a sleeve up the arm in the wrong direction in the middle of performance when putting on a shirt. She may also start off correctly aiming at the armhole, but go past it without noticing it. Thus when attempting to guide a paralyzed arm into the armhole by pulling the shirt first from over the arm and then from under the arm, she may pull past the hole. Pay attention to any indication of motor perseveration as described previously when this occurs. A patient may go past an armhole and put the arm through the neckhole. There may be difficulties matching buttons and buttonholes correctly. It is possible that a patient with these problems will attempt to put her hand into the distal end of a sleeve, instead of the proximal end. A pants' leg may be looped into the pants' waist without the person's realizing it or being able to correct it. The patient may also place both legs into the same leghole without realizing it, or a foot in the wrong leghole. Fig. 7-30 illustrates several examples of the manifestation of spatial-relations dysfunction during primary ADL. A patient, after putting a shirt on wrong, front to back, may attempt to turn it with the shirt on and both arms in the sleeves by pulling at the bottom of the shirt. Similarly, the patient may try to turn pants front to back, after placing one leg into the leghole, by pulling at the waist opening (Fig. 7-31). When this happens, there is a strong possibility of ideational problems, which should be checked out by questions regarding the plan of action. A spatial-relation disability may also manifest as a problem with learning to tie laces one-handedly, or an inability to do so. This may be the reason for refusing to learn the method.

Spatial-relations deficits often become evident during grooming activities. A patient may put glasses on by turning them upside down, or attempt to place the bottom dentures at the roof of the mouth (Fig. 7-32). Distances may be over- or underestimated. For example, a patient may reach out for a washcloth and end up with a glass, which may disrupt the whole plan (Fig. 7-33). A patient may also attempt to reach with the washcloth above instead of below the faucet for water. Spatial-relations problems may become so severe that the patient attempts to brush the teeth of the mirror image, or wash the mirror image (Fig. 7-34). In

this case, there is also a somatognostic problem, where the patient's body scheme is defective. This deficit will be outlined in detail later on in this section.

Spatial-relation difficulties may also manifest during transfer performance and mobility activities. There may be complications when a patient tries to orient his body in terms of directions according to the intended activity. He may lean forward instead of backward when assisting with getting out of bed (Fig. 7-35). When driving a one-handed drive hemiplegia wheelchair, the patient may grab onto the armrest on the sound side instead of the wheel, and push down on it. In this case one would have to check for a combination with ideational apraxia, as mentioned earlier. In severe cases combined with ideational apraxia, the patient may lie down sideways in the bed, as described previously under ideational apraxia. During feeding, this patient may over- or underestimate distances, for example, when reaching out for a cup or utensils, or when bringing them to the mouth (see Fig. 7-36).

Topographical disorientation. Topographical disorientation manifests itself in patients who have difficulty finding their way in space. It is composed of agnostic and amnestic problems (Siev et al., 1986; Walsh, 1987). Thus, there is either a recognition deficit, where a patient does not perceive the environment correctly, or a memory deficit. These patients may have problems finding their way in familiar surroundings, or have difficulties learning to find their way around the hospital. Map localization (both street maps and countries) have been used to evaluate this deficit. In ADL, lack of familiarity of the hospital environment, such as where the dining room and the washroom are located, may give an indication of this deficit. A patient's orientation in her room, such as finding her clothes in a closet, or objects in drawers by locating the closet and the drawers, can also be used as a clue to a deficit.

According to Walsh's review of neuropsychology, spatial-relation dysfunctions are most commonly associated with posterior lesions of the right, or nondominant hemisphere. However, one

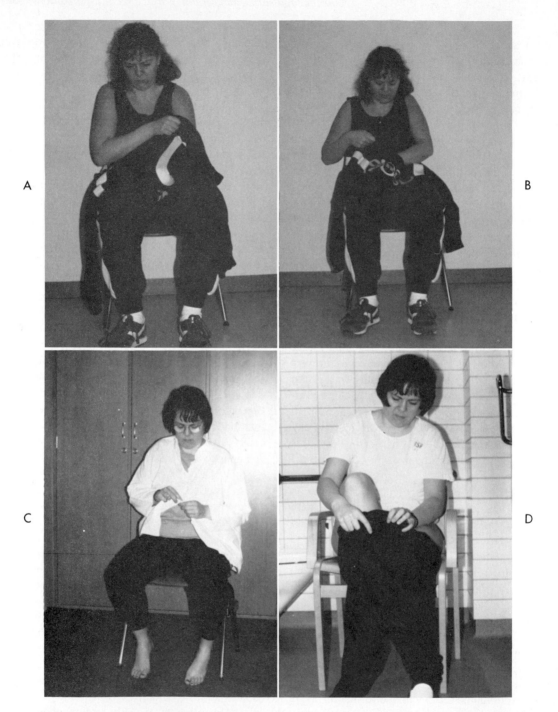

FIG. 7-30 Spatial-relation difficulties during dressing. **A,** The patient is unable to guide the paralyzed arm into the right hole. Pulling more on the shirt at the top of the arm than under it will result in the arm going past the right hole. This deficit can also be related to perseveration. **B,** The patient's arm goes through the neckhole instead of the armhole. **C,** The patient matches buttons incorrectly with buttonholes. **D,** The patient puts both legs through the same leghole.

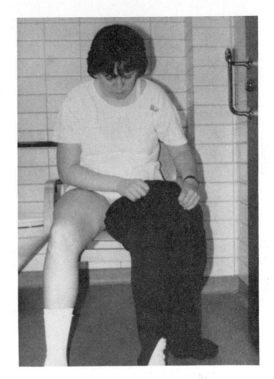

FIG. 7-31 Spatial-relation difficulties during dressing. The patient notices that the pants are turned wrong front to back, with the label at the front, and attempts to correct the mistake by turning the pants with the leg in the leg hole. Ideation also interferes with the patient's performance in attempting to correct for the error.

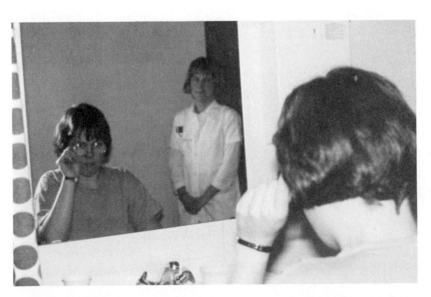

FIG. 7-32 Spatial-relation difficulties during grooming. The patient puts the glasses on upside down.

A

B

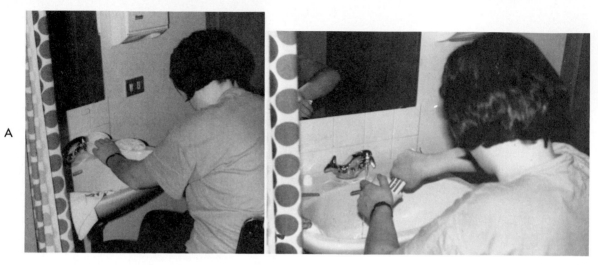

FIG. 7-33 Spatial-relation difficulties manifesting in underestimation of distance. **A,** The patient grasps a glass instead of a washcloth. **B,** This disrupts the whole plan of action, so that the patient ends up stirring with the toothpaste tube in the glass, forgetting about the intention to wash.

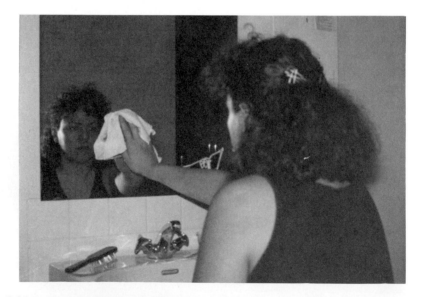

FIG. 7-34 Severe spatial-relation difficulties along with somatognostic problems. The patient attempts to wash the face of the mirror image instead of her own.

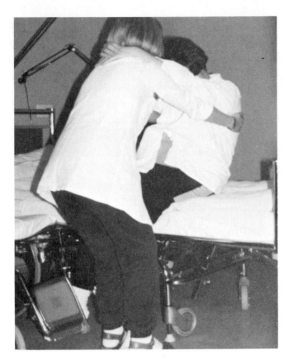

FIG. 7-35 Spatial relation difficulties and apraxia during transfers. The patient leans backward instead of foreward while the therapist is attempting to transfer her to a wheelchair. Such a patient can be dangerous for the therapist if she is unaware of the problem, as the patient's actions are unpredictable and often the opposite of what is expected.

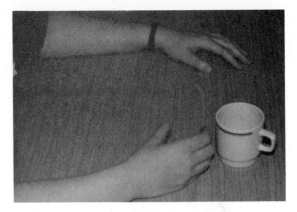

FIG. 7-36 Spatial-relation difficulties manifested in underestimation of distances when reaching for the cup.

needs to keep in mind that when a task requires verbal reasoning, this calls for action of the left hemisphere. When memory is a component of the task, as may be the case in topographical disorientation, one needs to keep in mind that memory for spatial relations is a function of the right temporal, rather than right parietal lobe.

Unilateral spatial neglect. Unilateral spatial neglect refers to inattention to, or neglect of, stimuli in the extrapersonal space contralateral to the lesion (Heilman et al., 1985; Siev et al., 1986; Walsh, 1987). Some authors have also reported that patients with unilateral spatial neglect may be able to attend to stimuli in the lateral extreme of the neglected visual field, according to Walsh's review of neuropsychology. There seems to be general agreement that this disorder occurs most com-

monly, and is most severe, when there is a lesion in the right inferior parietal area (Heilman et al., 1985; Siev et al., 1986; Walsh, 1987). However, left-side lesions and subcortical lesions of the thalamus and basal ganglia have also been reported (Walsh, 1987). In addition to the areas mentioned, Heilman et al. (1985) report that lesions in the dorsolateral frontal lobe and the cingulate gyrus may also lead to the deficit. The processing related to unilateral spatial neglect will be discussed further in the next chapter. These authors propose that hemispatial attention, intention, memory defect, and gaze defect, may all contribute to the deficit of unilateral spatial neglect. They further propose that the right hemisphere may be more important for promoting attention and intention than the left one. Stimuli in the left visual field may thus activate the right hemisphere, whereas stimuli in the right visual field may activate both the left and the right hemispheres. The right hemisphere can thus compensate for a left-hemisphere dysfunction, whereas the reverse is not true. This attention deficit may also occur with tactile and auditory stimuli, according to Heilman et al. (1985). Further, these authors report that the deficit may be manifested in spatial tasks that do not require vision.

Different methods have been used to evaluate unilateral spatial neglect. It is important to differentiate such neglect and inattention from the uni-lateral visual-field defects discussed in the section on dysfunction of the occipital lobes. According to Heilman et al. (1985), hemianopia may accompany neglect, but it cannot account for the severity of errors made by patients with neglect. Patients with a visual-field defect are usually aware of the dys-function and can compensate for it. A patient with neglect is not aware of the spatial defect, and even after numerous reminders, he may· not attempt to compensate for it. A patient with a unilateral spatial neglect may only draw half of a stimulus figure when asked to copy a drawing; the shapes of a house, a flower, and a clock are frequently used. The deficit can also be manifested in form drawings or writing in general. When writing, the patient will start to the right of the midline (Fig. 7-37). When reading the patient will start at the midline of the page instead of the left margin, and will thus not be able to comprehend the material. A test of line bi-section is commonly used to test for this deficit (Heilman et al., 1985; Siev et al., 1986; Walsh, 1987). Poor performance on a test where the patient has to circle specific letters, such as capital A, on a sheet taped down in front of him commonly in-dicates hemispatial neglect (Fig. 7-38). Further, movement of the examiner's fingers in the patient's visual field (presented either unilaterally or bilat-erally) is frequently used to test for this deficit (Heilman et al., 1985; Siev et al., 1986).

During daily activities a patient may not at-tend to a person approaching from the affected side, usually the left. When spoken to, the patient may answer questions presented by a therapist in the affected visual field, but will neither look at the therapist when listening to the question nor when answering it (Fig. 7-39). The patient may respond less well when instructed verbally from the affected side. During dressing, the patient may not pay at-tention to the clothes in the affected visual field, and may state that they are missing. Similarly, dur-ing grooming and hygiene activities, the patient may not use or attend to objects located in the affected visual field. She may even use objects incorrectly because of the deficit. For example, if a handle of a brush is located in the neglected visual field, she may grab the brush side and brush the hair that way (Fig. 7-40). During mobilization, the patient may walk into doorways or furniture located in the affected visual field. A patient in a wheel-chair may wheel into walls or furniture (Fig. 7-41). During feeding, the patient may not attend to food or utensils located on the affected side. When the meal is over, all the food located on the left side may be left, even though the patient is still hungry. The neglect may be so severe that not only eye and head movements are involved; the entire body may be turned away from the affected visual field while eating, and the plate pushed to the right side of the table (Fig. 7-42).

In general, the right parietal lobe seems to be more involved in the mediation of spatially re-lated behavior than any other cortical area inde-pendent of sensory modality, be it tactile or visual. Benton (1985a) points out that this common locale of spatial information does not imply, however, that spatial function can be attributed to the same neural mechanisms regardless of modalities. Thus, more than one mechanism may be involved, although the details of this are not yet known. Further, as stated in Chapter 4, the frontal lobe is important for attention, and thus unilateral neglect or inat-tention may also be related to frontal lobe dys-function on the right side, as will become evident in the next chapter.

Body-scheme disorders

Body-scheme disorders are related to deficits in the perception of body position and of the relationship of body parts to each other, according to Siev et al. Ayres (1985) describes body scheme as a pos-tural model on which movements are based. Knowledge of body parts and their relationship is necessary for deciding what to move, where, and how to perform. Siev et al. differentiate between body scheme and body image. According to them, body image is a mental representation of one's body based on visual memory, emotions, and thoughts. Benson (1985) hypothesizes about a spa-tially organized body model that provides a frame-work or basis for perceptual, motor, and judgment impulses directed towards the body. The body-

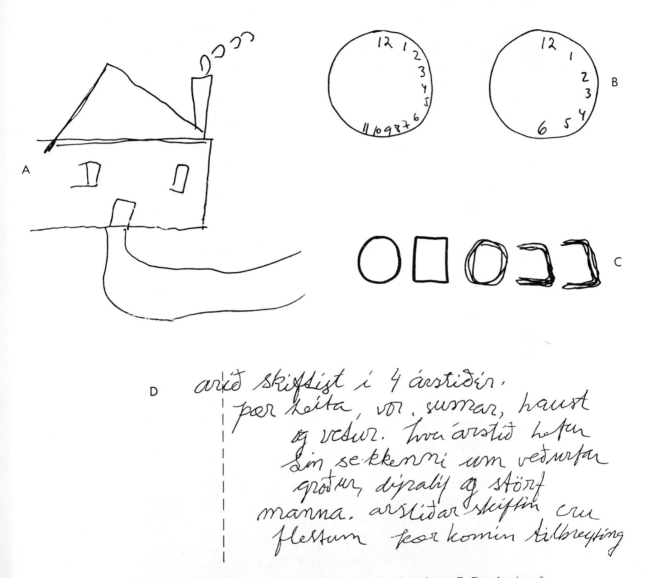

FIG. 7-37 Unilateral spatial neglect manifested in drawings. **A,** Copying a house. **B,** Free drawing of a clock. In the first clock, the patient has attempted to squeeze all the required numbers in one-half of the clock. In the second clock the patient stopped after the sixth numeral. **C,** The patient omits parts of the geometric shapes to be copied. Premotor perseveration is also evident. **D,** The spatial neglect becomes evident in the patient's writing. The dotted line indicates the midline of the visual field. The patient's writing is mostly to the right of the line.

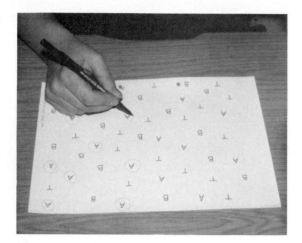

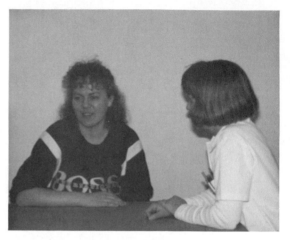

FIG. 7-38 Testing for unilateral spatial neglect. The sheet is taped down in front of the patient at the midline, so that it falls evenly into the two visual fields. The patient is instructed to draw a circle around each letter *A*.

FIG. 7-39 Unilateral visual-field neglect manifested during socialization (communication). The patient hears what the therapist says and speaks to her but does not visually attend to her.

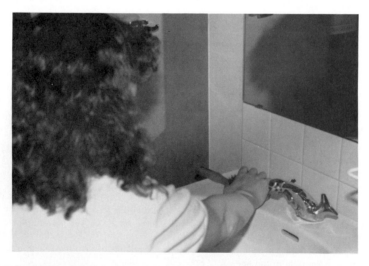

FIG. 7-40 Unilateral visual-field neglect manifested during grooming. The patient grasps the brush by the bristles, not the handle, which is out of her visual field. She may go on and brush the hair on the left side without noticing the handle.

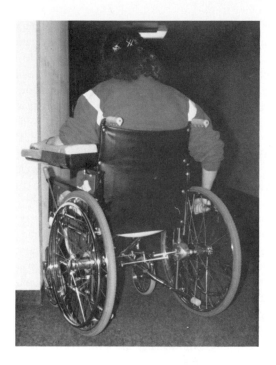

FIG. 7-41 Unilateral visual-field neglect manifested during mobility. The patient wheels into walls and objects on the left side of the environment without noticing them.

A

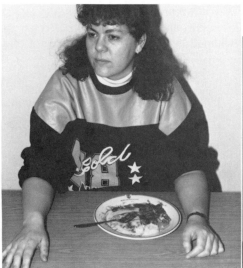

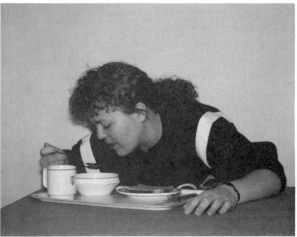

B

FIG. 7-42 Unilateral visual-field neglect manifested during feeding. A, The patient does not notice the food on the left side of the plate and may leave the dining area hungry, with considerable amounts of food left over. B, The neglect may be so severe that the patient's whole body turns over to the intact visual field, away from the midline of the table.

scheme disorders of the parietal lobes are unilateral neglect, anosognosia, somatoagnosia, finger agnosia, and difficulty with right-left discrimination (Siev et al., 1986; Heilman et al., 1985; Strub and Black, 1985).

Unilateral body neglect. Unilateral neglect was defined by Heilman et al. (1985) as the failure to report, respond, or orient to a unilateral stimulus presented to the side contralateral to a cerebral lesion. Siev et al. stated that this dysfunction more commonly affects the left side of the body, as unilateral spatial neglect usually affects the left side of the environment. Further, they relate it to a lesion located in the inferior parietal lobe of the nondominant hemisphere. Heilman (1979) differentiated between hemineglect and hemispatial neglect. He proposed two hypotheses for cause: the defective sensation hypothesis and the attention hypothesis. The attention hypothesis assumes that three brain areas are associated with the neglect syndrome, as stated in Chapter 4. These are the inferior parietal lobe with sensory and body scheme disorders, which is the most common lesion side, dorsolateral frontal lobe, and the cingulate gyrus, both of which are involved in attention. All these areas interconnect and all have access to one sensory modality, and the reticular formation. The reticular formation can thus also contribute to the symptom, according to Heilman (1979).

The body neglect may manifest in lack of or diminished spontaneous use of the left arm, as well as diminished sensory awareness. However, the impairment may at times be so severe that the patient may fail to accept extremities contralateral to cerebral lesion as their own, or refer to them as objects (Heilman et al., 1985). This impairment, as well as denial of paralysis and lack of insight with regards to the hemiplegia, has sometimes been termed specifically as anosognosia. Heilman et al. (1985) report difficulties in discriminating between hemianesthesia and somesthetic inattention in cases where the lesion site is unknown. However, if the deficit is due to inattention rather than primary sensory disturbance, the responses may improve if the patient's attention is directed to that body side. In testing for unilateral body neglect, traditional tactile tests have been used. Bilateral sensory stimulation, however, may be more informative than unilateral stimulation. Body puzzles and drawings have also been used (Figs. 7-43 and 7-44). During daily activities, the patient may not dress the affected body side, usually the arm. The unaffected arm will be dressed, and the patient will go on to the next task. In less severe cases the patient may dress all extremities, but may not pull the shirt all the way down on the affected side (Fig. 7-45). A pullover shirt may get stuck on the affected shoulder without the person trying to correct it or realizing what is wrong.

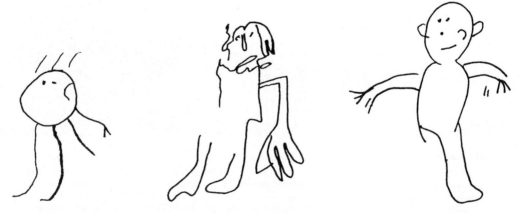

FIG. 7-43 Testing for unilateral body neglect with drawings. Different possibilities of manifestation.

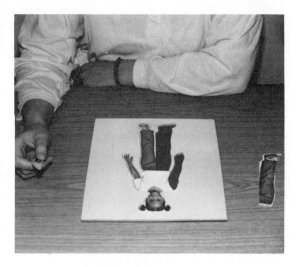

FIG. 7-44 Testing for unilateral body neglect with a puzzle.

During grooming and hygiene activities, the patient may only comb half the hair or shave half the body or the face. Further, a patient may not use the neglected hand for assistance in performing bilateral activities, despite sufficient strength. When there is inattention to the left hand, for example, the patient may attempt to use it at times, but may, for example, spill liquid from an aftershave bottle held by the affected hand, while the patient is looking at his own face in the mirror, as was mentioned earlier in relation to attention deficits of the frontal lobe.

During performance of transfers and mobility activities, the patient may not account for the affected side. When sitting up in bed in order to transfer out of bed, the blanket may be placed over the affected hand as if it was not there. The patient may also walk into doorways. When transferring over to a chair, she will only account for the unaffected side, the affected side or part of it may end up off the chair (Fig. 7-46). In more severe cases, a patient who is lying in bed may claim that the arm beside him is not his own but somebody

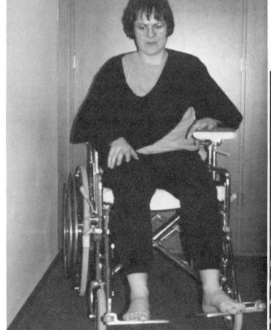

A

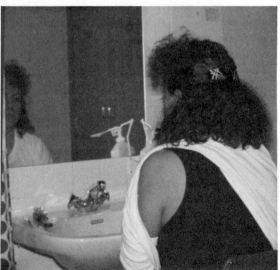

B

FIG. 7-45 Unilateral body neglect manifested during dressing. **A,** The patient has not pulled the shirt down completely on the affected side. In more severe cases of body neglect, the patient may not dress the affected side at all. **B,** The patient does not pay attention to the shirt being stuck on the affected shoulder.

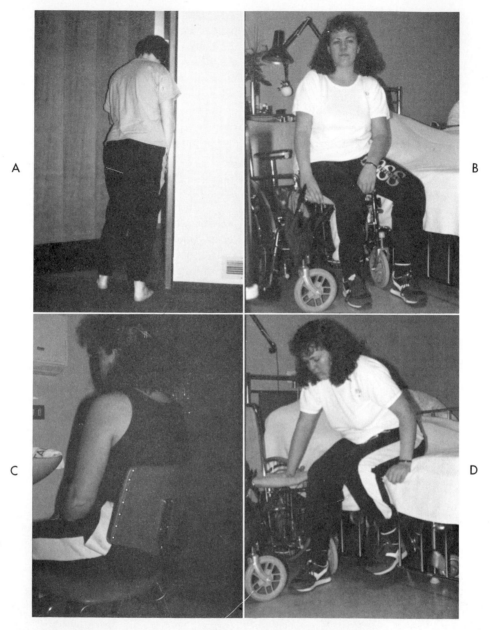

FIG. 7-46 Unilateral body neglect manifested during transfer and mobility. **A,** The patient walks into doorways, not accounting for her left body side. **B,** The patient, in transferring over to a wheelchair moves the right body side over to the chair but leaves the left body side off the chair. **C,** When sitting down, the patient leaves a part of the right side of the chair empty, not accounting for all of her left body side. **D,** During transfers, the patient neglects the left side and does not notice that the left foot has not been placed properly on the floor.

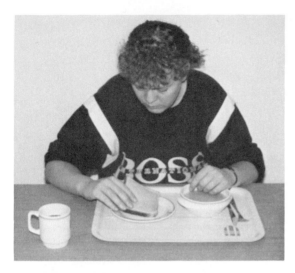

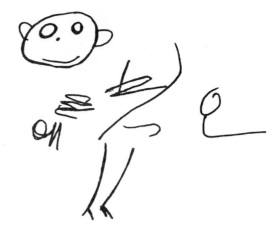

FIG. 7-48 Indications of somatoagnosia manifested in a patient's drawings.

FIG. 7-47 Unilateral body neglect manifested during feeding. The patient does not attend to the left hand, which is on its way into the soup dish.

else's. He may also refer to it as an object, such as an "old wreck of a car." Sometimes negative emotional terms will be attributed to an inattended arm. These neglect examples can be attributed to anosognosia. From some of the above examples it is evident that it can be difficult to differentiate between unilateral spatial inattention and unilateral body neglect when manifested in behavior, which includes both the body and extrapersonal space. It should be kept in mind that these deficits often occur together, and both can be related to similar cerebral locations, although possibly resulting from the disruption of distinct neuronal networks.

When eating, a patient may not attend to, or use an affected arm. This may result in the arm ending up in the soup dish or in awkward positions (Fig. 7-47).

Somatoagnosia. Somatoagnosia was defined by Siev et al. as "unawareness of body structure and the failure to recognize one's body parts and their relationship to each other" (p. 180). Patients with this deficit also have difficulties relating their bodies to objects in the external environment, according to the same authors. Thus the term seems to have different components, the main one being

body scheme. Another component concerns spatial relations. In addition to difficulties with perception of the relationship between body parts, patients may perceive their body or its parts as out of proportion, either bigger or smaller than they are in reality. Siev et al. include lack of awareness of body parts among the impairments caused by somatoagnosia, along with lack of awareness of spatial concepts in relation to body parts. According to these authors, the deficit is usually due to a lesion of the dominant parietal lobe. Commonly used tests for identifying somatoagnosia involve asking the patient to touch different body parts upon request, or to touch one part of his body with another, thus adding a language component to the test. An example of this would be, "Touch your knees" and "Touch your left eye with your right hand." A patient is sometimes asked to draw a man or to put together a puzzle with body parts (Fig. 7-48). The deficit can manifest as fragmentation of the body during washing, or as the washing of a mirror image (Fig. 7-49). Finger agnosia and difficulties with right-left discrimination can be considered subcomponents of somatoagnosia.

Finger agnosia. Finger agnosia has been defined as uncertainty about the fingers (Siev et al., 1986; Strub and Black, 1985). According to Siev et al., this disorder is due to a lesion located in the angular

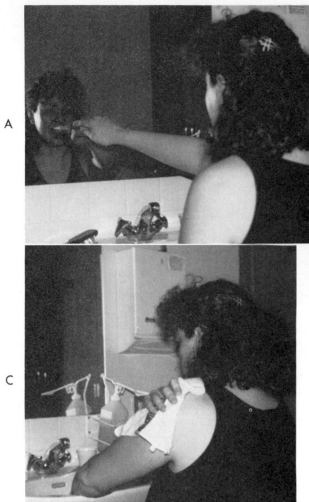

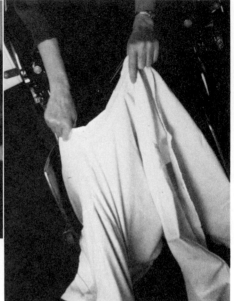

FIG. 7-49 Somatoagnosia manifested during washing and dressing. **A,** The patient brushes the mirror image of her teeth instead of her own. **B,** The patient attempts to dress by putting the legs through the armhole of the shirt. **C,** The patient fragments the body during washing. First one shoulder is washed completely and dried. Subsequently, the forearm is washed and dried and then the hand before the other upper extremity is washed. Neck, face, and body are also washed and dried separately.

gyrus of the dominant parietal lobe. Walsh, in his neuropsychological review, and Benton (1985b) claim that finger agnosia has many different components, including a verbal component for naming and comprehending instructions, a recognizing component through visual, verbal or tactile senses, as well as a localizing, discriminative component. Thus, lesions can be attributed to the inferior parietal lobe and the angular gyrus, as well as to

frontal and parietotemporal locations. Thus, presentation of a stimulus, be it verbal or nonverbal, may reveal the specific type of disorder, as well as more specific location, if the therapist attends to the details of the examination. According to Benton (1985b), aphasia and general mental impairment were accompanied by finger agnosia in the left hemisphere, whereas a general mental impairment accounted for the deficits on the right. Based on this fact, these authors conclude that finger agnosia does not have a specific localizing significance. Testing for this deficit includes naming of the fingers when touched or pointed to, identification of touch, and two-point discrimination.

Impaired right-left discrimination. Impairment of right-left discrimination was defined by Siev et al. as the "inability to understand and use concepts of right and left" (p. 65). It may manifest as a personal confusion, where a person cannot name or point to her own body parts according to the concepts of right and left, or extrapersonal confusion, including faulty discrimination of the examiner's right and left sides. According to these authors, these difficulties are due to a parietal lobe lesion on either side. Heilman (1979) stated that this deficit has three elements, as enumerated previously: verbal, sensory, and visuospatial. Thus, one would expect both the right and the left hemispheres to be possible lesion sites. Thus the presence of the deficit would not have a specific localization significance. This agrees with the findings of Sauget et al. (1971).

According to Walsh, right-left discrimination is a broad term. Benton (1985b) describes right-left orientation tasks as having four different components. One is a verbal component, pertaining to the concepts of left and right, and lateralization of these to the body sides and body parts. Another is a nonverbal component of tactile location of stimuli, or sensory discrimination. Also, a conceptual component is required for understanding the relativistic nature of the right-left concept when we use our lateralized body parts to identify lateral body parts of a confronting person. In addition, a visuospatial component is needed in order to identify left and right sides of objects and confronting persons. Because of the diverse components of the deficit, it is not surprising that it can manifest with right-hemisphere lesions where visuospatial abilities and body scheme are affected, and with left-hemisphere lesions where language abilities are affected. Language plays a role in both pure verbal tasks and in nonverbal tasks, and lateralization requires verbal mediation (Benton, 1985b).

Sauget et al. studied the relationship of body scheme to the hemispheric locus of lesion. They used verbal and nonverbal tests of right-left orientation, finger recognition, and body recognition for 80 patients with unilateral brain lesions of either hemisphere. They found that disturbances of body scheme are closely related to impairment of language comprehension in these patients, and therefore body-scheme disorders were more likely to be seen in patients with left-hemisphere diseases. However, when they excluded receptive language impairment from consideration, no essential relationship was found between the occurrence of these somatognostic defects and the hemispheric locus of the lesion. They reported also that although receptive language impairment was found to be closely related to failure on somatognostic tasks, it was not found to be a sufficient condition for such a failure. Sauget et al. reported these findings to be in agreement with those of the authors they reviewed for their study, that is, that verbal and nonverbal tasks involving finger recognition appear to be independent of each other. Failure in verbal identification is related to aphasic disorder, while failure in nonverbal identification is associated with many factors, the most frequent being mental deterioration.

In addition to the localization information provided by Sauget et al., they emphasized the importance of analyzing deficits into their most basic components. Seemingly identical deficits may be due to different mechanisms, which has been a source of confusion in the neurologic and neuropsychologic fields, according to the literature over the years, and requires clear definitions of deficits based on thorough analysis. Such analysis is obviously important if the information from assessments of such deficits is used to form treatment strategies geared toward specific processes within the CNS.

Aphasia

Other neurobehavioral deficits related to parietal lobe dysfunction are Wernicke's receptive aphasia, agraphia, alexia, and acalculia (Daube and Sandok,

1978; Siev et al., 1986). Wernicke's aphasia is a severe deficit in auditory comprehension, due to left temporal lobe lesion (Daube and Sandok, 1979; Liebman, 1979; Strub and Black, 1985; Werner, 1980). Wernicke's speech area reaches the border of the tertiary, overlapping cortical zones of the parietal and temporal lobes. According to Geschwind (1979a and b), speech may be phonetically or grammatically normal, but semantically deviant. Further, the speech of these patients often includes nonsensical syllables or words.

Benson (1985) describes Wernicke's aphasia as a profound comprehension deficit, accompanied by disturbed repetition. Verbally the patient is fluent, but paraphasias, indicated by the replacement of proper words by semantically related words, is present. Failure of comprehension may result in jargon speech, as the patient gets no feedback about his speech performance. Wernicke's aphasia is usually accompanied by defective reading comprehension. Conduction aphasia is thought to be a result of a white matter disruption in the arcuate fasciculus deep to the supramarginal gyrus. This deficit results in problems with repetition; speech is still fluent, although paraphasia with phonetic substitutions is present, and comprehension is relatively intact (Benson, 1985).

Luria (1980) states that patients with lesions of the left parieto-occipital structures have problems comprehending logical grammatical structures. Thus, inflections, prepositions, and conjunctions cause comprehension problems. An example of this, according to Luria, is a problem in following the command to "point to a pencil with a comb." Chapter 8 deals with deficits in language processing in more detail.

Agraphia

Siev et al. defined agraphia as a "disturbance in writing intelligible words" (p. 178). Strub and Black describe agraphia as an acquired writing disturbance. According to them, it refers to language errors, not to motoric errors in letter formation or poor handwriting. Roeltgen (1985) described many different kinds of agraphia, or writing disorders,

depending on the location of the lesion within the cerebral cortex. He differentiates between motor and linguistic components of the deficit. He described an agraphia associated with Wernicke's aphasia that involves severe spelling errors characterized by semantic and phonetic jargon. Agraphia accompanying conduction aphasia includes misspellings and overwriting, according to Roeltgen. Copying with paragraphia or repetitions of letters or words may be preserved. *Agraphia with alexia* is a term used to describe the deficit of poorly performed graphemes in writing and difficulties in spelling aloud. Roeltgen assigns this deficit to the parietal lobe. Apraxic agraphia, where there are formation difficulties with writing letters spontaneously, on dictation, or even by copying, is also a result of a "dominant" parietal lobe lesion. Spatial agraphia related to spatial-relation disorder is also related to the nondominant parietal lobe. Here the patient writes on the right side of the midline only, and may have problems writing on a horizontal line. Roeltgen's review of agraphia also reports that these patients may make spaces between graphemes and duplicate strokes.

Alexia

Friedman and Albert (1985) defined alexia as "an acquired inability to comprehend written language as a consequence of brain damage" (p. 49). Alexia has been related to both language and visual systems, according to its characteristics. Friedman and Albert differentiate between alexia without agraphia, and alexia with agraphia. Alexia with agraphia is further divided into agraphic alexia, or parietal alexia, and aphasic alexia. Patients with Wernicke's aphasia have a paralexic disorder. In parietal alexia, which has been associated with lesions of the dominant angular gyrus, there is both letter and word blindness (Friedman and Albert, 1985).

Acalculia

Acalculia is defined by Levin and Spiers (1985) as involving "acquired disorders of calculation" (p. 112). Siev et al. similarly defined acalculia as "a disturbance in the ability to solve simple or complex mathematical problems" (p. 178). According to Levin and Spiers, there are three types of acalculia. The first type is related to alexia and agraphia for numbers; the second is related to spatial disorganization of numbers; and the third is related to impaired calculation. All three types of acalculia have been related to parietal lobe lesions, as well as lesions in other lobes. The parietal lobe involvement applies to all the acalculia types, and is accompanied by only one or two of the other lobes at a time, if any. Both hemispheres have also been associated with acalculia. To some extent, it should be possible to attribute spatial acalculia to lesions in the right hemisphere, and acalculia related to alexia and agraphia to left-hemisphere or bilateral lesions. Because the assessment of agraphia, alexia, and acalculia is beyond the spectrum of the primary ADL evaluation proposed in this book, details regarding their localization within the cerebral cortex are not mentioned here.

In summary, parietal lobe lesions can result in loss of discriminative tactile sensation and localization of touch; apraxias (ideomotor, ideational, and constructional); agnosias (tactile, astereognostic, anosognostic, and visual-spatial); spatial-relation disorders (unilateral spatial neglect, spatial relations, and topographical disorientation); and body-scheme disorders (unilateral body neglect, somatoagnosia, right-left disorientation, and finger agnosia). Wernicke's receptive aphasia, agraphia, alexia, and acalculia can also be partially attributed to dysfunction of the inferior parietal lobes. In general the parietal lobes seem to play an important role in the mediation of many functions, including praxis, body scheme, spatial relations, and language. Table 7-2 provides a list of parietal lobe deficits in relation to their functional location within the lobe.

DYSFUNCTION OF THE OCCIPITAL LOBES

The occipital lobes house the primary and secondary visual areas. Unilateral lesions that affect the primary visual cortex of the occipital lobe cause a homonymous visual loss in the contralateral visual fields (Daube and Sandok, 1978). Lesions of the association areas of the occipital lobes can contribute to acalculia, agraphia, alexia, associative visual agnosia, color agnosia, constructional apraxia, prosopagnosia, receptive dysphasia, simultaneous agnosia, spatial relation deficits, topographical disorientation, and visual-object agnosia.

Primary visual cortex

Lesions of the primary visual cortex cause a visual-field defect (see Chapter 8 on variations in visual-field defects along the visual pathway). The visual-field examination is a part of the neurological examination. The subject usually has a blindfold on one eye, fixating with the other, for example, on the examiner's nose. The examiner moves her fingers in different parts of the visual field. The patient indicates verbally when movement is detected (Walsh, 1987). Zoltan et al. (1983) include an item for visual-field examination in their Perceptual Motor Evaluation. They use two white balls attached to wands instead of finger movements.

Visual association cortex

Topographical disorientation was described in the section on parietal lobe dysfunction as being a result of agnosia or a memory deficit. It manifests as a difficulty with finding one's way in space. Constructional apraxia was also described in the same section. Acalculia, agraphia, alexia, and comprehensive aphasia were all described under Dysfunction of the Parietal Lobes. Apractognosia and dressing apraxia were also described earlier in this review. As the last two deficits are composed of many subfactors, they are not included in the A-ONE terminology.

Visual agnosia

Walsh states that a number of deficits have been related to the category of visual agnosia, including prosopagnosia, visual-object agnosia, simultaneous agnosia, visual-spatial agnosia, color agnosia, and pure word blindness (agnostic alexia).

TABLE 7-2 Parietal Lobe Deficits

Cortical location of dysfunction	Deficit	Cortical location of dysfunction	Deficit
Primary sensory cortex	Somesthetic sensory dysfunction Impaired light-touch sensation Impaired proprioception	Inferior parietal association cortex—cont'd	Topographical disorientation Impaired depth and distance perception Impaired memory for spatial location Unilateral spatial neglect Spatial alexia Spatial acalculia Spatial agraphia
Superior parietal association cortex	Impaired somesthetic sensory discrimination Loss of discriminative tactile sensation and location of touch Loss of discriminative proprioception Impaired two-point discrimination Impaired sharp and dull discrimination Agnosia Impaired graphesthesia Astereognosis Motor impersistence		Body-scheme disorders Unilateral neglect Anosognosia Somatoagnosia Finger agnosia Impaired right-left discrimination Aphasia Paraphasia Conduction aphasia Defective comprehension of grammatical structures (Wernicke's receptive aphasia) (Jargon aphasia)
Inferior parietal association cortex	Apraxia Ideomotor apraxia Ideational apraxia Constructional apraxia Agnosia Apractognosia Visual-spatial agnosia Spatial-relation syndrome Foreground and background discrimination difficulties Impaired form constancy Impaired perception of position in space Spatial-relation disorders Constructional apraxia		Agraphia Spatial agraphia Spelling errors Paragraphia Apraxic agraphia Alexia Paralexia Agraphic alexia (letter and word blindness) Acalculia Spatial acalculia Alexic/agraphic acalculia Impaired calculation

Although questioning the validity of differentiating between the different categories of visual agnosia, Walsh claims that they are important indicators of occipital lobe lesions.

Visual-object agnosia. In addition to visual-spatial agnosia and tactile agnosia (discussed under Dysfunction of the Parietal Lobes) lesions of the association cortex surrounding the primary visual and auditory receptive areas will, according to Siev et al., cause visual-object agnosia and auditory agnosia. According to Bauer and Rubens (1985), "The patient with visual agnosia does not respond appropriately to visually presented material even though visual sensory processing, language, and general intellectual functions are preserved at sufficient levels" (p. 190). The recognition deficit is usually limited to visual stimuli. When tactile or auditory information is added, recognition with appropriate responses takes place. These authors state that visual agnosia has been subdivided according to the type of visual material underlying the recognition problem. One of these, according to them, is visual-object agnosia. Visual-object agnosia was defined by Siev et al. as the inability to recognize objects seen, although visual acuity and tactile recognition may or may not seem intact. Strub and Black describe this deficit as the patient's inability to recognize, name, and demonstrate the use of objects shown to them. They relate this deficit to distorted visual perception, which makes recognition of an object impossible. In describing this deficit, Luria (1980) uses as an example a person who cannot perceive a pair of spectacles, either in a drawing or the real object, because he cannot perceive an object as a whole, only its fragments. During the patient's analysis of the stimulus, two circles and a stick become a bicycle. When asked to demonstrate its use, the patient explains that it is used for riding, which is different from the answer given by a patient with anomia, who can describe the correct function. Visual-object agnosia has also been related to difficulties in discriminating a figure from its background. Black and Strub relate this dysfunction to bilateral damage of the visual association cortex. Goldberg (1989) relates it to dysfunction of the visual association cortex in the periphery of the occipital lobes and emphasizes the possibility of a left-sided unilateral lesion as well as bilateral lesions.

An example of the manifestation of visual-object agnosia during daily activities occurs when a patient looks around the sink for an electric razor in order to shave. The patient moves his head while looking, so that visual-spatial neglect can be ruled out. The patient tells the therapist that he cannot find the razor. Then he reaches with his hand by the sink along the same area he had looked at. His hand stops on the razor, and he states, "Here it is."

Prosopagnosia. Strub and Black defined prosopagnosia as the inability to recognize familiar faces, despite the fact that recognition by voice is possible. Walsh states that this deficit may account for an inability to recognize one's own face in a mirror as well. According to him, prosopagnosia is an inability to differentiate between items in the same category. This can occur in other categories than faces, such as cars and animals. According to Geschwind (1979a and b), this impairment results from a deficit in the inferior occipital lobes on both sides, extending forward to the inner surface of the temporal lobes. Bauer and Rubens (1985) agree on this location. In Walsh's review of neuropsychology, a lesion that dissociates "perceptual analysis from memory processes" (p. 267) may be the cause of prosopagnosia.

Associative visual agnosia. According to Strub and Black, there are two major categories of visual agnosia: visual-object agnosia, discussed above, and associative visual agnosia. Associative visual agnosia occurs when there is adequate visual perception, but the visual cortex is disconnected from the language area or visual memory stores. Clinically, an object can be recognized and its use demonstrated, but it cannot be named (Strub and Black, 1985). The objects can even be copied by accurate line drawings or matched to sample items during tests, although they cannot be named. Pointing to named objects works better than does a verbal explanation (Bauer and Rubens, 1985).

The lesions producing this condition are either bilateral, cortico-subcortical disconnections located at the inferior temporal-occipital junction, or infarcts that destroy the left medial occipital lobe, the posterior corpus callosum, and possibly temporo-limbic connections (Bauer and Rubens, 1985; Strub and Black, 1985).

Simultaneous agnosia. Simultaneous agnosia refers to the inability to recognize or abstract the meaning of a whole, because only one element of the stimulus can be appreciated at a time (Bauer and Rubens, 1985; Walsh, 1987). Luria (1980) claims that people with this disorder have problems perceiving more than one object at a time visually. According to him, optic ataxia accompanies this deficit. The patient with this deficit has trouble perceiving pictures and tracing, for example, around specific forms. Identifying a figure contaminated by lines or embedded figures becomes difficult. Walsh considers the analysis and integration of information required for this type of perception to be composed of many factors. These include, according to him, "visual, perceptual, oculomotor, attentional, and cognitive factors" (p. 263). He relates this process to occipito-frontal connections and states that either occipital or frontal lesions can disrupt it.

Color agnosia. Color agnosia was defined by Strub and Black as the inability to recognize colors because of an acquired cortical lesion. They described two types of color agnosia: the color-naming disturbance associated with alexia and agraphia, resulting from "a disconnection of visual input from the language area" (p. 150) without damage to the primary language area; and the color-recognition disturbance, which is a deficit in color perception caused by bilateral inferior temporooccipital lesions.

In summary, dysfunctions of the occipital lobes can result in visual-object agnosia, associative visual agnosia, prosopagnosia, simultaneous agnosia, and color agnosia. Table 7-3 provides a list of occipital lobe deficits, according to location of the dysfunction within the lobe.

TABLE 7-3 Occipital Lobe Deficits

Cortical location of dysfunction	Deficit
Primary visual cortex	Homonymous hemianopsia, or visual-field defect

Visual association cortex	Visual agnosia
	    Prosopagnosia
	    Visual-object agnosia
	    Simultaneous agnosia
	    Visual-spatial agnosia
	        (including spatial acalculia, spatial agraphia, constructional apraxia, and topographical disorientation)
	    Associative visual agnosia
	    Color agnosia
	    Pure word blindness (agnostic alexia)

DYSFUNCTION OF THE TEMPORAL LOBES

As stated in Chapter 3, the temporal lobes play an important role in auditory, memory, learning, emotional, and visual functions. They house the primary receptive area for hearing, as well as secondary and tertiary association cortices.

Primary auditory cortex

Because of bilateral representation for hearing in the cerebral cortex, a unilateral lesion involving the primary auditory cortex on one side causes diminished acuity of hearing in both ears. The loss is greater in the ear opposite to the lesion. The impairment, however, is slight, and it is difficult to detect it by clinical tests (Barr and Kiernan, 1983).

Auditory association cortex

Lesions of the auditory association cortex, or posterior portion of the left superior temporal gyrus cause receptive, or Wernicke's aphasia, described previously in this review, which is a comprehension deficit caused by a severe auditory processing deficit resulting in the inability to understand spoken language. Luria (1980) uses the term *acoustic agnosia* to describe a similar deficit of phonemic hearing and impaired ability to discriminate between phonemes in the absence of elementary hearing loss or primary articulation deficit. The speech produced by patients with such deficits can be difficult or impossible for others to comprehend. The patient answers questions inappropriately and is unaware of the mistakes (Strub and Black, 1985). A lesion of the right hemisphere in the superior temporal gyrus causes impaired comprehension of tonal sequences and timing of sounds, as well as of sound modulation. This manifests in the patient's speech as a result of impaired feedback regarding his own performance (Kaupfermann, 1985a). Alexia and agraphia are also associated with the disorder, as outlined in the section on parietal lobe dysfunction (Strub and Black, 1985; Siev et al., 1986). Lesions of the anterior temporal lobe are reported to cause transient dysphasia (Walsh, 1987).

Walsh describes lateralization in the secondary temporal association cortex. According to him, the analysis of speech sounds takes place in the left hemisphere, whereas the nondominant language hemisphere mediates nonverbal auditory perception. Perception of music is a function of the right temporal lobe, and thus amusia, which is a deficit in auditory perception of music, is attributed to a lesion of the right temporal lobe.

According to Walsh, auditory discrimination of phonemes is a function of the left auditory association cortex. Writing is also heavily dependent on auditory discrimination, until it becomes automatic. Walsh reports that the middle temporal gyrus is more concerned with verbal memory than auditory discrimination. Thus, damage in this area

results in an inability to repeat verbally presented word series. Anomia for objects can result from a temporal lobe lesion, a deficit that is related to visual association. To overcome this, the patient may use lengthy explanations, known as *circumlocution.*

Auditory agnosia was defined by Siev et al. as "the inability to recognize differences in sounds" (p. 95). This inability affects words as well as nonword sounds, according to these reviewers. Bauer and Rubens agree with this definition, but state that the literature's use of the term is confusing; in addition to being used to describe agnosia of both verbal and nonverbal sounds, it has also been used to describe a recognition deficit in nonverbal sounds only. They thus suggest a subdivision of the term to *auditory sound agnosia,* referring to nonspeech sounds only, and *auditory verbal agnosia. Amusia,* as previously mentioned, refers to an inability to perceive musical characteristics (Bauer and Rubens, 1985; Siev et al., 1986).

According to Bauer and Rubens, impairment in the recognition of speech sounds and amusia accompany impaired recognition of nonverbal sounds. They report, in agreement with the authors reviewed above, that the right hemisphere is important in the processing of music and nonverbal sound patterns, whereas the left hemisphere is dominant in the processing of verbal information and temporal sequencing material of any kind, including music. However, bilateral impairment may be the cause of auditory sound agnosia, according to these authors.

Auditory verbal agnosia has also been termed *pure word deafness* (Bauer and Rubens, 1985). Patients with this deficit cannot comprehend spoken words, although both spontaneous speech and hearing are intact. Reading and writing are also intact.

Visual-field defects of upper quadrants can result from temporal lobe lesions, due to the structure of the visual pathway (Daube and Sandok, 1978; Walsh, 1987). A lesion of the left temporal lobe may result in a right-field deficit, whereas a lesion on the right side may produce deficits in both right and left visual fields, according to Walsh. Further, the temporal lobes are important for the integration of visual experiences with input from all the other senses.

Limbic association cortex of the temporal lobe

The medial temporal region is directly associated with memory processes in humans, according to Butters (1979). Further, lesions of the left temporal lobe result in difficulties with learning and retaining verbal material that is presented either visually or aurally. Butters also reported that lesions of the anterior sector of the left temporal lobe result in anterograde amnesia, which is a storing problem resulting in a recent memory deficit. Lesions of the posterior, or temporo-parietal region, on the other hand, produce retrograde memory problems in which the patient cannot remember what happened previously. Further, processing of nonverbal material was associated with lesions in the right temporal lobe. Such patients may have difficulty remembering if they have previously seen an unfamiliar geometric pattern. They are also impaired when it comes to learning visual tactile mazes (Butters, 1979).

According to Geschwind (1979a and b), the temporal lobes are involved in the long-term memory process. He stated that "the nature of the impairment is a matter of controversy" (p. 113): it may result from a failure in transferring information from short-term to long-term storage or from an inability to review the stored information. Geschwind, however, agreed with Butters regarding the location of verbal memory on the left side, in contrast to the ability to remember spatial locations, abstract visual patterns, faces, and melodies, which according to Geschwind is located on the right side. Walsh, in his neuropsychological review, supports this differentiation of the function of the two temporal lobes.

Strub and Black acknowledged that memory is commonly subdivided into three types, according to the time span between stimulus presentation and retrieval of memory. These are immediate, recent,

TABLE 7-4 Temporal Lobe Deficits

Cortical location of dysfunction	Deficit
Primary auditory cortex	Diminished acuity of hearing

Auditory association cortex and posterior tertiary association area	Aphasia
	    Wernicke's aphasia
	    Impaired auditory discrimination of phonemes
	    Verbal memory disturbance
	    Anomia
	    Circumlocution
	    Paraphasia
	Agnosia
	    Auditory-sound agnosia
	    Auditory-verbal agnosia
	    Amusia
	Agraphia
	Acalculia
	Higher order visual impairment

Limbic association cortex	Memory
	    Verbal memory deficit
	    Visual memory deficit
	    Short-term memory deficit
	    Long-term memory deficit
	    Retrograde memory loss
	    Anterograde memory loss
	Emotional disorders
	Personality disorders

Note: The definitions of some of the terms in this table overlap.

and remote memory. These authors claimed that the time span on which these concepts are based is not well defined for clinical use. Immediate memory, or short-term memory, "refers to the recall of a memory trace after an interval of a few seconds" (p. 78) and is often tested by repetition of a series of digits. Recent memory refers to the "capacity to remember day-to-day events . . . the ability to learn new material and to retrieve that material after an interval of minutes, hours, or days" (p. 78). Remote memory, on the other hand, refers to earlier events, including recall of events that occurred before the onset of a recent memory defect, in the case of CNS patients. These authors defined *anterograde* amnesia as "the inability to learn new material" (p. 79) from the time of the event, and *retrograde* amnesia as loss of memory for events that occurred before brain insult in CNS patients. Butters and Miliotis (1985) relate retrograde amnesia to difficulties with retrieval from long-term memory.

As mentioned in Chapter 3, the anterior temporal pole is a part of the limbic association area. Lesions of this area or its connections can result in emotional disorders. These were mentioned in the section on dysfunction of the frontal lobes, and will be expanded upon in the next chapter.

In summary, the temporal lobes are involved in acuity of hearing, Wernicke's aphasia, alexia and agraphia, amusia, and memory loss. They may also play a role in acalculia and body scheme disorders, as there is a language component in some components of body scheme. Table 7-4 presents a list of temporal lobe symptoms according to their location within the lobe.

CONCLUSION

In conclusion, the cerebral cortex is specialized in function: specific parts of the brain are more efficient than others for particular functions. Thus, lesions of primary receptive areas produce identifiable functional deficits. Lesions of secondary as-

sociation areas usually produce unimodal deficits or impaired processing of information from one sensory modality only, whereas lesions of tertiary areas result in deficits that depend on the combined function of more than one cortical location. This chapter attempts to match some common neurobehavioral deficits with dysfunctions of specific functional areas. It also attempts to relate the deficits to the way they manifest during the performance of daily activities, as opposed to how they appear in the more common specific testing situations. The test manual in Part II provides a summary table of the localization of neurobehavioral deficits, based on this literature review, as well as neurobehavioral deficits and their manifestation as impairments during daily activities. Definitions of neurobehavioral deficits are provided in the Glossary at the end of the book. Cortical connections play an important role in processing of function and related deficits. A lesion in a specific location may result in a functional deficit of a remote area, due to lack of input from the lesioned area necessary for processing in the remote area. Further, the same cortical area, especially the higher order association areas, depend on functional input from many areas, and different types of functions take place in the association areas. Thus a lesion of a multimodal area may produce many types of deficits, some of which have similar components. Thus it may be difficult at times to differentiate between some similar deficit types involving similar components, although they may be a part of different but adjacent neuronal networks. The next section describes some defects in processing that result in neurobehavioral deficits. These deficits, and their detection and the choice of the most effective treatment to diminish them, are the principal concerns of the therapist working with this type of CNS patient. Thus, the ability to predict processing deficits and to understand CNS mechanisms may give the therapist clues as to the most appropriate treatment for a particular dysfunction.

CHAPTER
8

Processing Dysfunctions Leading to Neurobehavioral Deficits

With the evolution of knowledge, it has become evident that neurological deficits are not necessarily a result of localized damage in a one-to-one relationship. Rather, they can result from damage to different CNS areas, all of which contribute to the processing that must take place to produce a particular behavior or emotion. This processing relates to discrete areas of the brain and how they connect, as indicated in Chapter 4. Faults anywhere along the processing path can lead to neurobehavioral impairment, regardless of whether processing is simultaneous or parallel, or whether it depends on electrical current or "pattern recognition." Defective processing thus disrupts the holistic synchronized function of the brain. This section reviews the literature on neurobehavioral impairment, focusing specifically on processing deficits rather than discrete localization, which was reviewed in the previous chapter. The introduction will touch upon basic components of this approach, as well as functional examples in relation to the functional view provided in Chapter 4. Some theories and studies related to the topic of processing deficits will be reviewed, and some considerations related to the treatment of patients with neurobehavioral dysfunction will be mentioned.

As indicated in Chapter 4, processing can be viewed as both a sequential and parallel activity. Numerous pathways are responsible for sensory, motor, and mental functions, according to Kandel

(1985c). Thus, damage to one pathway can be partially compensated for by the other pathways. When this occurs, however, some lack of precision in performance can often be detected. As stated by Kandel, "damage to a single area need not lead to the disappearance of the function; or, if the function does disappear, it may partially return because the remaining parts can either assume the function or rearrange themselves to accomplish the primary task" (p. 11). Kandel continues his comments on sequential and parallel processing, stating that one cannot view the "anatomical basis of the localization of related functions . . . as a series of functional links in a single chain, an arrangement in which all related functions would stop if the chain breaks" (p. 11). Rather, as a result of the parallel processing of related functions by many individual chains, "the break of a single link will interrupt one chain, but this need not interfere permanently with the performance of the whole system" (p. 11). Further, one should keep in mind the frequently quoted thoughts of Hughling Jackson regarding behavior and CNS lesions. The observed behavior is not a result of the "missing or damaged tissue" (Heilman, 1983). According to Heilman (1983), the observed behavior is produced by the remaining brain "in the absence" of the damaged tissue. Heilman goes on to state that "Lesions may change behavior because they not only interrupt a critical system but also affect other areas, which under physiologic conditions may be either inhibited or facilitated by the area in which the lesion lies" (p. 2). Heilman's view is in agreement with Kandel's (1985c), in that other unaffected cortical areas may be able to compensate for the functions of a lesioned area, thus preserving some of the behavior for which that area was responsible.

In Chapter 4 an activity analysis of a self-care task based on neurobehavioral principles was provided. Processing of different sensory information related to the task leads to the integration of information at different CNS levels on the basis of previous experiences, resulting in behavioral responses. These behavioral responses can be both motor movements and emotions, which are modified via a continuous feedback mechanism. When the neurobehavioral responses that result from this process in individuals with CNS dysfunction are analyzed, they can reveal neurologic and neurobehavioral deficits such as perseveration and apraxia, as well as lability, depression, apathy, and aggression. These deficits can be subsequently traced back to brain function.

As stated in Chapter 4, the cortical locations and the processing that takes place as a result of cortical function can be conceived in terms of a road map and traffic. One could even go further and identify chemical or hormonal functions as the fuel on which the "traffic," or electrical conductance reflected from activated neurons, depends. But the CNS is not designed to function in internal isolation. It is designed as an executor and control system of behavior, promoting survival in the external environment and the quality of life relative to potential independence and functional success. Behavior is thus a reflection of how the nervous system works and can be observed and measured by an ADL instrument. This behavior is an indicator of CNS integrity.

Using the "road map and traffic" analogy, we can see the relationship of behavior to a damaged structure or defective processing. If, for example, a car was supposed to deliver an object from Place A to Place B on the map, and Place A has had such an earthquake that it no longer exists, there

will be no delivery. If the "delivery place" was in the cortical motor area of the hand, there would be paralysis or weakness of hand function. If it were in the primary sensory cortex, there would be no sensation, and thus no tactile and proprioceptive feedback to affect further behavior. Some instances of road obstruction may prevent a car that is supposed to pick up items for a delivery from different places from reaching them all, so it can make only a partial delivery. In neurological terms, there will be a behavioral response, but it will not be of the same quality as if the "car" had been able to take the most direct route. Speech, for example, may be produced despite parieto-occipital or temporal "road obstruction," but some of the words may be missing (as in anomia), or some of the words may be replaced by other words (as in paraphasia).

Now, if there had been a snow bank or snow drift on the road, the car would be stuck. Attempts to proceed would be impossible; the car would "spin its wheels" and get nowhere. A similar event in the premotor zone of the nervous system would be reflected in the behavioral deficit of perseveration, described in Chapter 7.

Thus, behavior can be considered as "mirroring" the CNS, but it is a two-way mirror, because the CNS needs feedback from its product, behavior, and the way it affects the external world in order to work most effectively. If a behavior is not effective, the CNS will attempt to adjust or make corrections. The more feedback about how behavior affects the external world, the more adjustment it can make, resulting in a better chance that the desired effect will occur. Thus the mechanism of nervous processing and neurobehavior is one of a complex stimulus-processing-and-response interaction path.

DISRUPTED LANGUAGE PROCESSING

In this section the previously mentioned disconnection approach to language dysfunction based on the work of Wernicke and Geschwind will be reviewed, as well as Luria's neuropsychological analysis of factors underlying the different language deficits and their cortical location. Luria's "functional system" approach refers to complex neurological processes that are responsible for integrating the work of different areas necessary for the existence of complex psychological function (Walsh, 1987). Thus in a functional system, the performance of a specific task depends on various factors. According to Walsh, "damage in any part of a functional system may lead to disruption of a psychological process" (p. 24). Further, "damage to different parts of a system will impress a different character on the complex of symptoms and signs which result from the damage" (p. 24). It is therefore important to consider the qualitative aspects of a psychological function that has been affected by cortical damage. A functional system is based on structural CNS areas and cortical as well as subcortical fiber connections between these areas, which need to work in harmony to allow task performance as a product of a functional system (Walsh, 1987).

The disconnection approach is based on the assumption that different cortical areas have specialized cells for particular functions. Fiber pathways connect different primary cortical areas with adjacent association areas, which in turn connect to other areas. The transmitting connections thus run to and from specific "decision" points, forming a network of communication. The decision points are areas responsible for making specific decisions. Interruption of either input or output from these areas will result in impaired task performance (Walsh, 1987).

Luria and Thomas Hutton (1977) disagree with the disconnectionists regarding the reasons for language deficits, but not with their clinical description of impairments. They criticize the idea of language centers, and offer a spectrum of locales that are responsible for similar but not identical symptoms. Thus, according to these authors, manifestations of slightly differentiated impairments depends on the exact location of damage, and its relation to adjacent functional areas, be they auditory, visual, or motoric.

Geschwind's model for language processing was described in Chapter 4. According to that

model, Wernicke's area and the Broca's area are connected by the arcuate fasciculus. Further, the visual cortex is connected to Wernicke's area by connections in the angular gyrus.

According to Geschwind (1979b), a lesion of Wernicke's area leads to a comprehension deficit. A lesion in Broca's area results in nonfluent speech, characterized by impaired articulation and slow speech that requires effort. Further, although speech may be sensible, it may be telegraphic, lacking the necessary grammatical sentence structure, including inflection of verbs. A lesion of the face area in the primary motor cortex leads to weakness or paralysis of facial muscles, resulting in dysarthria. Geschwind states that Wernicke's aphasia reveals speech defects in addition to comprehension problems. Here speech may be "phonetically and even grammatically normal" (p. 4), although "semantically deviant" (p. 4). Thus, despite recognizable sentence structure, the words are inappropriate and may include "nonsensical syllables or words" (p. 4).

The processing pathway from Wernicke's area to Broca's area with connections to the visual area is vulnerable to lesions anywhere along this pathway, according to Geschwind (1979a and b). A lesion in the arcuate fasciculus that disconnects Wernicke's area from Broca's area will, for example, manifest in fluent but semantically defective speech, according to this model, because information from the comprehension area does not reach the motor speech area. Comprehension will, however, be close to normal, because Wernicke's area is intact. Further, damage to the angular gyrus connecting the visual and auditory cortices will result in impaired comprehension of written language.

Luria and Thomas Hutton provided neuropsychological descriptions of what they term "basic forms of aphasia." These include, according to these authors, sensory or acousticognostic aphasia; motor aphasia, including both afferent, or kinesthetic, and efferent, or kinetic, aphasia; nominative, or amnestic, aphasia; transcortical motor aphasia; and conduction aphasia.

According to Luria and Thomas Hutton, sensory aphasia is caused by lesions of Wernicke's area. They claim that Wernicke's area is responsible for phonematic hearing. This requires the ability to "qualify" sounds according to a "system of phonemes," phonemes being the "basic units of speech" according to these authors. The sounds received by the primary auditory cortex must be isolated and analyzed according to their phonematic characteristics; subsequently, they are organized into phonematic categories. A lesion of Wernicke's area thus leads to comprehension deficits as a result of impaired phonematic hearing (Luria and Thomas Hutton, 1977). This impairment can manifest in the repetition of isolated sounds, inability to comprehend the meanings of words, and problems in understanding simple sentences or sentences based on more complex logical-grammatical structure. Defective phonematic hearing leading to impaired understanding of the meanings of words is related to the anterior temporal aspects of Wernicke's area, whereas lack of grammatical meaning, including spatial relationships, is due to a more posterior lesion in the left parieto-occipital area or the angular gyrus. Here meaning becomes restricted to a narrow context, with loss of information provided by prepositions and conjunctions (Luria, 1980). The right temporal lobe is important in perception of rhythms, according to Luria (1980).

Luria (1980) also described receptive speech deficits as a result of fronto-temporal or pure frontal dysfunction in the left hemisphere. This affects comprehension of the order of sound sequences or sequences of words. There appears to be a perseveration or inertia related to the meanings of words, which has been termed *paragnoses*. During repetition of words, the same word will be repeated rather than shifting over to the following word in the sequence.

Luria and Thomas Hutton describe a secondary deficit related to sensory aphasia. Their description of this speech impairment, which occurs as a result of defective phonematic analysis, is in keeping with the view of Geschwind (1979a and b). This patient speaks fluently but "confuses pho-

nematic characteristics," resulting in so-called "word salad." Thus, many paraphasias occur because of incorrectly organized speech due to loss of phonematic structure. A writing dysfunction may also accompany the sensory aphasia, as the person does not know how to put phonemes together to form a word.

According to Luria (1980), the formulation of an idea is a necessary precursor to verbal communication. From a general idea, the next step in the language process is a stage that Luria terms *internal speech*. At this stage the previously mentioned idea or plan begins to take the form of a verbal expression, which evolves to verbal communication. Luria claims that a reversal of this process takes place during speech comprehension. Here speech sounds are converted to a meaningful idea after passing through a stage of internal speech. According to Luria, lesions located in the posterior frontal lobe or the temporo-frontal areas disrupt the internal-speech process responsible for the "verbal plan of communication."

Luria and Thomas Hutton described two forms of motor aphasia as a result of a lesion of either side of the primary motor area for speech functions. These are kinesthetic and kinetic motor aphasia. A lesion in the lower postcentral gyrus results in kinesthetic motor aphasia, including a lack of sensory information from the speech musculature, which affects organized speech movements, despite an intact motor cortex. The result is a specific form of oral apraxia, where the sounds produced are similar in articulation, although they sound different. When writing, a person with articulatory disorders confuses sounds that are close in articulation, resulting in specific paraphasias.

Kinetic motor aphasia, on the other hand, refers to the lack of sequential organization of movement. Such organization is responsible for the smooth interchange of separate movement components, which have been labeled "kinetic melodies." This deficit results from a lesion in the lower premotor cortex and manifests as an "inertia of motor stereotypes," which refers to an inability to switch from the first sounds, once initiated, to subsequent sounds, resulting in the difficulty of changing from one syllable to another, or in motor perseveration of speech sounds.

In amnestic aphasia, the patient has difficulty recalling the names of objects. According to Luria and Thomas Hutton, this is a complex form of aphasia resulting from different sources. A parietooccipital lesion can result in visuognostic impairment. Here the necessary visual characteristics of an object cannot be isolated, resulting in anomia, or lack of the desired word. A lesion of the second left temporal gyrus will result in impaired auditory retention of word structure. Thus, as auditory traces for the word are poorly preserved, its meaning cannot be found. Amnestic aphasia can further result from a temporo-parieto-occipital impairment, in which the patient exhibits difficulty in selecting the required word because all possible alternatives of words belonging to a particular category have an "equal probability of being selected" (p. 144), resulting in paraphasia of words.

There are two variations of the previously termed "transcortical motor aphasia" (Luria and Thomas Hutton, 1977, p. 146). One occurs when spontaneous speech is impaired despite intact repetition ability, naming, and understanding of single words. Luria and Thomas Hutton related this deficit to "pathological inertia," or perseverative aphasia, which affects the sequencing of word series but not the sequencing of syllables. It refers to either "repeating, naming or understanding a series of objects" (p. 146). This is usually accompanied by other perseverative and sequencing errors that manifest during functional performance of activities in general, as a result of anterior frontal dysfunction.

Another form of the traditionally termed *transcortical aphasia* has been termed *dynamic aphasia*. According to Luria and Thomas Hutton, this defect results from a lesion of the "posterior frontal, or fronto-temporal, sections of the left hemisphere" (p. 146). Spontaneous speech cannot be performed without assistance. However the ability to repeat words and phrases is intact, as well as naming of objects and comprehension. These authors relate this deficit to impairment of internal speech. Such patients, according to them, are unable to convert an initial conception to the scheme necessary to produce a statement, resulting in an inability to use the "retained speech possibilities" (p. 147). These authors quote a patient who stated, "Other people have Friday after Thursday, whereas, I have nothing" (p. 147). The internal speech and ideation necessary to language has a lot in common with the ideation necessary for praxis.

Luria and Thomas Hutton described a patient with conduction aphasia as one having difficulty in repeating words despite unimpaired ability to speak, name objects, and understand speech. The repetition difficulty resulted in phonemic paraphasias. Here the sound structure of one word is analyzed but retained ineffectively due to a failure to inhibit irrelevant associations. The repetition thus includes a word from the same category of, for example, common birds or flowers, but not the exact type. Such a deficit is also likely to manifest during spontaneous speech, although not as prominently as during repetition.

Luria and Thomas Hutton based their description of language disturbances on neuropsychological observations, which they related to CNS processing in different areas of the brain that contribute to a functional language system. Many of the language disorders described above are used in the Árnadóttir OT-ADL Neurobehavioral Evaluation (A-ONE) instrument.

Boller et al. (1978) evaluated the effect of delayed auditory feedback in normal control subjects as compared to nonfluent and fluent aphasics. Delayed auditory feedback refers, according to these authors, to a "person's own voice" being returned to his or her ears "with an artificially induced delay" (p. 212) which disturbs subsequent speech: speech usually becomes louder and slower, and qualitative changes take place, including "phonemic substitutions and syllable repetitions." For the study, two different delays in the presentation of auditory stimuli were used: 180 ms and 360 ms. The results indicated that some delay in auditory feedback was present in all subjects, including all of the fluent aphasics. The effect was less in "fluent aphasics" than in "nonfluent aphasics." Subjects with conduction aphasia were found to have the least-impaired auditory feedback. The smaller effect observed in "fluent aphasics" compared with the other subjects supports the authors' view that these patients have a disturbance in auditory feedback; thus, they are less affected by the experimental conditions.

Boller et al. hypothesized, on the basis of their findings, that delayed auditory feedback results from changes in two different systems. Changes related to intensity of speech appear to be unaffected by aphasia, whereas "duration and qualitative changes in speech" (p. 225) are affected differently depending on the pathology that produces the aphasia. This study supported the processing theory of CNS function, because auditory impulses affect speech output.

Mayeux and Kandel (1985) support the Geschwind model of language processing. According to them, conduction aphasia is the result of a lesion of the supramarginal gyrus in the left parietal lobe or the posterior superior temporal area of the same side. They state that this deficit is often accompanied by apraxia of facial or limb movements and, further, that transcortical aphasia usually results from a vascular dysfunction affecting the cortex of the lateral side of the left hemisphere. They differentiate between two types of transcortical aphasia (as discussed in Chapter 7): transcortical motor aphasia and transcortical sensory aphasia (as well as a combination of the two). In the first type involving a motor deficit due to a lesion anterior or superior to Broca's area in the frontal lobe, repetition of speech is possible, but not "unprompted speech." In the sensory type, as a result of a brain lesion at the parieto-temporo-occipital junction, repetition is performed but difficulties are manifested in auditory memory, reading, and writing.

Mayeux and Kandel point out that language has emotional components, including prosody, or "musical information of speech." According to the authors, and in agreement with Kaupfermann (1985a) and Luria (1980), these processes depend on the right hemisphere. Patients with lesions of the anterior part of the right hemisphere cannot express affective content verbally, whereas patients with lesions located posteriorly in the hemisphere have defective comprehension of affect (see Fig. 8-1 for an outline of deficits due to disrupted language processing).

Before leaving the subject of language processing, it should be pointed out that aphasic impairments have been reported with lesions of the left thalamus, putamen and caudate, according to Brown and Perecman (1986). These include mutism, transcortical aphasia, and jargon, with left thalamic dysfunctions. These authors point out that some aspects of subcortical aphasia might be non-linguistic in origin but related to deficits in short-term memory, motor initiation, or attention.

DISRUPTED PROCESSING OF PRAXIS

Geschwind (1975) defined apraxias as "disorders of the execution of learned movement which cannot be accounted for either by weakness, incoordination, or sensory loss, or by incomprehension of or inattention to commands" (p. 188). Geschwind explained apraxias according to his model of motor processing (described in Chapter 4, where neurological processing related to cerebral function was reviewed). He proposed that Wernicke's area in the left hemisphere and the premotor region of either hemisphere (depending upon which hemisphere controls the body side to be moved), as well as the primary motor areas are involved in the performance of movement on command. The corpus callosum is also involved if information needs to be carried to the right premotor region, which controls the left side of the body. Lesion anywhere along this pathway will result in limb apraxia. The apraxic manifestation is unilateral or bilateral, depending on where in the processing path the lesion occurred. According to Geschwind (1975), damage to the pathway between Wernicke's area and the premotor region on the left side is usually accompanied by conduction aphasia, but not paralysis. These patients are unable to perform correct movements with either hand, as the instructions do not

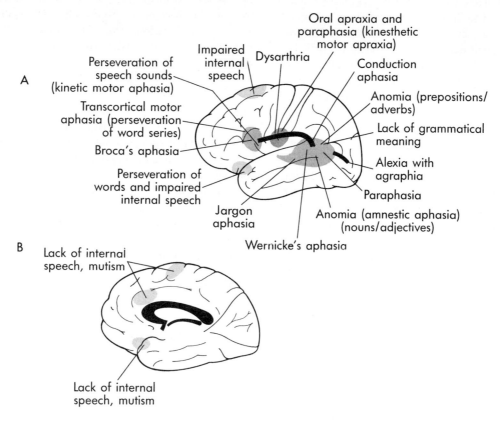

FIG. 8-1 Disrupted language processing. **A,** Lateral view of the left hemisphere indicating areas associated with different language impairments. The dark arrows indicate association fibers. **B,** Medial view of the left hemisphere.

reach the left and subsequently the right premotor cortical areas via the corpus callosum.

According to Geschwind (1975), most apraxic individuals also show difficulties in imitating movements where language comprehension is not required. Further, patients with an unaffected right hemisphere may present with apraxia of the left body side, because destruction of the left premotor area affects motor learning significantly. A patient with left premotor lesion shows poorer motor performance with his left arm than an adult who does not have a CNS lesion that deprives him of

access to the "store of motor skills" located in the left cerebral cortex. On the basis of observation of some patients performing when they see the actual objects, as opposed to performing imaginary tasks, Geschwind suggests that the right hemisphere possesses storage of motor learning that is only accessible when much more information is provided, as compared to the "easy" activation of the more accessible memory engrams in the left hemisphere.

Geschwind (1975) points out that although the flow of information to the pyramidal motor system has been disconnected, axial movements are preserved, and it appears that the extrapyramidal system can be used to perform "crude approximations" of individual limb movements.

Chapter 4 reviews a processing model of praxis described by Heilman and Rothi (1985). This model assumes that visuokinesthetic motor engrams are stored in the left parietal lobe, and that information from this area activates the premotor cortex in the left and subsequently the right hemispheres via connections in the corpus callosum.

Heilman et al. (1982) suggested two types of ideomotor apraxia based on this model. One results from damage of the left posterior hemisphere or the supramarginal and angular gyri where, they proposed, visuokinesthetic motor engrams for the programming of motor acts are stored. The other type of ideomotor apraxia results from lesions located in the more anterior part of the hemisphere, "disconnecting" the visuokinesthetic motor engrams in the posterior-inferior parietal areas from the motor areas in the frontal lobes. They hypothesized that patients with either type of ideomotor apraxia would have trouble performing skilled movements both on command and by imitation. However, patients with disconnection in which motor engrams were preserved should be able to discriminate between correct and poor task performance, according to this hypothesis. A patient with damage of the parietal lobe resulting in destroyed motor engrams would not, on the other hand, be able to differentiate between acts that were well or poorly performed.

Heilman et al. (1982) conducted a study on 20 patients who were divided into four groups based on anterior or posterior lesion location as well as the presence or absence of apraxia. The subjects' assignment was to differentiate between correct and poor task performance and recognition of gestures. The findings supported the authors' hypothesis regarding the two possible forms of disconnection of the anterior hemisphere from the visuokinesthetic motor engrams. One is by lesions in the left hemisphere, which result in bilateral motor apraxia. The other is due to callosal lesions, resulting in failure of correct performance with the left hand only. Heilman et al. also comment on the role of visual and auditory messages in performance. Defective performance can result if Wernicke's area is damaged, as emphasized by Geschwind, resulting in a lack of understanding of verbal instructions. Damage to the visual association pathway can further result in defective performance when imitating gestures as a result of a lack of visual information necessary for performance.

This information regarding the different cortical origins of unilateral and bilateral apraxic impairments is valuable for therapists when hypothesizing regarding a lesion site. Awareness of the different nature of the sensory information that is provided with instructions and the type of such information necessary for successive performance is also important. Heilman and Rothi (1985) state that the fact that apraxic patients with lesions of the left parietal lobe have more difficulty consolidating memory than do other apraxic patients and "normal" subjects supports the hypothesis regarding the storage of visuokinesthetic motor engrams in that locale.

Ragot et al. (1982) provided support for the differentiation of ideational and ideomotor apraxia. They studied event-related cerebral potentials and reaction times in two right-handed patients with parietal lobe lesions, including ideomotor apraxia, and compared them with seven control subjects. Their results did not indicate an increase of P300 latency (which is the late positive evoked-potential component) in the apraxic patients as compared to control subjects. According to the authors, the P300 is related to cognitive information processing, especially to the identification of a stimulus when a response choice is required. Reaction time latency, on the other hand, was increased. According to the authors, these results suggested that the "motor execution stage is impaired" in ideomotor apraxia, but the "decision making process is left intact," which supports Ayres's (1985) ideas of ideomotor and ideational apraxia.

De Renzi et al. (1982) examined the relationship between apraxia and the nature of the stimulus used to elicit required gestures. They had 220 right-handed patients imitate movements and demonstrate object use. Information was presented to subjects through the three sensory modalities; vision, audition, and tactile sense. Most patients either passed or failed both of the tests. However, 13 patients showed considerably poorer performance when demonstrating as compared to imitating, which was considered to be a result of ideational rather than ideomotor apraxia. Although many patients had deficits spanning more than one sensory modality, 23 apraxic patients with left-hemisphere lesions had test scores that were considerably affected by presentation of a particular sensory modality. These were usually either visual or auditory modalities, and occasionally (but rarely) tactile. The authors interpreted the results as supporting the hypothesis that apraxia results from disconnection of the information-processing area from the movement-programming area presented by previously mentioned authors. Multimodal sensory apraxia was considered to be due to either destruction of the programming area or interruption of pathways that connect it with sensory information areas. However, isolated lesions may disconnect the programming area from one type of sensory information processing center, resulting in the patient's inability to execute gestures elicited by a particular sensory center, but leaving her able to perform when instructed via other sensory modalities, according to the researchers.

This study supported the processing of movements as set forth by Geschwind (1975) and modified by Heilman and Rothi (1985), who proposed that motor engrams for movement are stored in the left hemisphere. Destruction of this region or disconnection of it from other important areas will result in apraxia, the type depending on the site and the extent of the lesion within the processing pathway. It also supported the view of Heilman et al. (1982) that lesions affecting different sensory modalities (visual or auditory) may affect task performance differently.

Kimura (1977) examined the acquisition and performance of manual skills requiring hand movements in patients with both right- and left-hemisphere damage. She used the Manual Sequence Box Test of manual skill, a measure of hand strength, timing, and finger tapping, to gather data. Her results indicated that patients with left-hemisphere damage, whether aphasic or not, were impaired in task acquisition, as compared with those with right-hemisphere damage. The aphasics, however, were found to be most severely impaired. Error analysis indicated that perseverative errors and unrelated movements differentiated the left and the right groups, these errors being associated with lesions of the left hemisphere, whereas sequencing errors did not.

Kimura's findings supported the view that apraxia is more often due to lesions of the left hemisphere, and that language is associated with the severity of apraxia. Her conclusion suggested that tests of finger tapping, speed, and grip strength are not sufficient to assess function. More complex movements and more functional movements, as well as tests, are needed to detect such deficits. The results also point to the fact that patients are at very different levels of function. Some severely apraxic patients may not be able to participate in tests such as those used in Kimura's study. However, it might be possible to detect apraxic deficits on a self-care evaluation. One could, on the other hand, speculate as to whether apraxia in some of the least-affected patients would be detected by an ADL evaluation. In return, one could further question the importance of detecting such deficits for the treatment of the patient, if they do not interfere with functional skill performance.

Kimura's results also supported the view that errors in sequencing can result from a lesion in either hemisphere. This agrees with the views of Geschwind (1975) and of Heilman et al. (1982), described earlier in this chapter. They believed that the disconnection of the right motor and premotor areas from the left hemisphere, where the motor engrams for movement are stored, would result in unilateral apraxia on the left body side. A lesion of the left hemisphere, on the other hand, would result in bilateral apraxia.

Roy (1983) takes a wider perspective regarding movement than do the authors previously reviewed. He agrees with Luria (1980) in that the cerebral cortex is composed of highly differentiated areas, and that functional performance is based on interaction of these areas. Praxis depends on a functional neurobehavioral system of the integrated activity of such areas, and lesions in any of its components, be they cortical areas or links between such areas, may result in apraxia. He found support in the writings of Roland et al. (1980) (reviewed in Chapter 4) based on blood-flow studies of the contribution of different cortical regions to motor performance which showed that this contribution was dependent upon the nature of the task. Roy describes apraxia as a disruption of one or more factors in a "cognitive, information-processing system." According to him, planning is disrupted by lesions in the frontal and parieto-occipital areas. Execution of movement is, on the other hand, disrupted by lesions in the premotor areas, which affect the sequence of movements, or by sensory-motor area damage, which affects control over the sequence of isolated movements.

Roy's model of limb praxis proposed that the actions of two subsystems are required for an action. These are a conceptual system and a production system. The conceptual system provides the necessary knowledge base for actions, be it perceptual or linguistic. It has three components: knowledge of the functions of objects; knowledge of actions; and sequences of action steps. In other words it includes ideation, object use, and the sequencing of action. The production system provides the necessary mechanisms for generating action. These could be classified as planning and execution of movement, if one uses Ayres's (1985) terminology. To ensure a correct action sequence, attention becomes crucial. Roy outlines the errors

that may become evident during performance of movement, and these exceed the errors usually associated with apraxia. According to him errors can be seen in the sequence of action. This includes the omission of steps or components, repetitions, or perseverations, disturbed sequencing of movements, inertia of terminating movements, and difficulty in coordinating the limbs in time and space. Errors may also show up in the performance of movement elements in a particular action sequence. This can be seen in lack of smoothness, jerky movements, lack of fine finger control, or spatial misalignment of the movement, according to Roy.

Roy suggested that the problem with object use in apraxics may be a result of conceptual rather than motor-production disorder. Errors of spatial misalignment, on the contrary, are related to production problems. According to Roy, in agreement with Kimura (1977), damage in the left hemisphere leads to more perseverative errors than does a lesion in the right hemisphere. Further, aphasic patients had a higher order of perseverations than did those without aphasia. Roy concluded that perseverations seemed to have a motor, not a conceptual, origin. The sequencing of action steps, however, was related to a dysfunction of the conceptual system, this being related to attention.

According to Roy, detailed error analysis in relation to the environmental conditions under which tasks were performed is important in order to understand the nature of apraxia. For example, when assessing the production system, various dimensions of performance, such as timing of action components or movements and performance accuracy should be considered. Error analysis would, according to Roy, provide suggestions with respect to the nature of disrupted processing necessary for motor control, and these clues can be used to provide treatment geared toward the specific problem. Thus, one would expect such treatment to be more effective than unspecified treatment.

Roy presented a global view of apraxia, including both ideational and ideomotor aspects, as well as perseverations, which are not usually in-

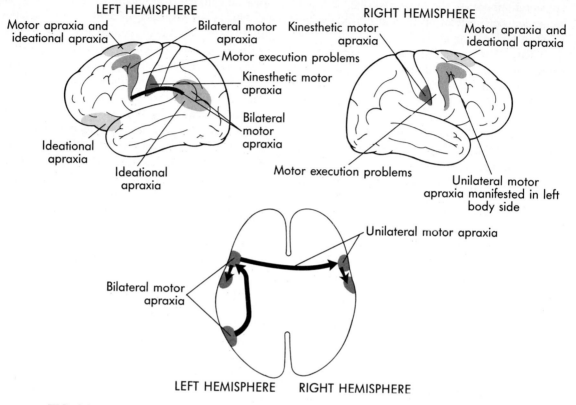

FIG. 8-2 Disrupted processing of praxis. **A,** Lateral view of the hemisphere. Lesion at the praxic sites of the left hemisphere, where the kinesthetic motor engrams are stored, can produce bilateral motor apraxia, whereas lesion of the praxic sites in the right hemisphere can produce unilateral motor apraxia. **B,** Transverse view of the praxic areas, including association and commissural fibers thought to be involved in the process.

cluded in discussions of apraxia. He stressed the importance of analyzing errors. This is in accord with the purpose of the A-ONE, which emphasizes analysis of deficits. Roy's view of bilateral versus unilateral apraxia, as well as lesion location within the left hemisphere or primary motor area of the right hemisphere, is in agreement with the previously reviewed authors.

Roy's idea of two subcomponents of the "action system," in which ideation appears to be linked with conception, perception, attention, and language, whereas motor apraxia refers to the planning of movements and execution, seems realistic. See Fig 8-2 for processing deficits related to praxis.

LANGUAGE AND PRAXIS PROCESSING NETWORKS

Kertesz et al. (1984) studied the relationship between aphasia and apraxia in 177 left-hemispheric stroke patients. A strong association between the two was in agreement with the report of De Renzi et al. (1980) and was considered to support the view that aphasia and apraxia share an origin in some of the same anatomic structures, despite functionally independent networks, resulting in association with both functional and structural components. Thus, certain areas were considered to be important for both praxic and language functions, although the neuronal networks upon which integrated function depends are thought to be distinct. A structural association was related to the fact that aphasia and apraxia are commonly caused by left middle-cerebral artery occlusion, which damages language as well as praxis areas, both of which are dependent on the middle cerebral artery for blood supply.

The results from this study suggested that the apraxic network may, more often than language, have bilateral hemispheric representation in neuronal networks. This conclusion is based on the observation that praxis was spared in some of the aphasics, which in turn suggested the sparing of motor engrams in the right parietal lobe.

De Renzi et al. (1980) studied apraxia during imitation of movement and its association with aphasia in a large group of patients. The incidence of apraxia was considerably higher in patients with left-hemisphere lesions as compared to those with right-side lesions. Apraxia was also more severe in patients with left-hemisphere lesions, and was usually associated with aphasia.

On the basis of the findings it was suggested that discrete neuronal networks exist in the left hemisphere, involving the frontal, parietal, and temporal lobes. They also supported the previously mentioned view that the nature of the stimulus, be it auditory or visual information, and the environment in which a movement was provoked were crucial for the performance of sequential organization of a motor program.

DEFECTIVE PROCESSING OF SOMESTHETIC SENSORY INFORMATION

As reviewed in Chapter 4, somesthetic sensory information is conducted by a pathway from peripheral sensory organs via subcortical structures and the thalamus to the primary sensory cortex in the parietal lobe. From the primary sensory cortex, information is processed on its way through secondary association areas to tertiary association areas. Lesions of the primary sensory cortex in this pathway lead to unilateral sensory deficits of the body side contralateral to the lesion. Lesions of the

cortical association areas of the pathway may lead to unilateral inattention to or neglect of a body side. Another pathway is from the reticular activating system, via thalamic nuclei and limbic structures, including the cingulum, to the somesthetic association areas in the parietal lobes and the dorsolateral frontal lobes. A disruption of this pathway leads to sensory inattention. As the right hemisphere is considered to be dominant for attention, lesions to the cortical processing pathway on the right side lead to unilateral inattention to the left side. Lesions to the left processing pathway, on the other hand, will not cause any definite deficits (Heilman and Van Den Abell, 1980). Specific tactile memory processing of somatosensory information related to this pathway take place in the association areas and the cingulate gyrus of the limbic system. These have sometimes been termed *haptic* memory. (See Fig. 8-3 for somesthetic processing deficits.)

The deficit of motor impersistence, which was described in Chapter 7, can be related to the processing of somesthetic sensory information. It refers to defective feedback to the sensory cortex, affecting motor movement.

Dee and Benton (1970) studied the involvement of tactile and visual factors in spatial deficits on constructional tasks in patients with lesions of either hemisphere. They found that patients with constructional apraxia showed an additional defect in tactile kinesthetic form perception in the hand ipsilateral to the lesion, and defective visual perceptual ability. These defects were not found to be related to associated neurological defects, nor to the lesion site, although there seemed to be a tendency for patients to have lesions in the parietal area. A definite relationship of constructional apraxia with aphasia, motor deficit, sensory impairment, or visual-field deficit was not present. The authors concluded that a general spatial factor underlies function in both the tactile and visual sensory spheres. They further assumed that spatial perception can be analyzed into "partial" functions and that hemispheric differences might be found in such functions. In keeping with that, the right hemisphere plays a special role in the realization

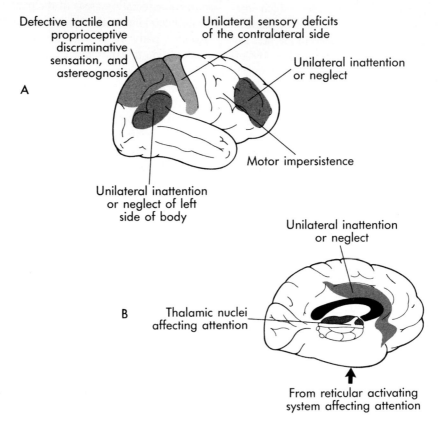

FIG. 8-3 Somesthetic processing deficits. **A,** Lateral view of the right hemisphere, indicating areas associated with defective tactile and proprioceptive information, astereognosis, unilateral inattention, and neglect, as well as motor impersistence. **B,** Medial view of cortex as well as thalamic nuclei affecting attention and resulting in inattention to sensory stimuli.

of depth perception, whereas the nature of possible other lateralized components is unknown so far.

Dee and Benton's study supported the more frequent occurrence of constructional apraxia in the parietal lobes, where convergence of sensory information from different modalities takes place. Their report of the right hemisphere and parietal lobe as dominant locations for the analysis of spatial information is in agreement with the authors reviewed earlier in this chapter. The study indicated that constructional apraxia can originate in either hemisphere, which agrees with results from the experts who validated the localization table in the

A-ONE test manual in Chapter 12. It also suggests that the deficit may be analyzed further and, by doing so, that hemisphere-specific differences might be detected.

DEFECTIVE VISUAL PROCESSING

The processing of visual information was traced from the retina to the occipital lobes as well as to several other cortical areas in Chapter 4. Fig. 8-4 summarizes visual deficits due to lesions in the processing pathway from the optic nerves, via the optic chiasma and the optic tract, to the primary visual cortex in the occipital lobes. From the pri-

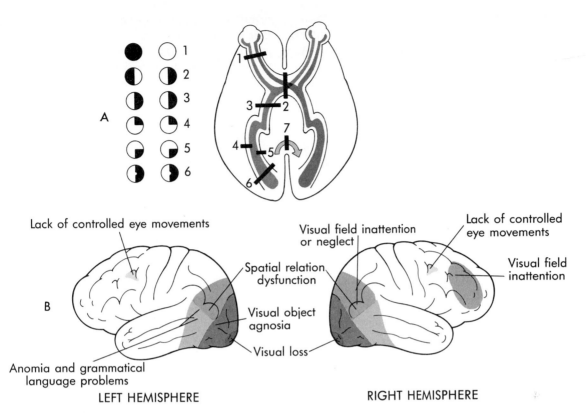

FIG. 8-4 Visual processing deficits. **A,** The visual pathway viewed from the base of the brain (inferior view). The dark bars indicate lesions at different sites in the pathway. The numbers refer to visual-field disturbances according to location of the lesion: *1,* lesion of the optic nerve, leading to blindness in the corresponding eye; *2,* lesion of the optic chiasma, leading to bilateral temporal field defect; *3,* lesion of the optic tract, resulting in complete loss of visual field on the contralateral half of the visual field, or *homonymous hemianopsia; 4,* lesion of the optic tract in the temporal lobe, resulting in loss of vision in the upper quadrant of the contralateral visual field in both eyes; *5,* lesion of the optic track in the parietal lobe, resulting in loss of vision in the lower quadrant of the contralateral visual field in both eyes; *6,* lesion in the occipital cortex, leading to visual loss in the contralateral visual hemifield with macular sparing; *7,* lesion in the posterior corpus callosum, resulting in a disrupted route, causing pure word blindness, or alexia without agraphia. **B,** Lesion sites that can produce visual-spatial relation problems, or anomia and grammatical language problems related to spatial relations. Unilateral visual neglect is related to dysfunction of the inferior parietal lobe, cingulate gyrus, and dorsolateral frontal lobe, especially on the right side.

mary visual area, information travels to the visual association area in the occipital lobe, where further analysis of the visual information takes place. As reviewed in Chapter 4, a pathway continues from the occipital visual association cortex to the parietal lobe, contributing to spatial analysis as well as to the perception of movement and attention to stimulus components. Many of the spatial-relation problems reviewed in Chapter 7 can be related to lesions affecting information from this pathway. Visual-field neglect can occur as a result of damage to the parieto-occipital association area or to other areas important for attention to visual information. Another pathway travels from the visual association area in the occipital lobe to the inferior temporal lobe, which is involved in the perception of form and color, as well as in visual recognition of objects. Lesions affecting this pathway may thus result in anomia and grammatical language problems. Further, the left posterior hemisphere was reported to play a superior role in the registration of verbal-visual stimuli, whereas the right posterior hemisphere was reported to be important in the registration of nonverbal stimuli. The memory processes that take place in relation to visual stimuli have been referred to as *iconic memory* by some authors (Little, 1987). This form of sensory memory is claimed to be of very short duration. A breakdown of iconic memory is thought to result in attention deficits, as well as visual perceptual problems (Little, 1987). As was further outlined in Chapter 4, the frontal lobes also play an important role in simultaneous visual processing, as they are important for control of eye movements, attention to the stimulus, information retrieval, decision-making, and task organization (Roland and Skinhøj, 1981). Thus a lesion affecting the functions of the premotor and prefrontal areas may affect visual processing and the attention necessary for such processing.

PROCESSING DEFICITS IN ATTENTION AND INTENTION

Heilman and Van Den Abell (1980) suggested, on the basis of their study of 12 normal subjects who were given lateralized visual stimuli during EEG readings, a right-hemisphere dominance for attention. According to them, neglect is an "attention-arousal-intention defect" caused by lesions that interrupt a corticolimbic-reticular processing loop. Further, each hemisphere has its own corticolimbic-reticular loop. They suggested, as stated earlier, that the right hemisphere dominates in the mediation of attention, because neglect is seen more frequently with right-hemisphere lesions. They postulated that the left hemisphere attends to stimuli from the contralateral side, whereas the right one attends to stimuli from both sides. Thus, in the case of a left parietal lobe lesion, the right parietal lobe would compensate for the lesion by continuing to attend to ipsilateral stimuli from the right side. Right parietal lobe lesions, on the other hand, would result in profound inattention to contralateral stimuli because the left parietal lobe is not able to attend to ipsilateral stimuli. These authors further proposed that the right hemisphere is dominant for intention, including preparation for action, or readiness to respond. As indicated in the section on sensory neglect, attention is important for processing information from the sensory modalities. Further, as indicated in the section on motor praxis and practic deficits, intention is an important component for movement.

According to Gronwall (1987), there is a controversy regarding whether attentional problems in head-injured patients result from under- or over-arousal. He further states that the reduced rate of information processing in head-injured individuals may be caused by dysfunction of the "attentional control system" (p. 368).

PROCESSING DEFICITS AFFECTING EMOTION

As outlined in Chapter 4, the processing of emotion depends on a path from the hypothalamus, via the medial forebrain bundle to the orbitofrontal cortex, and via the cingulum to the parahippocampal gyrus of the temporal lobe. According to Kaupfermann (1985b), lesions of the lateral hypothalamus result in emotional placidity, whereas lesions of the medial hypothalamus produce aggressive behavioral responses. Kaupfermann (1985a) reports that orbitofrontal cortical damage in primates reduces normal aggressiveness and emotional responses. According to him, such findings were responsible for the application of frontal lobotomies and other surgical procedures applied to the limbic association cortices and their connections in aggressive patients. However, such treatment, in addition to reducing aggressiveness and anxiety, also resulted in personality changes, including a lack of inhibition, or lack of initiative and drive. Further, Kaupfermann (1985b) reports that animal studies involving the removal of temporal lobes in monkeys have indicated abnormal placidity, emotional flattening, and hypersexuality. Temporal lobe epilepsy, on the other hand, produces the opposite effects, that is, hyposexuality and heightened emotionality.

Gainotti (1972) studied emotional behavior in relation to the hemispheric side of lesions in 160 patients with left- and right-hemisphere lesions. He used a neuropsychological test battery to analyze the emotional reactions of patients faced with failures. He reported, on the basis of his findings, that an anxious-depressive mood orientation, termed *catastrophic reaction,* was more frequent in patients with left-hemisphere damage, chiefly in patients with severe aphasia. This was associated with repeated failures in verbal communication. The severity of the catastrophic reactions was further related to the anterior-posterior location of the lesion within the left hemisphere. Emotional reactions were found to be particularly sharp in Broca's aphasics; slowly increasing anxiety attacks were the most evident of the catastrophic reactions in the amnestic group, whereas Wernicke's aphasics showed less-frequent anxiety, no tendency to weep, and 25% of them seemed unaware of their language disturbance. However, swearing and curses were most frequent in this group of patients. Patients with lesions of the right hemisphere, on the other hand, had "indifference" reactions and a tendency to joke. These reactions correlated significantly with unilateral neglect, or inattention to body or visual field, and were considered to be a result of defective nonverbal synthesis of sensory information, according to the authors. The authors provided support for the view that the functional or-

ganization of sensory information may be different in the two cerebral hemispheres. In the left hemisphere, sensory information undergoes a "complex conceptual elaboration" based on language, whereas sensory information is processed in a *more primitive way* with rich affective value in the right hemisphere (p. 53).

Although this study supported the idea of processing differences between the two hemispheres, one could argue with regard to which processing mechanism is more "primitive" as compared to "complex." The findings agree with Geschwind's (1979a and b) review, which reported that depression is more associated with left-hemisphere lesions, whereas patients with right-hemisphere lesions are more frequently unconcerned with their condition. It also suggested a possible lateralization effect of emotional discharge. Kaupfermann (1985a) further stated that some studies of the results from sodium amytal tests have indicated that injection on the left side produces a brief depression, whereas a right-hemisphere injection produces brief euphoria. In the view of the information obtained previously from Kaupfermann (1985a and b) regarding temporal lobe lesions, one would speculate whether the temporal lobe lesions did not contribute to the unawareness of disability and lack of "expected" anxiety in Wernicke's aphasics. Patients with the more anterior language disturbances may have had an intact limbic cortex, including the temporal lobe and the orbitofrontal cortex. Thus they would have more "normal" reactions to their frightening condition. Gainotti did not consider the anterior-posterior dimension or the exact lesion location in the right-hemisphere group, but only the presence or absence of unilateral space or body neglect. Unilateral neglect and inattention have three possible cortical locations, according to the literature reviewed in the section on "Processing Involved in Attention" in Chapter 4, and the section on "Processing Deficits in Attention and Intention" earlier in this chapter. These are the inferior parietal association cortex, the dorsolateral frontal area, and the cingulate gyrus. Thus, the location of lesions could affect simultaneously the neuronal substrate of the networks for attention and emotion, which would contribute to the association of these impairments. Thus, conceptual elaboration based on language may not be the only explanation for the different emotional reactions of the patients in Gainotti's study.

In summary, this section has so far been based on the concept of neurological processing, which takes place between different CNS locations. Many of these locations are identified in the localization table in Chapter 12, as well as in Chapter 7. Although behavior has been dissected into impairments, and these have been related to specific processing paths and CNS locations, one must remember that *each process is a partial function of a larger system*, in which different processes are activated at the same time. Thus, it is not enough to dissect the information; one must consider re-synthesizing it into the "whole" functional system: an individual.

In terms of language, the authors reviewed agreed that different deficits can be related to the location of the lesion along the CNS processing pathway for language functions. This pathway extends from Wernicke's area in the left temporal lobe via the arcuate fasciculus through the left parietal lobe to Broca's area in the left frontal lobe. However, they disagreed about the exact mechanisms responsible for the deficits. According to Heilman et al. (1982), an additional connection from the visual cortex in the occipital lobe to the language processing path is important, for example, in the comprehension of written language.

The review of the literature on ideomotor apraxia revealed an emerging model, with each author adding to the ideas of previous authors. The most complete model thus suggests that storage for motor engrams is situated in the left posterior supramarginal or angular gyrus. A pathway runs from this area via the left premotor area across the corpus callosum to the right premotor area. The premotor areas on each side provide information to the primary motor areas. Pathway disruption in the left hemisphere, except for the primary motor area, results in bilateral apraxia. A lesion in the corpus callosum or in the right hemisphere results in unilateral apraxia of the left body side.

Ideational apraxia is caused by a lesion in the frontal or parieto-occipital areas; it is considered to result from a disruption in a neuronal network that is separate from the network involved in ideomotor praxis.

Two pathways have been identified for the processing of somesthetic information. These include the primary sensory areas and the secondary and tertiary association areas, all in the parietal lobes, as well as the areas responsible for attention to the stimuli. The attention areas include the frontal lobe and cingulate gyrus, in addition to subcortical structures. Lesions of these pathways are responsible for deficits such as unilateral neglect of body or space, somatoagnosia, impairments of tactile discrimination, and motor impersistence. A lesion in the right hemisphere produces some deficits, such as neglect, more frequently than does a lesion in the left hemisphere.

Spatial perception was considered to be a product of the convergence of information from different sensory modalities, including both visual and tactile input. Thus, the posterior teritary association area, including the inferior parietal lobes, was determined to play an important role in such perception and in deficits related to their dysfunction, such as constructional apraxia. Further, the right parietal lobe was considered to play a special role in depth perception.

Lesions producing defective visual fields can occur on the visual pathway from the retina to the primary visual cortex in the occipital lobe. The nature of the deficit depends on the exact location of the lesion on this path. Visual information is processed by different pathways, one leading to the inferior parietal lobe, the other to the posterior temporal lobe. Lesions of these pathways may result in visuospatial deficits, and language deficits related to color or the spatial order of visually based verbal output, respectively. Lesions of the right-hemisphere pathway produced more spatial-relation disorders, including visual-field neglect, whereas lesions of the pathway in the left hemisphere were related to language deficits. Further, lesions of the frontal lobes may affect visual processing.

In terms of attention, it is suggested that each hemisphere has its own corticolimbic-reticular formation loop, or processing pathway. The right pathway is dominant for mediating attention, the right parietal lobe receiving bilateral input, whereas the left parietal lobe receives only contralateral input. The right hemisphere also seems to be dominant for intention. Disruption of these pathways results in inattention and defective intention related to the body or to different types of sensory stimuli in the extrapersonal space.

Emotion is processed on a pathway that connects the limbic structures, including the hypothalamus and the limbic cortex. Lesions of this pathway may result in emotional deficits, such as irritability, aggression, apathy, emotional flattening, and lack of motivation and drive, as well as in personality changes.

IMPLICATIONS RELATED TO EVALUATION AND TREATMENT

There are many different ideas for the treatment of patients with neurobehavioral dysfunctions. Although treatment methods are beyond the spectrum of this book, it is worthwhile to review some of the ideas discussed in this section, because of their relation to treatment. However, regardless of which approach we choose for treatment, we need to be able to identify the disrupted behavior, measure it, and understand its origin and nature. Only then can we speculate regarding the most suitable treatment methods for a particular condition. Only after reliably measuring the neurobehavioral dysfunction and how it affects functional independence can therapists begin to evaluate the effectiveness of their treatment. The A-ONE provides therapists with a clinical tool that enables them to make clinical inferences about structures and functions on the basis of behavior. This is in agreement with Devor (1982) who stated that "in trying to understand recovery of function, one must know what, in essence, was lost" (p. 44). The purpose of the A-ONE is to provide a tool that could aid therapists in determining what processes contributing to behavior and independence have been lost. ADL task performance depends on many different parame-

ters. Thus it is not enough to examine performance-skill dysfunctions when setting treatment goals; dysfunctions of performance components must also be considered. These must be identified before they can be localized. The following considerations should be of further value for speculation regarding treatment after identifying neurobehavioral dysfunction. These include demographic information, degree of laterality, parallel processing, "dormant" cerebral areas, diaschisis, and plasticity of the nervous system.

As mentioned previously, Kandel (1985c) emphasized that isolated damage does not necessarily result in functional loss. Further, if function disappears, it may be regained, to a degree, as other areas of the brain may be able to take over the function. Returning to the analogy of processing pathways resembling the links in a chain, higher mental function is, according to Kandel, dependent on the connections of many chains arranged in parallel; thus, the breaking of a single link does not necessarily interfere permanently with the performance of an entire functional activity. Thus, after identifying particular deficits, therapists should keep the processing patterns in mind and the areas that might be able to resume some of the lost function. Moore (1986) emphasizes the therapeutic consideration of alternate pathways, including parallel processing at different levels of the CNS, as well as the potential use of bilateral pathways. According to her, the secondary neocortical sensory motor centers are an example of the existence of such bilateral pathways, as these centers are capable of receiving input from both body sides.

Moore describes parallel pathways as several pathways with synaptic relay centers at different CNS levels. In such pathways, newly integrated signals are fed forward from one center to another. Similarly, integrated information is fed backward to the centers from which the initial information originated. According to Moore, synchronous use of such systems provides, for example, dynamic postural tone, emotional tone, and memory. Further, it is responsible for the planning and programming of sequential behaviors, in accordance with incoming sensory information in the form of feedback. The interruption of signals between the centers at the various CNS levels and locations disrupts the timing, sequencing, and stimulus intensity of the information, affecting the whole system. If enough parallel pathways remain intact, these could be utilized for functional retraining or compensation of function, according to Moore.

According to Devor, functional loss refers to the fact that the undamaged cortex cannot perform a particular function without the contribution of the lesioned area. The importance of the contribution of a lesioned area may vary from being a minor one, such as setting the excitability level for another cell group, to a major one, including the responsibility of specialized cell groups for organizing the sequence of neuronal impulses for a particular function. A minor contribution refers to the depression of neural mechanisms, sometimes termed *diaschisis* (Devor, 1982). Moehle et al. (1987) refer to diaschisis as a temporary dysfunction resulting from an abnormal "systematic climate." The abnormality results from edema, metabolic disturbance, and decreased blood perfusion, according to these authors. In the case of damage to a major functional circuit, Devor feels that plastic changes, such as the substitution of processing by parallel activity, or "mobilization of redundant capacity," may contribute to rehabilitation. He further describes the concept of "silent synapses," which are relatively ineffective synapses under normal circumstances, and claims that there are numerous such contacts in the adult nervous system. These synapses may be silent for different reasons. CNS dysfunction of a particular location may result in reinforcement of the synapses that survive partial deafferentation. This can be a result of increased sensitivity of the postsynaptic membrane. Synaptic replacement is, on the other hand, rare in the mature CNS. Further, different types of "sprouting" may occur as a result of a CNS lesion, according to these authors. These are reactive sprouting, which refers to the growth of adjacent fibers that are intact; regenerative sprouting, in the case of a cut fiber; and compensatory sprouting, which refers to the sprouting of an axonal branch, where the

distal end of the axon has been damaged. These authors point out that the connections that form as a result of damage to the CNS can be both "correct," referring to the ability to compensate for lost function, and "anomalous," referring to inappropriate regeneration. Further, regardless of the quality of the desired responses, both types have behavioral consequences. Moehle et al. classify axonal regeneration and collateral sprouting under regrowth theories.

Geschwind (1979a and b) supports the idea that a specific function of a lesioned area may be "substituted" for by a function of an area that remains dormant until dysfunction of the dominant hemisphere for a particular function occurs. Thus, despite the existence of specialized functional locations within the brain, there may be some flexibility of the location of functional performance under the circumstance of dysfunction. An example of such substitution given by Geschwind (1975) would be the ability of the right hemisphere to take over some language functions in the case of left-hemisphere dysfunction. Similarly, the anterior commissure can take over some transmission of visual information in the case of a lesioned corpus callosum. Further, Geschwind implies that the non-pyramidal system can possibly be trained to take over some functions of a defective pyramidal system. As mentioned previously in this chapter, Geschwind believes that the two motor systems belong to distinct neuronal circuits. Moehle et al. classify this view of the substitution of analogous neurophysiological processes for lost function to achieve the same behavioral result as *Substitution Theory*.

Heilman and Watson (1978) suggest the possibility of affecting the deficits involving neglect by using tasks that influence hemispheric arousal. They report that stimuli that activated a lesioned right hemisphere, such as visuospatial tasks, reduced the neglect, whereas stimuli that activated the intact left hemisphere, such as language, increased the neglect.

Kertesz (1985) in his review of neuropsychological recovery and treatment, acknowledges the substitution theory mentioned previously, the phenomenon of diaschisis, hierarchical rerepresentation, and the theory of equipotentiality. According to him, equipotentiality refers to that learning of brain lesioned animals correlates positively with amount of remaining intact cortex after the lesion. Moehle et al. (1987) relate this to a mass action of remaining intact nervous tissue. In agreement with Devor (1982) Kertesz describes diaschisis as a state of shock, where damage to a particular location of the nervous system results in a deprivation of normal stimulation in other cortical areas. However, with time, these undamaged areas resume their normal function. Hierarchical rerepresentation, on the other hand, seems to have a lot in common with parallel processing at different CNS levels, mentioned previously. This phenomenon is described as compensation of lower levels, as a result of a release from inhibition due to a lesion at higher levels.

Kertesz (1985) agrees with the authors previously reviewed in that plasticity influences recovery, although he believes that this plasticity is limited in the adult CNS. He relates the reduction of plasticity in adults to possible effects of hormonal changes in the teenage period, with subsequent limitation of the adaptability of a particular cell group. Other factors influencing recovery, according to Kertesz, are handedness and the degree of hemispheric laterality, which has been discussed in Chapter 3, and the nature of the lesion, for which the reader is referred to Chapter 5. The extent of damage also played a role in recovery. However, age was reported to be of contradictory importance in the literature, according to Kertesz.

Kertesz acknowledges diaschisis, plasticity, and regeneration, including sprouting, as physiological changes that accompany functional recovery, and thus agrees with Devor. He also mentions the phenomenon of central denervation hypersensitivity, where intact remaining fibers "produce a greater effect on the denervated region" (p. 485), thus enhancing recovery.

In addition to the previously mentioned neuronal recovery factors, Kertesz describes functional compensation as an aspect of behavioral recovery.

According to him, this refers to the development of new solutions to functional problems by use of residual structures. He includes for example, Luria's functional reorganization of the CNS in his approach. Moehle et al. claim that Luria's model seems to be the foundation for neuropsychological rehabilitation of brain injury. It is based on his theory of hierarchical functional systems, which relies on a dynamic structure, mentioned earlier in this part of the book. Complex function or behavior is made possible by numerous connections between different areas. The goal of the theory is, according to Moehle et al., to account for the creation of new functional systems to overcome dysfunctions. Kertesz further pointed out that motivation is an important behavioral factor that affects recovery.

Siev et al. describe the functional treatment approach utilized in occupational therapy in the rehabilitation of stroke patients as a "repetitive practice of particular tasks" (p. 14). According to them, these tasks are usually related to ADL and aim at increasing the functional independence of a particular patient. They further state that this treatment approach is aimed at the impairment and not at the origin of the dysfunction. Thus the functional approach is used to affect impairments of occupational performance skills rather than dysfunctions of performance components. These authors subdivide the functional treatment approach into two categories: compensation and adaptation. Compensation refers to making the patient aware of a particular problem and teaching specific strategies to overcome it. This would include, for example, encouraging the patient to use diaries, time schedules, and note books to compensate for memory problems and the instruction to "look to the left" in a case of unilateral spatial neglect and environmental set-up which requires that the patient look to the left side for successful task completion. Adaptation, on the other hand, refers to environmental changes to reduce the effects of the disability. Referring again to the deficit of unilateral spatial neglect, when applying this treatment approach utensils would have to be placed at the right side of the patient, on the side of the unneglected visual field. The furniture in the patient's room would be arranged so that all important items would be on the unneglected side and so socially the patient would be approached from that side. Thus, for this deficit, functional compensation and functional adaptation refer to contradictory approaches, and therapists may disagree as to which is more "correct" for which cases. Siev et al. state that the functional approach is favored by occupational therapists over specific perceptual-training approaches, which need to be "transferred" on a neuronal level if they are to affect functional independence. They also point out that the method is supported by practice rather than empirical studies.

In the literature review made by Siev et al., four treatment approaches used by occupational therapists in the treatment of patients with CNS dysfunction are acknowledged. These are the sensory-integrative approach; transfer-of-training approach; functional approach, which was outlined previously; and neurodevelopmental approach. The sensory-integrative approach developed by Ayres (1972) refers, according to Clark et al. (1985), to the "process of organizing sensory information in the brain to make adaptive responses" (pp. 372–373). The approach uses controlled sensory input with the aim of eliciting goal-directed, purposeful, adaptive responses. Adaptive responses affect sensory integration, as they increase the ability of the nervous system to organize sensory information from the environment, thus enhancing the individual's behavioral ability to meet environmental demands. Motivation is recognized as an important factor in enhancing integration (Clark et al., 1985). Although the sensory-integrative treatment approach, which is a neurobehavioral approach, was originally developed for the treatment of children, many of its principles apply to the treatment of adults with CNS dysfunction. According to Siev et al., its use with stroke patients has been justified by studies in the field of aging, environmental effects on CNS functioning, and brain plasticity.

In addition, I believe, based on my clinical observations, that controlled vestibular stimulation can play an important role in affecting the reticular activating system (see Ayres, 1979, for anatomical connections of vestibular and reticular systems) in CNS-damaged adults with a lowered level of consciousness and that it subsequently increases cortical tone, which is a necessary prerequisite for introduction of any other forms of neurobehavioral treatment.

The transfer-of-training approach refers, according to Siev et al., to the assumption "that practice in a particular perceptual task will affect the patient's performance on similar perceptual tasks" (p. 13). Thus, if a patient practices building with blocks, this should improve defective performance in dressing caused by neurobehavioral impairments. Many of the newly developed "popular" computer training approaches can be classified under this approach. Such training emphasizes drilling of certain exercises related to, for example, memory functions, and attention to affect performance in general. However, such transfer of training has not been demonstrated yet. In such a computerized cognitive retraining approach to treatment, visual stimuli dominate, whereas in sensory-integrative treatment, a combination of tactile, proprioceptive, kinesthetic, vestibular, visual, and auditory input, as well as feedback from motor responses is emphasized to generate an adaptive response.

According to Siev et al., neurodevelopmental treatment approaches are primarily used to affect recovery of motor function. However, they have also been utilized as a means of restoring a "normal body scheme," according to the same authors.

In addition to the above-mentioned treatment approaches, behavior modification has been used to reduce many of the psychosocial impairments that accompany cerebral dysfunction. These include irritability, aggressive outbursts, and egocentric behavior. According to Sbordone (1987), such maladaptive behavior should be extinguished and behaviors that are of benefit to the patient and his family should be reinforced. Positive reinforcement for desirable behavior and shaping, where successive approximations to desired response, for example, social behavior, is reinforced, starting with a simple response and progressing to a more complex response, are commonly used to affect low levels of motivation, impaired attention, and participation in functional task performance. Chaining of activity steps where cues are used to chain one step to the next has also been used by therapists in the treatment of CNS-damaged patients.

Moore's excellent article, in which she reviewed the recovery potentials following CNS lesions, encouraged therapists to make use of new principles in their treatment of neurological patients. Her article emphasizes brain plasticity and the existence of parallel processing. Moore further stresses the effects of repeated use of neurons in order for them to regain their functional potentials. She acknowledges the existence of what she terms *polysensory cells,* which, according to her, synapse with multiple motor and sensory cells. A lesion that affects one or more of these synapses may result in a functional imbalance. The previous balance may be regained to a degree by repeated functional use, accompanied by altered strength of neuronal signals from the surrounding intact synapses. Functional recovery may further depend on restoring the balance between the remaining neurotransmitters that act upon a polysensory neuron. Moore, in agreement with Kertesz, stresses the importance of individual differences, be they a result of genetic, or environmental factors, when considering treatment.

Bergland (1985), as opposed to many of the authors reviewed, emphasizes hormonal therapies for restoration of the "whole" brain. He believes that "hormonal harmonies regulate both the brain and the body" (p. 160). Thus hormonal analysis of cerebral spinal fluid in the ventricles becomes a crucial issue for determining appropriate treatment for brain illness. Such analysis may shed light on some of history's myths related to healing. Further, it could explain how certain behavior, such as laughing, affects the hormonal balance and subsequently produces a change in other behavioral components of well-being. According to Bergland, acknowledging hormonal harmonies as regulators of the brain as well as the body, as opposed to the earlier view of an electrically driven brain, provides a more holistic view of the individual. Thus the new hormone-based paradigm will allow for explanation of previous myths, because they fit "the scientific facts of the new paradigm" (p. 160).

I agree with Moore that awareness of information regarding neuronal processes and recovery is a prerequisite for the choice of effective treatment. Further, it is essential that therapists have the ability to evaluate the neurobehavioral dysfunction that interferes with independence, as well as the ability to relate this information to the CNS function for individual patients. In addition to aiding therapists in clinical reasoning regarding choice of treatment, evaluation instruments become essential for evaluation of treatment efficacy. The treatment forms viewed above all have in common the lack of research studies to support the efficacy of the particular treatment. I also agree with Kertesz that spontaneous recovery of neuronal function is often underestimated in efficacy studies, and that neurobehavioral dysfunction is a dynamic process that calls for reevaluation and reconsideration. This is necessary, both in terms of treatment approaches and the status of functional independence. As stated previously, detailed treatment suggestions or guidance are beyond the scope of this book. Its purpose is to guide the therapist in detecting the patient's dysfunction, including dysfunction of performance skills as well as performance components, and by so doing to provide an aid to clinical reasoning. With the information provided in the previous chapters, a therapist should be able to make independent speculations on which to base treatment considerations. It is important to identify deficits early, before treatment decisions are made, in order to affect potential neuronal plasticity and compensatory processes or strategies in a constructive way.

PART

II

The Árnadóttir OT-ADL Neurobehavioral Evaluation(A-ONE) Instrument

The need for an occupational therapy ADL instrument to evaluate neurobehavioral impairments that also has the potential of relating such impairments to cortical CNS dysfunction on the basis of observed neurobehavioral deficits during task performance was established in the previous chapters. In this part, the background for the development of an instrument that would combine occupational therapy principles with neurobehavioral theory is reviewed. This is a clinical evaluation that has some research potential in relation to occupational therapy. The evaluation manual presented in the different chapters of this part includes information on the administration of the instrument and the scoring and interpretation of the information obtained. Further, results from research studies that have been performed to provide preliminary validity and reliability for the evaluation instrument are reviewed.

CHAPTER
9

Introduction to the Árnadóttir OT-ADL Neurobehavioral Evaluation (A-ONE) Instrument

Therapists involved in the assessment and treatment of patients with neurobehavioral dysfunctions have an ethical responsibility to assure themselves that they are using the most effective methods. As Zoltan, et al. (1983) state, "we need to refine our tools" and justify our treatment methods "if we wish to continue to improve the quality of life for our clients" (p. 2). Therapists also have to demonstrate the efficacy of their assessments and treatments, as do other health professionals, because of financial cutbacks in the health-care system and the call for quality assurance regarding the services offered (Smith et al., 1986; Yerxa, 1983; Zoltan et al., 1983). To establish the effectiveness of evaluation and treatment, valid and reliable tools are necessary (Trombly, 1983; Yerxa, 1983; Zoltan et al., 1983). Such tools are also necessary in order to identify the dysfunctions that cause impaired independence, which is a prerequisite for goal formation and for choosing the most pertinent treatment. After establishing goals and implementing treatment programs, it is clinically important to be able to detect any change in a patients' performance. Studies performed to investigate which behavioral factors changed and the reasons for the change could generate new knowledge regarding methods and prognosis, which could possibly be used in the treatment of neurological patients.

As stated in the Introduction, an instrument is an essential component of a paradigm, or the accepted practice pattern of a profession. According to Kuhn (1970), standard tests and instruments are necessary for science, and although they restrict the investigation field, they provide the method necessary for research. Further, new instruments based on technological advances may necessitate a paradigm change, affecting both the "procedures and expectations" of a particular scientific community.

It is necessary to test theoretical statements through research, in order to explore whether they can be confirmed or not. Such research can generate knowledge. Research requires valid and reliable instruments capable of measuring the variables under study. Most evaluations used by occupational therapists are clinical instruments, developed to meet practical needs at different locations. Most of these tools lack reliability and validity and are therefore not suitable for research purposes. However, an instrument can be developed and used to operationalize concepts from a theory. Such an instrument with established reliability and validity is better suited to testing a theory's relational statements than are tools developed

FIG. 9-1 Constructional apraxia.

Possible error components
Spatial-relation difficulties

Perseveration of color

Perseveration of spatial fragment

Unilateral spatial neglect

Comprehension problem

Ideational problem

Motor apraxia

Attention deficit

Lack of motivation or cooperation

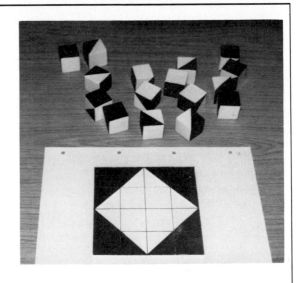

for other purposes, which do not necessarily address the theory's concepts (Yerxa, 1983). The purpose behind the Árnadóttir OT-ADL Neurobehavioral Evaluation (A-ONE) instrument was to develop an ADL instrument by operationalizing concepts from the discipline of occupational therapy to aid therapists in clinical reasoning and decision making. It was hoped that through future improvement and subsequent research studies, the instrument would be capable of contributing to knowledge development within the field of occupational therapy.

PRESENT OCCUPATIONAL THERAPY EVALUATIONS

A variety of occupational therapy evaluation methods for neurobehavioral dysfunctions are being used across occupational therapy settings (Siev et al., 1986). However, according to Zoltan et al. (1983), few of these have established reliability and validity. The occupational therapy assessment tools that are presently used with neurological patients seem to address either neurobehavioral dysfunction or functional independence, not both simultaneously. Traditionally, ADL evaluations report functional independence. None of the published ADL instruments address neurobehavioral dysfunction as such, either in terms of assessment or treatment aims, although such dysfunction often interferes with functional independence. However, if evaluations of dysfunction are to be used to provide information for treatment considerations, it is important that they be sensitive to the exact variables that cause the dysfunction. Further, occupational therapy assessments of cognitive function do not usually include structured observations of performance in activities of daily living (ADL), although, according to Ottenbacher (1980), ADL assessments are among the tools most often used by occupational therapists to assess occupational role performance in CVA patients.

To evaluate neurobehavioral deficits, therapists traditionally work from categories of dysfunction, such as constructional apraxia, and test for each category separately. The A-ONE empha-

FIG. 9-2 Putting on a shirt.

Possible behavioral deficits interfering with function
Premotor perseveration: pulling up sleeve

Spatial-relation difficulties: differentiating front from back on shirt

Spatial-relation difficulties: getting an arm into the right armhole

Unilateral spatial neglect: not seeing shirt located on neglected side (or a part of the shirt)

Unilateral body neglect: not dressing the neglected side or not completing the dressing on that side

Comprehension problem: not understanding verbal information related to performance

Ideational apraxia: not knowing what to do to get shirt on or not knowing what the shirt is for

Ideomotor apraxia: having problems with the planning of finger movements in order to perform

Tactile agnosia (astereognosis): having trouble buttoning shirt without watching the performance

Organization and sequencing: dressing the unaffected arm first and getting into trouble with dressing the affected arm; inability to continue the activity without being reminded
Lack of motivation to perform

Distraction: becomes interrupted by other things

Attention deficit: difficulty attending to task and quality of performance

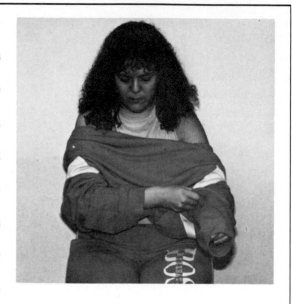

Irritated or frustrated when having trouble performing or when not getting the desired assistance

Aggressive when therapist touches patient in order to assist her (tactile defensiveness)

Difficulties recognizing foreground from background or a sleeve of a unicolor shirt from the rest of the shirt

sizes a different approach, in which many deficits can be detected simultaneously from observation of performance in a single activity, such as a primary ADL task. Fig. 9-1 indicates how various deficits can be detected by this method through the use of a traditional cognitive test. Fig. 9-2 indicates how the same method can be used to detect neurobehavioral deficits from an ADL activity. Illustrations of the examples listed can be found throughout Part I of the book. These deficits are then classified and related to their potential origin within the CNS.

When looking at the roots of the measures used by occupational therapists for testing neuro-behavior, it was obvious that cognitive perceptual tests with items originating within the discipline of occupational therapy are not available. Rather, the items used appeared to be "borrowed" from the disciplines of neuropsychology or neurology. However, it is very important for professional identity and the autonomy of any profession that the instruments used be based on the profession's concepts and theories. It is also important that a profession use instruments that originate within the knowledge base of that profession if its members are not to be misled and moved away from the profession's goals.

According to Ayres (1985), praxis, except

for constructional praxis, is evaluated "out of context," because "an assessment creates an artificial environment" (p. 6). Unfortunately this is true for many other neurobehavioral deficits, which means that the information provided by such tests does not reflect functional capacities in "real-life situations."

The results from cognitive-perceptual assessments have only rarely been compared to functional performance in daily living (Siev et al., 1986). Such comparisons have led to suggestions such as this: since a relationship between constructional dysfunction and dressing dysfunction has been demonstrated, transfer of training from practice in block-building (constructional praxis) will take place, benefitting the performance of ADL (e.g., dressing). This is a cause-and-effect extrapolation from two related factors, an error that is all too easy to fall into, yet which is without empirical basis. Therapists wanting to make direct use of the functional information obtained from ADL observations of neurological patients must acquaint themselves with the comparative studies. Then separate ADL evaluations must be performed in addition to the cognitive-perceptual evaluation in order to determine the functional status of the particular patient. Such methods are cumbersome, and they may be misleading. Further, only one of these methods addresses the heritage of occupational therapy. I reasoned that occupational therapists need more direct and functionally oriented measures of impairments to establish more precise evaluations and more effective treatment methods. The use of ADL seemed to be a far more reasonable approach.

The Árnadóttir OT-ADL Neurobehavioral Evaluation (A-ONE) instrument was constructed on the basis of this identified need. This new instrument tests ADL and neurobehavioral components simultaneously and thus should be less cumbersome for therapists than the previously described procedures. The A-ONE should reveal more direct information regarding the dysfunctions of neurobehavioral performance components and how they interfere with functional performance of

skills, as well as how they relate to the localization of lesions and of processing sites that underlie the CNS dysfunctions.

In summary, occupational therapists need to change their method of evaluating patients with neurobehavioral dysfunctions. The A-ONE was developed for that purpose.

Although occupational therapy curricula include information on evaluating cognitive and perceptual dysfunction, many entry-level therapists feel insecure about their skills in evaluating such dysfunction, interpreting the results from the assessments, and applying them to treatment. They feel a lack of professional guidelines in this area. Similar problems were identified by Geschwind (1985) in the profession of medicine. He points out that the examination of the mental status of neurologically damaged patients seemed to be different from the examination methods used in other fields of medicine. The difference is that mental status examinations are more diffuse and indirectly related to diagnostic categories. He further claims that there is a lack of direct correlation between the items used in clinical assessments and disorders of structure and physiology, which hinders the perception of relationships between abnormal clinical findings, physiology, and anatomy.

It was obvious that therapists are not always prepared for the complex responsibilities that follow neurobehavioral evaluation and its interpretation in providing the most effective treatment. Most occupational therapy expertise in this area has been developed by "trial and error." It is time to reconsider the teaching strategies used in occupational therapy for the development of neurobehavioral expertise.

The difficulties that occupational therapists encounter in evaluating neurobehavioral dysfunction in the absence of guidelines also affects their use of ADL observations for detecting neurobehavioral deficits. This is unfortunate, as neurobehavioral dysfunction can be the underlying cause of the lack of functional independence in a particular activity. It is easy for therapists to focus only on general function and not to take the underlying neurobehavioral dysfunction into account; thus at times they may ignore the basis for the problem and perhaps limit the treatment. However, if therapists are guided through the first steps of translating clinical observation data into neurobehavioral information, they can master the required skills for accurate evaluation and detection of impairments, which is a prerequisite for choosing the most effective treatment. In connection with the development of the A-ONE, I propose that therapists can be trained in a short time to use effective and meaningful strategies to evaluate patients with neurobehavioral dysfunctions. The training would include the effective use of evaluative information to understand how the neurobehavioral deficits interfere with function as well as the nature of the patients' dysfunction. Such training might subsequently result in more effective treatment, as therapists identify the impairments that interfere with functional independence and understand the CNS origin of these impairments. Problem identification and knowledge regarding the source of a problem are basic to speculation about whether a problem can be affected by treatment, and if so, how.

A systematic occupational therapy evaluation of ADL such as the A-ONE can be used to detect neurobehavioral dysfunction in addition to its role in assessing ADL skills. In addition, guidelines to interpret the evaluation in order to relate specific neurobehavioral deficits are included with the evaluation to make it accessible to most therapists, not only the neurobehavioral specialists. The new instrument should provide more direct information regarding impairments, how they interfere with functions, and how they relate to the location of lesions and the processing mechanisms that underlie the dysfunction. This information should be valuable during consideration of treatment strategies because it should identify the cause of the dysfunction interfering with independence and provide ideas regarding the CNS origin of the dysfunction. Thus, by use of the A-ONE's identification of the components of a dysfunction, treatment can be geared toward reducing skill dysfunction or improving performance components,

or toward affecting the CNS processes that cause the deficit through the use of carefully selected sensory stimuli. Even a compensatory treatment approach could be more carefully selected when based on such an evaluation.

In selecting the A-ONE's form of standardization, I attempted to achieve a balance between the flexibility of clinical observations and the rigidity of standardized methods, keeping in mind the conflicting views put forth in the neuropsychological literature. Although standardization is important for determining psychometric qualities, it should not be so important that the assessment loses its sensitivity for the aspects it was designed to measure.

Let us examine the concept of balance further. Obviously, it is possible to become a therapist who is expert in detecting neurobehavioral deficits through behavioral observation; however, this takes many years of practice and continued study. With standardized assessments, therapists who are not experts can use specific procedures in a reliable way to test and obtain results. However, there is the danger of losing important information that is not included in the standardization frame, because the test cannot be adapted to the needs of each individual patient. Such adaptation requires a skilled examiner. As the A-ONE is a clinical evaluation, it was considered more important to train therapists to use clinical reasoning to evaluate the endless possibilities in a patient's behavior than to provide them with an evaluation that has such rigid standardization criteria that important clinical information gets lost. However, one must trade clinical flexibility for lower reliability; it is hard to obtain high reliability when standardization is sacrificed for clinical flexibility. Thus a therapist's training becomes an important factor in the reliability of the A-ONE.

The A-ONE was designed to address this balance issue. It aims for a balance between flexibility and standardization, and by doing so provides a guided process that therapists may use to evaluate patients with neurobehavioral dysfunctions. It requires an understanding of the subject matter as well as "adaptability" and "critical thinking skills." The guided process should be introduced in a seminar on the theoretical base of the A-ONE instrument and its assessment procedures, followed by repeated use of the evaluation. This process can provide expertise in a relatively short time and allows increased reliability in using the evaluation.

THEORETICAL BASE

As stated earlier, the discipline of occupational therapy needs to develop evaluation methods founded on the principles of occupational therapy. Therefore, I have attempted to combine the neurobehavioral literature with principles of occupational therapy in order to develop a theory that relates factors from these two sources. It was hoped that therapists could subsequently base and develop their treatment methods on this factor-relating theory. Chapter 1 reviewed this theoretical base. Statements proposing a relationship between the behavior of the individual with CNS damage and the structural and neurobehavioral abnormalities caused by CNS damage were selected to test the new theory and to contribute to its development. It was also proposed that by using the A-ONE to evaluate the behavior of a patient with CNS damage, therapists could speculate regarding the structural damage or information-processing dysfunction within the brain. Both of these statements, if further supported, may become important in identifying the specific problems underlying a patients' dysfunction. In addition, they may contribute to the development of new treatment methods for neurobehavioral dysfunctions. Increased understanding of the CNS processes involved in dysfunctions and in the improvement of such dysfunctions will facilitate speculation regarding how these processes can be affected by, for example, carefully analyzed and selected sensory stimuli that subsequently affect behavior.

DESCRIPTION OF THE INSTRUMENT

The A-ONE instrument is a clinical test intended for the evaluation of patients who have neurobe-

havioral dysfunctions of cortical origin and are more than 16 years old. The test format involves the primary ADL with items that address neurobehavioral deficits. The evaluation yields objective scores regarding functional independence and neurobehavior.

The evaluation is composed of two parts. Part I is used to assess functional level and neurobehavioral dysfunction. It includes the Functional Independence Scale and the Neurobehavioral Impairment Scale. The Neurobehavioral Impairment Scale is composed of two subscales: the Neurobehavioral Specific Impairment Subscale and the Neurobehavioral Pervasive Impairment Subscale. Part I indicates the level of ADL independence and the types of assistance needed as well as the types and severity of the neurobehavioral deficits that interfere with function. Part II is used to convert the results from Part I to reveal information regarding dysfunctions within the CNS. This information should aid in goal-setting and treatment planning for patients with neurological dysfunctions.

INSTRUMENT DEVELOPMENT

The development of the A-ONE followed the steps described by Benson and Clark (1982). The developmental process included all of the following: planning, construction, quantitative evaluation, and further validation.

Planning

The purpose of the instrument was to detect neurobehavioral dysfunctions as well as the functional levels of CNS damaged patients via an ADL assessment. The test domain was determined to be ADL. The literature on the test construct was reviewed. The construct was primary ADL performance defined as the self-care components of dressing, grooming and hygiene, transfer behavior and mobility, feeding, and communication, and their relation to brain structure and function.

Open-ended questions were provided from the author's previous experience with patients with CVA, head injuries, brain tumors, brain atrophy, and cardiac problems. These questions were modified in order to form objectives that were developed into neurobehavioral impairment checklists and scales (Neurobehavioral Specific Impairment Subscale and Neurobehavioral Pervasive Impairment Subscale) to be used to detect neurobehavioral deficits during ADL performance (see Chapter 10). The item format was ADL evaluation, including primary ADL skills.

Construction

A table of specifications was developed according to the objectives. Content validation for both Parts I and II of the evaluation had two components. The literature provided a content validation for the instrument. Further content validation was provided by expert opinions obtained from four experts within the field of neurology and occupational therapy.

Quantitative evaluation

The instrument was initially prepared for a pilot study using 65 subjects. Interrater reliability was established for both Parts I and II of the evaluation. These and other research studies related to the development of the A-ONE are reviewed in Chapters 11 and 12.

Validation

As mentioned previously, content validation was provided for both parts of the evaluation. The literature review in Part I of this book serves as a content validation of the instrument, including the Localization Table in Chapter 12. Expert opinions were used as additional content validation. Concurrent validity was provided for patients with CVA. The comparison of results from the A-ONE to neuroimaging was also examined for further validation of the instrument. Results from these studies are reviewed in the following chapters.

The A-ONE is only starting its developmental course as an instrument. Refinements have been made according to presently available research studies on the instrument. However, much work is still ahead in terms of establishing further reliability and validity.

LIMITATIONS OF THE EVALUATION

It is vital for therapists using the A-ONE to be familiar with the test manual and the standardized instructions for administration. It is also necessary for therapists to have attended a training seminar in the use of the evaluation instrument, so that they will be thoroughly familiar with the theory behind it, and to have the required knowledge of neurology, neurobehavior, and occupational therapy principles. The reliability of the A-ONE is conditioned by these requirements.

CHAPTER
10

The A-ONE: Part I

There are two parts to the Árnadóttir OT-ADL Neurobehavioral Evaluation (A-ONE) instrument. Part I contains items that determine functional skill performance and detect specific components of neurobehavioral dysfunction. This part includes the primary ADL domains of dressing (putting on a shirt or dress, pants, socks, shoes, and manipulating fastenings); grooming and hygiene (washing face and upper body, combing the hair, brushing teeth, shaving, continence, and bathing); transfer behavior and mobility (sit up in bed, get out of bed, maneuver around, transfers to toilet and tub); feeding (drinking from a mug, using fingers for sandwich, using fork, spoon, and knife); and communication (speech and comprehension). The components in each domain are reported with the use of two scales. The Functional Independence Scale is a multiscore scale ranging from independence to dependence, scored 4 to 0 respectively. The item scores can be summed for a Functional Independence Score for each ADL domain if required.

It was assumed that while observing the patient's performance on the functional components, the therapist could also detect neurobehavioral impairment. Therefore the ADL task was analyzed into components relative to neurobehavioral deficits. Part I of the A-ONE thus includes the Neurobehavioral Scale, which is composed of two subscales. The Neurobehavioral Specific Impairment Subscale is a multiscore scale with item scores ranging from no deficits to severe deficits, scored 0 to 4. Here the specific impairments are

scored separately for each ADL domain. The Neurobehavioral Pervasive Impairment Subscale is a dichotomous scale that measures the presence or absence of items that may be obtained from observations in any of the ADL domains.

ADMINISTRATION
Population

The instrument is intended to be used with people with CNS dysfunctions of cortical origin, especially where neurobehavioral deficits are suspected. The causes of such dysfunction are diverse and include the following: vascular disorders, metabolic disorders, head injuries, infections, toxins, brain tumors, and degeneration of the nervous system. The evaluation is constructed for people more than 16 years of age who have already developed the neurological processing strategies needed to perform the items chosen for the evaluation instrument.

Location

The A-ONE should be performed at the patient's bedside in any setting where occupational therapy is provided. A sink is needed either in the patient's room or at a location close to it. The evaluation should be performed in the morning, at realistic times for the activities, and in keeping with the daily routine. Clinically, in terms of location, one should weigh flexibility against rigid standardization criteria. Novelty in the location requires more from a patient than does an environment in which the patient has learned to function automatically. This could be used as a criterion worthy of notice for evaluating progress over time.

Materials

ADL items such as a shirt, pants, socks, shoes, towel, washcloth, soap, toothbrush, toothpaste, razor, deodorant, comb, fork, knife, spoon, glass or cup, plate, and breakfast are needed. Some flexibility is appropriate for a realistic adaptation of the situation. Patients should generally use their own clothes and equipment. Again the therapist should keep in mind that a novel object requires more processing than does a familiar object that the patient may even use automatically.

All aids that the patient needs or uses should be within reach. These include such items as hearing aids, glasses, dentures, walking aids, wheelchair, and self-care aids.

Administration time

According to results from a questionnaire filled out by therapists who have used the evaluation, the time for administering the A-ONE is the same as it takes to administer traditional clinical ADL evaluations. Interpretation and scoring of Part I of the evaluation (including the checklists) was completed in 25 minutes, on the average, by therapists who had scored no more than five protocols. One would expect this time to be reduced with experience.

General procedures

It is possible to administer parts of the instrument at different times, if fatigue is a problem. The therapist can assist the patient verbally or physically, according to the minimum of assistance required, but should be able to differentiate between physical and neurobehavioral dysfunctions, as well as their severity. The type of assistance needed for performance, whether it is physical, pantomime, or verbal, should be recorded, as well as the reason for the assistance, that is, neuromotor or neurobehavioral deficits.

Before beginning the evaluation, the therapist should elicit responses that reveal information regarding language functions, judgment, and memory. This should be done in casual introductory communication: patients may be asked questions related to their medical problems, social situation, and length of stay in the hospital. Questions regarding temporal orientation (time of day, date, month, season) should also be addressed. If there is any indication of memory loss or confabulations, more specific questions should be asked regarding specific events, such as how last weekend was spent, what the therapy schedule was the previous day, or the nature of the last meal. If language problems are indicated, when possible the therapist should simplify his or her language or use pantomime because of the nature of the scoring. Further, note should be made of whether the patient can name concrete things or repeat words. This information is important for the rest of the evaluation. The concepts of left and right in relation to the patient's body parts should also be introduced at least once in the therapist's instructions during the evaluation. A note should be made of the patient's responses on the Neurobehavioral Pervasive Impairment Scale.

In general, items used should be placed within the patient's reach, on both sides of his or her body. It is not necessary to have exactly the same items for all patients as long as they are items that the patient uses. Additionally, patients need not perform all the items to reveal neurobehavioral deficits. Tub and toilet transfers, bathing, and incontinence are thus frequently left out of a pure neurobehavioral evaluation. However, for a complete functional assessment, the person should attempt all the items, if capable.

The therapist should keep in mind important variables such as that long sleeves are harder to put on than short ones, and fastenings behind the back are harder to manage than front fastenings. Also, it is possible to make items more difficult for persons who have questionable presence of impairments; one sleeve could be turned inside out to see how the patient deals with that situation. Further, the familiarity of an item makes the activity easier, even "automatic." To clinically increase task difficulty, an unfamiliar activity should be provided, or an activity in an unfamiliar location. This is an

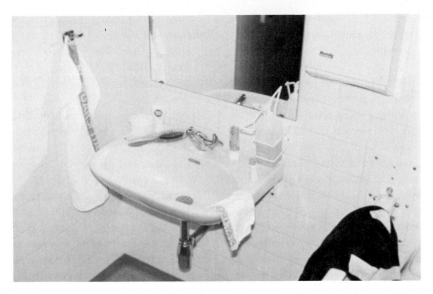

FIG. 10-1 Environmental Setup for the Evaluation. All items needed for performance should be located within the patient's reach. Items should be divided between the right and the left sides of the sink area.

important consideration when reporting progress. It is not enough for a person to get used to a set environment; the optimal level is not to be able to perform an activity automatically but to be able to carry the skills over to different situations. For this reason too much rigidity is discouraged for this evaluation. Note however, that if the evaluation is to be used for research purposes, more stringent criteria should be used for the procedures, and they should be reported with the results.

Specific item procedures

The ADL assessment should be administered in the following sequence. The therapist brings a washcloth, towel, soap, toothbrush, toothpaste, and a comb, as well as a razor, deodorant, and any lotions that belong to the patient, and places them on both sides of a sink before the patient gets up. The patients' clothes, and helping aids, should also be within reach. It is important to place the items on both sides in order to check for unilateral spatial neglect; doing the placement of items within the vision of the patient will provide extra clues (see Fig. 10-1). Before the patient gets up, she is in-

structed about the procedures. The patient is told to get out of bed, wash, comb her hair, brush her teeth, and dress, performing these activities as they would normally be done, by the sink, and then to go over to the breakfast area and eat. The patient is instructed to do as much as possible independently, and as normally as possible, and is informed that assistance will be provided when needed throughout the performance. If further guidance for performance is needed, the following procedures are used.

Verbal instruction is provided before physical assistance. The therapist instructs the patient who is lying in bed to get out of the bed to a chair or a wheelchair, offering physical assistance if the patient's disability requires it. The patient can dress the lower body part at this point, if desired. The patient maneuvers over to a sink with instructions and assistance as needed. If the patient is able to and wishes to stand by the sink, that is also acceptable.

The therapist asks the patient to take off the pajama jacket, and wash the face and the upper body.

The therapist asks the patient to comb the hair, brush the teeth, or shave (if the patient is a man), if these activities are not performed automatically.

The therapist brings the patient's attention to any lotions or cosmetics owned by the patient if the patient does not use them automatically.

The patient is instructed to complete the dressing.

The therapist asks the patient to move toward a table where breakfast has been located. Food and utensils have been placed on both sides within the patient's reach.

The following qualities of the therapist are important parts of the administration procedures for the A-ONE instrument: (1) the therapist's knowledge of neurobehavior and the performance of daily activities; (2) the therapist's sensitivity to the patient's responses and needs; (3) the therapist's ability to analyze responses and the sensory information that provokes the responses, which is provided and controlled for by the therapist; and (4) the therapist's familiarity with the items necessary for activity performance. Thus, for reliable results it is crucial for the therapist to be thoroughly familiar with the theory behind the evaluation and to have obtained the training required for administration of the A-ONE.

SCORING AND INTERPRETATION

There are two scales for scoring the evaluation. The Functional Independence Scale focuses on the traditional functional level of independence. The Neurobehavioral Impairment Scale measures the number and type of neurobehavioral deficits that interfere with function. The scoring should ideally be based on two or three ADL observations. This allows the therapist to form ideas during one observation and then test more specifically for suspected problem areas. Note that it is absolutely necessary to observe the patient's performance. The A-ONE should never be used as a questionnaire. If information on specific items is not clear, this is indicated by the entry *not tested* (NT) on the scoring sheet. As the level of assistance needed for the performance of daily activities is an important rehabilitation concept, this enters into the scoring criteria. The independence level is scored from 4 to 0 in the following way:

4 Indicates that the person is functionally independent.

3 Indicates that the person is independent physically but needs supervision or reminding in order to engage in a task or for safety reasons.

2 Indicates that the person needs verbal assistance to perform.

1 Indicates that the person needs minimum or moderate physical assistance to perform and that he or she actively participates in the task.

0 Indicates that the person is unable to perform and is totally dependent on assistance.

Thus, the higher the functional score, the more independent the patient is. The use of helping aids does not enter the scoring, but the aids should be listed. It is the premise of this test that if a person is independent, he or she should not get a different score (presumably lower) for using helping aids.

The measures on the Neurobehavioral Specific Impairment Scale are scored from 0 to 4. In this case, the lower the score, the less severe the interference with function. The scoring is partially based on an analysis of which type of stimulus provokes the necessary neuronal processing to elicit the desired performance and overcome or diminish the effects of neurobehavioral dysfunction, be it verbal, tactile, proprioceptive, or visual. The scoring is performed in the following way:

0 No neurobehavioral deficits are observed during performance.

1 The patient is able to perform without additional information, but some neurobehavioral deficits do appear during the observation.

2 The patient is able to perform with additional verbal assistance, but neurobehavioral deficits do appear during the performance. Thus, the patient is capable of processing verbal information.

3 The patient is able to perform with demonstration and minimal or moderate physical assis-

tance. Thus, the patient is able to utilize visual, tactile, and proprioceptive information to perform.

4 The patient is unable to perform due to CNS dysfunction.

Thus, the two scales of independence and neurobehavioral impairment should be inversely related. The scoring on both scales indicates the type of assistance needed and which processing mechanisms the patient is able to utilize for performance. Assistance should be provided only if the patient does not give any indication of an intention to perform within 2 to 3 minutes, or if the patient is performing incorrectly and cannot get back on the right track, as the patient must have an opportunity to show the dysfunction.

If the patient has manifested neurobehavioral deficits for example, started washing the face a second time and then realized the mistake, stopped the activity, and begun another activity, a score of 4 would be given on the function scale and 1 on the neurobehavioral scale. Similarly, if a person has turned the comb wrong, but then realized it on his or her own and corrected it without any information in addition to the feedback from the activity, a score of 4 is given for independence and 1 for the presence of neurobehavioral deficits.

Verbal information may be needed in order for a patient to perform. The assistance will not be standardized because flexibility is needed to meet the needs of individual patients, and the therapist should, after attending a training course for test administration, have the adaptability to provide just sufficient information and to determine to which category that information belongs. An example of verbal information may be, "You already washed your face, now wash your hands" (if the patient perseverates when washing the face), or "The toothpaste is on your left side" (if the patient seems to be looking around for it and does not see it because of unilateral spatial neglect). This information will result in a score of 2 on both scales. A score of 2 is also given if the patient needs frequent reminders or step-by-step guidance for organizing an activity.

Although the person may need to be reminded once, for example, to brush the teeth, this would not be scored as a verbal assistance after the other activities are complete. The therapist needs to be flexible. A patient may, for example, not be accustomed to brushing his teeth in the morning before breakfast. Therefore, he should not be marked down for not doing that automatically. The testing situation may also make the person a little nervous, and this should be taken into consideration.

Patients can also ask for verbal responses from the therapist. These should be evaluated before they are rated. For example, if the patient asks where the toothpaste is, and it is on the left side of his visual field, she is asking for verbal assistance to deal with visual-field neglect, which would be rated as 2. If the patient, on the other hand, asks, "What do you want me to do next?" or "Is there anything else?" (after finishing a particular activity), or "Do you want me to comb my hair, too?" this should not necessarily be rated as verbal assistance needed to cope with neurobehavioral deficits if there are no other indications for organization problems.

For physical assistance, the therapist must differentiate between physical assistance needed because of actual muscle-tone problems, such as paralysis or spasticity (or lack of coordination due to subcortical lesions), and physical assistance needed because of neurobehavioral dysfunction. Physical impairment should be recorded in pertinent areas on the evaluation, and the reason for physical assistance should be noted in the Comment sections throughout the evaluation, and on the Neurobehavioral Pervasive Impairment Subscale. Physical assistance needed to overcome interference from neurobehavioral deficits includes, for example, showing the patient how to pull the shirt sleeve in a specific direction in order to put on a shirt. This results in a score of 1 on the independence scale and a score of 3 on the neurobehavioral scale. Another example of physical assistance would be taking the patient's hand and placing it to wash the chest when the patient persists in washing the face over and over again. These acts are scored as 1 on the independence scale and 3 on the neurobehavioral scale. Note that both visual processing, when a patient is shown how to perform, and tactile-kinesthetic processing, when a patient is guided through movements, are included in this scoring category. Therapists should be alert with respect to which of the processing forms is more meaningful to the patient and make a note of that in the Comment section, although on the basis of present reliability studies, this information has been grouped under one category.

A score of 0 is given on the Functional Independence Scale if the therapist has to provide maximum physical assistance in order for a particular ADL item to be performed, and the patient provides very little or no contribution to the performance. This results in a score of 4 for the pertinent item on the Neurobehavioral Specific Impairment Subscale. Note that more than one type of neurobehavioral deficit can interfere with functional performance, and these should all be recognized, if indicated by the observation. Of course, if the patient is totally unable to perform because of paralysis, for example, it may be impossible to evaluate the presence and severity of other deficits. In this case a patient does not get a score of 0, indicating no deficit. Rather, no score is indicated,

and the clarification *not tested* (NT), along with the reasons, is indicated in the Comment section. See Fig. 10-2 for different levels of assistance.

Assistance on the independence scale is scored according to the type of assistance needed to complete an activity, regardless of its cause, be it a physical disability or a neurobehavioral dysfunction. For further information, see the following section on detailed examples for scoring.

According to results from research studies, it is possible to add up the independence scores within each subcategory on the Functional Independence Scale, although it is not necessary and not recommended except for specific purposes. For such exceptions the total scores for dressing (max 20), grooming and hygiene (max 24), transfers and mobility (max 20), feeding (max 16), and communication (max 8) would be obtained. It is further possible to obtain a percentage score for each category by multiplying the scores by 100 and dividing by the maximum scores in each domain. Grooming and hygiene scores would thus be divided by 24, dressing and transfers by 20, feeding by 16, and communication by 8. It is important to note that any items labeled *Other* under the different ADL domains do *not* enter the total scores. They need to be commented on separately in the Comment section. Note that the total scores across

---

FIG. 10-2 Different Levels of Assistance Important for Scoring. (a) No motoric apraxia is observed when the patient brushes the hair independently. The right upper extremity is paralyzed, so the patient uses the left hand for the task. (b) A clumsy grasp is noticed when the patient moves the brush from the left to the right side of the hair, but she is able to correct it without interference from the therapist and complete the task independently. Thus, the patient combs independently, but motor apraxia is observed. (c) The patient, after moving the brush from the left to the right side, turns the bristles of the brush away from the hair because of lack of sequencing and flexibility in movements, or motor apraxia. The patient does not correct this until the therapist verbally guides the action. Thus the patient needs verbal assistance to complete the combing task, as well as to overcome the motor apraxia. (d) Verbal assistance is not sufficient for the patient to perform, and the therapist needs to physically interfere and turn the brush correctly. Thus, some physical assistance is necessary in order for the patient to complete the activity (score of 1 on the Functional Independence Scale) and to overcome the motor apraxia (score of 3 on the Neurobehavioral Specific Impairment Scale). (e) The patient is unable to brush the hair because of a complete inability to sequence the different movements necessary for the activity. Thus a score of 0 on the Functional Independence Scale is given for the *Combing* item, and a score of 4 is given on the Neurobehavioral Specific Impairment Scale.

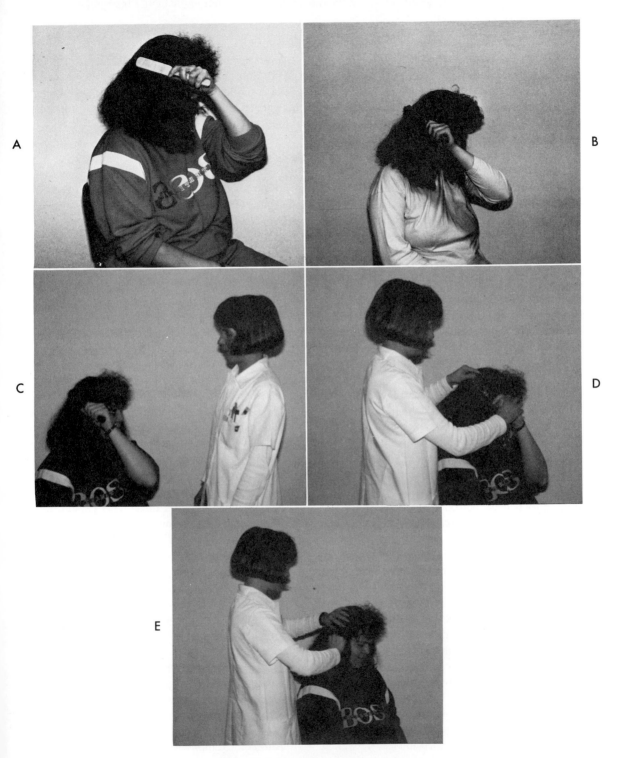

FIG. 10-2 For legend see opposite page.

domains should *not* be added up, as the categories are not additive. Patients can, for example, be independent in dressing, grooming, feeding, and transfers, although they cannot express themselves verbally or comprehend specific instructions. Further, the categories are not evenly weighted, and the intervals between the rank-ordered scores within the categories are not necessarily even. It is felt that the most frequent scores throughout the evaluation are much more informative in terms of independence level and assistance needed than are total scores. Comments regarding performance are thus preferred to total scores as conclusions.

The neurobehavioral impairment scores are transferred to a summary sheet, and the most frequent score for each neurobehavioral dysfunction component across the different functional domains can subsequently be determined. This score indicates the level of processing at which the patient should be approached in treatment. Fig. 10-3 shows the evaluation forms for the Functional Independence Scale, and the Neurobehavioral Specific Impairment Subscale in Part I of the A-ONE.

The scores on the Neurobehavioral Scale are not additive. Each deficit is identified, and its severity is evaluated and reported independently in the different domains. The most frequent score across domains for a particular impairment is much more informative in terms of treatment planning than is a total neurobehavioral score that has lost all important specific information for such purposes.

Note that the A-ONE is an evaluation instrument and not a treatment format. It is intended to assess functional performance, regardless of what methods are used to perform. Thus it does not require any specific procedures, such as standing up, by using Bobath procedures, or approaching a patient with some form of neglect from a particular side (there is a controversy among therapists as to which side)—methods whose effectiveness is judged differently by different therapists. However, in cases such as neglect it is important to provide an opportunity for the deficit to appear. Thus the patient should be approached from both sides, and

a note should be made of any neglect or inattention that may manifest. For the remainder of the evaluation the therapist may, at times, choose to approach the inattentive patient from the side that is not neglected to be better able to get information across to the patient.

CRITERIA FOR SCORING
Functional Independence Scale

Score each item separately. The following examples are only intended for guidance.

Dressing (shirt, pants, socks, shoes, and fastenings)

4 The person is completely independent in getting dressed. That is, no physical assistance is needed, no verbal assistance is needed, and the person does not need to be reminded to dress or to turn the clothes correctly (inside out or front to back). This person is able to carry performance over to different situations or environments.

3 The person is able to perform the activity of dressing but needs supervision from another person to perform. This person may lack the motivation or judgment to get dressed in the morning or to undress at night. This person might go to a dining room in a pajama jacket that he had slept in, or may need to be reminded to change clothes when they get dirty. This person might also need to have things located at specific sites in order to approach them and would, for example, not be able to get clothes from closets or gather other items needed. The score of 3 thus indicates that, although the person is able to perform, he or she may not do so without being monitored or supervised. This score gives an indication for and may justify the need for social services.

2 The person needs verbal assistance in order to complete an activity, for whatever reason. Examples would be, "You need to dress your other arm first" (in the case of a paralyzed person who has started by dressing the unaffected arm first). Another example would be, "Look, the shirt

A-ONE Part I
Functional Independence Scale and
Neurobehavioral Specific Impairment Subscale

Name_____   Date_____

INDEPENDENCE SCORE (IP):

4 = Independent and able to transfer activity to other environmental situations.
3 = Independent with supervision.
2 = Needs verbal assistance.
1 = Needs physical assistance.
0 = Unable to perform. Totally dependent on assistance.

LIST HELPING AIDS USED:

NEUROBEHAVIORAL SCORE (NB):

0 = No neurobehavioral impairments observed.
1 = Patient is able to perform without additional information, but some neurobehavioral impairment can be observed.
2 = Patient is able to perform with additional verbal assistance, but neurobehavioral impairment can be observed during performance.
3 = Patient is able to perform with demonstration or minimal to moderate physical assistance.
4 = Patient is unable to perform due to neurobehavioral impairment. Needs maximum physical assistance.

PRIMARY ADL ACTIVITY   SCORING   COMMENTS AND REASONING

DRESSING	IP SCORE					COMMENTS AND REASONING
Shirt (or dress)	4	3	2	1	0	
Pants	4	3	2	1	0	
Socks	4	3	2	1	0	
Shoes	4	3	2	1	0	
Fastenings	4	3	2	1	0	
Other						

NB IMPAIRMENT	NB SCORE					
Motor apraxia	0	1	2	3	4	
Ideational apraxia	0	1	2	3	4	
Unilateral body neglect	0	1	2	3	4	
Somatoagnosia	0	1	2	3	4	
Spatial relations	0	1	2	3	4	
Unilateral spatial neglect	0	1	2	3	4	
Abnormal tone: Right	0	1	2	3	4	
Abnormal tone: Left	0	1	2	3	4	
Perseveration	0	1	2	3	4	
Organization/Sequencing	0	1	2	3	4	
Other						

GROOMING AND HYGIENE	IP SCORE					
Wash face and upper body	4	3	2	1	0	
Comb hair	4	3	2	1	0	
Brush teeth	4	3	2	1	0	
Shave, makeup	4	3	2	1	0	
Continence/toilet	4	3	2	1	0	
Bath	4	3	2	1	0	
Other						

Note: All definitions and scoring criteria for each deficit are in the Evaluation Manual.

FIG. 10-3 Functional Independence Scale and Neurobehavioral Specific Impairment Subscale. (Copyright © 1988 by Guðrún Árnadóttir.) Please see order form on page following the Index for ordering test pads.

Continued.

	SCORING	COMMENTS AND REASONING

NB IMPAIRMENT (grooming)	NB SCORE					COMMENTS AND REASONING
Motor apraxia	0	1	2	3	4	
Ideational apraxia	0	1	2	3	4	
Unilateral body neglect	0	1	2	3	4	
Somatoagnosia	0	1	2	3	4	
Spatial relations	0	1	2	3	4	
Unilateral spatial neglect	0	1	2	3	4	
Abnormal tone: Right	0	1	2	3	4	
Abnormal tone: Left	0	1	2	3	4	
Perseveration	0	1	2	3	4	
Organization/Sequencing	0	1	2	3	4	
Other						

TRANSFERS AND MOBILITY	IP SCORE					
Sitting up in bed	4	3	2	1	0	
Transfers to/from bed (chair)	4	3	2	1	0	
Maneuver around	4	3	2	1	0	
Toilet transfers	4	3	2	1	0	
Tub transfers	4	3	2	1	0	
Other						

NB IMPAIRMENT	NB SCORE					
Motor apraxia	0	1	2	3	4	
Ideational apraxia	0	1	2	3	4	
Unilateral body neglect	0	1	2	3	4	
Spatial relations	0	1	2	3	4	
Unilateral spatial neglect	0	1	2	3	4	
Abnormal tone: Right	0	1	2	3	4	
Abnormal tone: Left	0	1	2	3	4	
Perseveration	0	1	2	3	4	
Organization/Sequencing	0	1	2	3	4	
Topographical disorientation	0	1	2	3	4	
Other						

FEEDING	IP SCORE					
Drinking from a mug	4	3	2	1	0	
Use fingers/sandwich	4	3	2	1	0	
Use fork or spoon	4	3	2	1	0	
Use knife	4	3	2	1	0	
Other						

NB IMPAIRMENT	NB SCORE					
Motor apraxia	0	1	2	3	4	
Ideational apraxia	0	1	2	3	4	
Unilateral body neglect	0	1	2	3	4	
Spatial relations	0	1	2	3	4	
Unilateral spatial neglect	0	1	2	3	4	
Abnormal tone: Right	0	1	2	3	4	
Abnormal tone: Left	0	1	2	3	4	
Perseveration	0	1	2	3	4	
Organization/Sequencing	0	1	2	3	4	
Other						

FIG. 10-3, cont'd

Functional Independence Scale and Neurobehavioral Specific Impairment Subscale continued.

SCORING   COMMENTS AND REASONING

COMMUNICATION	IP SCORE					COMMENTS AND REASONING
Comprehension	4	3	2	1	0	
Speech	4	3	2	1	0	

NB IMPAIRMENT	NB SCORE (0 = absent, 1 = present)					
Wernicke's aphasia	0	1				
Jargon aphasia	0	1				
Anomia	0	1				
Paraphasia	0	1				
Perseveration	0	1				
Broca's aphasia	0	1				
Dysarthria	0	1				
Other						

Results from specific sensory and motor tests:

Comments:

FUNCTIONAL INDEPENDENCE SCORE (optional)

FUNCTION	TOTAL SCORE	% SCORE
Dressing		
Grooming and hygiene		
Transfers and mobility		
Feeding		
Communication		

FIG. 10-3, cont'd

turns inside out" (when a person with a spatial-relation deficit attempts to put on a shirt without turning it right).

1 The therapist needs to physically assist or interfere with the patient's activity to get the desired outcome. This score indicates that the therapist has to use pointing or physical guidance in order to show the patient how to perform. An example would be the therapist pointing to a sock and then guiding the patient's hand with the sock to the patient's foot when the patient does not get the idea that she is to put on the sock. Another example would be pointing at a patient's shoulder where a shirt has gotten stuck when dressing, or guiding the patient's hand to the shoulder. This score also indicates that the therapist needs to assist the patient a little, or some, but that the patient does show *active participation* during performance. An example of this would be pulling down a shirt that has gotten stuck on the patient's shoulder, or physically stopping a person who persists in pulling on one sleeve, showing him that the shirt has gone far enough up the arm, and assisting in bringing the shirt behind the patient's back to the other side, so that the patient can proceed to dress the other arm.

0 The therapist must give a lot of assistance or completely dress the patient because of neuromuscular weakness or neurobehavioral deficits. An example of this would be a person who has just started sitting up in a chair and dressing the upper body but does not have the endurance or balance to dress the lower body (socks and pants).

Note: If a patient does not wear clothes with fastenings, it is possible to use the O.T. testing frames with buttons, zippers, and laces if required by the patient's habits. Do not give a patient credit for something that has not been tested. In many settings laces are changed to Velcro fastenings, or shoes with Velcro are purchased rather than laced shoes. The scoring of the item of *Fastenings* should take into account the individual patient's needs and habits. Some patients never wear clothes with zippers, thus, the ability to manipulate zippers does

not interfere with their independence. If a patient can button, but not zip up, and both are required by the patient's needs and habits, the lower score is indicated with comments. Some patients do wear clothes without fastenings. Note that many patients wear jogging suits without fastenings in the hospitals, but would not use this kind of clothing elsewhere. Use the item of *Fastenings* also to indicate the patient's ability to put on braces if this is pertinent. The *Socks* item refers to both socks, and thus the scoring targets the lower or more impaired performance elicited by putting on socks.

Common scoring mistakes. If a patient needs physical assistance when standing up to pull up trousers, this assistance is scored under *Dressing*, not under *Transfers.*

Grooming and hygiene (wash face and upper body, comb hair, brush teeth, shave/makeup, continence/toilet, and bathe)

4 The person is totally independent and will perform without any reminders. The outcome is acceptable, and the person is able to carry the performance over to new situations or environments.

3 The person is physically able to perform the components of grooming, but may not perform without supervision. This person may not consider combing the hair in the morning before going for treatment sessions or to the dining room. The person may lack memory, judgment, or motivation. The person may further not be able to organize which grooming items to use, or to gather these items if they are not laid out for him or her. Further assistance may be needed to clean up the sink area afterwards and make sure everything is in order.

2 The person needs verbal assistance in order to complete the activity. An example would be, "You already washed your face, now wash your body" (when a person perseverates in the former movements). Another example would be, "Your toothpaste is on your left side" (when the patient obviously keeps looking for the toothpaste without luck, in order to brush the teeth). A third

example would be, "You have not turned the water off yet" (when the person keeps the water running while dressing or even after leaving the sink area).

1 The therapist needs to physically assist or interfere with the patient's performance to obtain the desired outcome. An example would be when the therapist has to pantomime combing the hair, or physically guide the patient's hand towards the hair, in order for the patient to understand that he is to comb the hair. Another example would be when a therapist has to physically stop a patient who perseverates in washing the face, and move her arm over to another body part. A third example might be the therapist washing an unaffected arm for a person with a completely flaccid arm who is just starting ADL training.

0 The therapist must give a lot of assistance or completely perform the activity. An example would be the therapist holding both the patient's hands while the patient attempts to brush dentures or the therapist having to take over the activity when the patient looks as if he will not succeed. A third example would be the therapist having to wash a person completely because of the patient's apathy, or because the patient only touches the face or arm once with the washcloth.

Note: A score of 3 indicates that supervision is needed. If a patient is able to complete the shaving activity but needs assistance to plug in the electric cord, this becomes a score of 3 for shaving, not 1 (the razor could be left plugged in at the patient's home, or a battery-driven razor could be purchased that only had to be charged every now and then). Further, if a patient is able to wash her face, hands, underarms, and the front of her body but wants assistance for washing her back, this is given a score of 3, not 1. Many people do not wash their backs daily by a sink but do so only in the shower or a tub. Thus, this inability should be marked down for *Bathing,* but not for *Washing face and upper body.* Use the item of *Other* to indicate the ability to manipulate glasses and hearing aids when pertinent, with comments. If the inability to put on glasses interferes with independence, it is possible to score this inability under the item of *Makeup,* so it will be included in the total scores. **Common scoring mistakes.** *Transfers* is a separate category in the evaluation. *Continence* refers to whether the patient is continent and does not include the ability to get to and from the bathroom (mobility) or onto or off of the toilet (transfer). Similarly, bathing refers to the ability to bathe, not the ability to transfer into a tub. Note that bathing and continence are considered items on the functional scale only; they are not required for the neurobehavioral evaluation. The shades in the grooming and hygiene domain on the evaluation forms are intended to highlight this point.

Transfer behavior and mobility (sitting up in bed, transfers to and from bed/chair, maneuver around, toilet transfers, and tub transfers)

4 The person is completely independent in transfer behavior and moving around in the environment. This person knows his way and does not get lost.

3 The person may be able to transfer from a wheelchair independently at times, but supervision is required for safety reasons, as the person is not reliably consistent in successful transfer, or may be barely able to transfer.

2 The person needs verbal assistance to perform. For example, she may be instructed to place the unparalyzed arm on the armrest of a chair to push up, or to make sure that the chair is in the right place behind the patient before she lowers down to it during transfers.

1 The patient needs physical instructions or assistance in order to perform. An example would be the therapist placing the patient's arm on the armrest if the patient does not quite understand what to do, or giving a little physical assistance in order for the patient to get up from the bed or from a chair. The therapist could also allow the patient to pull on the therapist's arm as a physical assistance in order to get up. Further examples would be walking by the patient and giving him guidance and a little support when he is ambulating, or helping the patient to wheel straight ahead or to correct the wheelchair po-

sition after the patient has wheeled into the wall (possibly because of unilateral spatial neglect).

0 The patient needs full physical assistance to transfer and maneuver around. The patient does not have the endurance or understanding to move in a wheelchair. Another example would be when the therapist must transfer the patient from a bed to a wheelchair with minimum assistance from the patient, whether due to physical handicap or neurobehavioral deficits.

Note: This domain refers to ambulation indoors and on one level only. If needed, the item *Other* can be used, for example, to indicate the ability to maneuver on stairs if this is required by the patient's environment. The ability to get around outdoors and use public transportation is classified as a secondary ADL function in the A-ONE. Toilet and tub transfers are important components of an ADL evaluation, but they are not necessary to detect neurobehavioral deficits. This is indicated by shading on the evaluation forms.

Feeding (drink from a mug, use fingers/sandwich, use fork, spoon, and knife)

4 The patient is totally independent in feeding and will recognize the need to eat and the appropriate amounts of food to be ingested.

3 The patient needs supervision. This patient may forget to eat or may not be motivated to eat, although physically able to perform the activity. This person may also have a tendency to eat at all times, without remembering it, thus requiring supervision to control the amount of food intake.

2 The patient needs verbal assistance to perform. For example, "Your spoon is located on your left side on the table" (when a patient does not see the spoon she is looking for) or "Turn the other side of the knife down" (when the patient turns the knife wrong). Another example would be the therapist's asking the patient to use both hands to hold a cup that he cannot manage with one hand.

1 The patient needs minimal physical assistance, or the therapist must pantomime or physically interfere with the patient's activity. An example

would be pointing to the spoon (which the patient had not seen) by keeping the patient's attention on the therapist's hand. It might also be physically turning the patient's head so that she sees the spoon, or bringing the spoon into the patient's visual field. The therapist might assist the patient by guiding the first movements for eating and then have the patient take over.

0 Full assistance is needed for performance of task. The patient needs assistance to cut because he has a paralyzed arm and cannot yet manage a one-handed approach. Another example would be if the person does not know what to do with the food and starts poking or "playing" with it. This score is also given if a patient has to be fed because she is physically unable to perform.

Note: Under the item *Other* in the feeding section, the ability to open containers could be checked in hospitals where a patient's tray includes such things. Such performance can reveal neurobehavioral information, such as problem-solving strategies. These objects can further provide additional information in a clinical evaluation when they are available. However, they do not enter into scoring, as food preparation is considered a secondary ADL function in the A-ONE. The item *Use of knife* refers to both buttering and cutting. A score of 4 is only given when the patient is independent in both tasks. A score of 1 indicates the need for partial physical assistance in either or both tasks.

Communication (comprehension and speech)

4 The person can understand the therapist's verbal messages without any additional cues, and can be understood by the therapist (it is assumed that the therapist does not have problems).

3 This score is used for the speech category when a patient can make himself understandable, but the therapist notices signs of disarticulation, anomia, or slow speech production. This score is rarely used for the item of *Comprehension*.

2 The person needs additional verbal assistance to understand the verbal message; for example, sentences may have to be repeated, or broken down into fewer and shorter sentences. This

score also applies to speech if the therapist must repeat the patient's words to verify that the patient's message was understood correctly. Other examples would be when the therapist needs to correct words that have been altered or misplaced, or to add words that are missing in order to obtain the meaning.

1 Physical indications, such as pointing or pantomime, are needed in addition to verbal modification in order for the person to understand the therapist. This score is also used for speech, if the person needs to point or use pantomime in order to communicate.

0 For the *Speech* item, the patient is not able to communicate at all, by any means. For *Comprehension,* the patient cannot comprehend information provided by other individuals in the environment.

Common scoring mistakes. Where there is a comprehension deficit, so that the patient needs to be guided through movements or shown how to perform, a score of 2, which indicates verbal assistance, is impossible. (This refers to the entire evaluation, not just the two items on *Communication*.)

  Note: If the person uses communication tables instead of verbal output, a score of 1 would be given for expression through pointing or pantomime. This only affects the communication scores, since verbal output from the patient is not required elsewhere during the evaluation. This is because expression is not evaluated throughout, but the level of processing of information from the therapist and the environment does enter scoring.

**The Neurobehavioral Specific
Impairment Subscale**

In general, if the therapist notices any problems during the patient's ADL performance, these should be commented on and included in the evaluation report. For an example, obvious disability or neurobehavioral deficits may be noted when a patient takes off a pajama jacket, although putting on a shirt can be completed without problems. Be aware of automatic performance as compared to active use of planning and ideation. Small alterations in procedures may be needed to assess performance more fully when deficits are suspected or vague. Remember to give the patient a chance to show the deficit. Do not jump in too fast to assist without giving some thought to what the problem is.

  Scoring examples for the main categories follow in the next section. These are examples, but not complete criteria for scoring. Because this is a flexible clinical evaluation to assess behavior that has endless possibilities and combinations, the examples are to be considered as guidelines for therapists who have the skills to apply this information in other situations. Examples for each impairment do not span all the ADL domains. Note that a score of 0 is always given if no neurobehavioral or neuromotor impairments are observed during performance. Please refer to Chapter 7 for ADL examples of neurobehavioral dysfunctions and photographic illustrations.

Motor apraxia (ideomotor apraxia)

Motor apraxia refers to impaired planning and programming of action, due to disrupted processing of visuokinesthetic motor engrams, which manifests as clumsy inflexible movements even though the idea and purpose of the task are understood. Rule out pure executive motor disorders and pure sensory deficits.

0 No neurobehavioral deficits occur during performance.

1 Clumsiness in movement is observed, but the person is able to complete the activity without the therapist's intervention. An example might be holding a spoon or a comb with an awkward grasp. The right-hemiplegic patient may, for example, comb the left side of his hair well, but will show difficulty when attempting to adjust his grasp on the comb in moving on to comb the right side with the left hand.

2 The patient holding a comb with an awkward grasp needs verbal assistance in order to correct the grasp.

3 The therapist must physically assist the patient

who is holding a brush with an awkward grasp. The bristles of the brush may be turned away from the patient's head, and the patient's movements may not be flexible enough to turn the brush around although she understands what she is supposed to do.

4 The therapist must brush the patient's hair if the activity is to be completed properly.

Note: Fig. 10-4 presents the Neurobehavioral Specific Impairment Checklist, which contains behavioral examples for different neurobehavioral deficits. The checklist is used for teaching purposes during the therapist's training as a guideline for identifying types of neurobehavioral impairments. **Common scoring mistakes.** Do not confuse motor (ideomotor) apraxia with ideational apraxia.

Text continued on p. 245.

Name_____   Date_____

ACTIVITIES OF DAILY LIVING (ADL) FUNCTIONS	NEUROBEHAVIORAL IMPAIRMENT SCORE		
DRESSING	PRESENT	ABSENT	COMMENT

MOTOR APRAXIA

1. Has difficulties related to motor planning. May grab a shirt or a sock, but has trouble adjusting the grasp according to needs.   ☐   ☐

2. Difficulties with buttons or fastenings because of clumsy hand movements: R/L side?   ☐   ☐

IDEATIONAL APRAXIA

1. Does not know what to do with shirt, pants, or socks.   ☐   ☐

2. Misuses clothes. Starts to put leg into armhole or arm into leghole.   ☐   ☐

(a) Other apraxia: ☐   ☐

UNILATERAL BODY NEGLECT

1. Does not dress the affected body side.   ☐   ☐

2. Does not pull down shirt all the way on the affected side, or shirt gets stuck on the affected shoulder without the person's trying to correct it or realizing what is wrong.   ☐   ☐

NOTE: All definitions are in the Evaluation Manual

FIG. 10-4 Neurobehavioral Specific Impairment Checklist. (Copyright © 1988 by Guðrún Árnadóttir.) Please see order form on page following the Index for ordering test pads.

ADL FUNCTIONS	NEUROBEHAVIORAL IMPAIRMENT SCORE		
DRESSING (continued)	PRESENT	ABSENT	COMMENT

SOMATOAGNOSIA

1. Starts putting legs into armholes or arms into legholes. ☐ ☐

(b) Other body-scheme disorders: ☐ ☐

SPATIAL-RELATION DISORDERS

1. Unable to find armholes, legholes, or bottom of shirt. ☐ ☐

2. Pulls sleeve in the wrong direction. ☐ ☐

3. Unable to differentiate front from back or inside from outside of clothes. ☐ ☐

4. Aims correctly at armholes but misses it without noticing. ☐ ☐

5. Matches buttons and buttonholes incorrectly. ☐ ☐

6. Puts hand into sleeve through distal instead of proximal opening. ☐ ☐

7   Legholes end up inside of pants at the top opening without the person realizing it or being able to correct it. ☐ ☐

8. Puts arm through neckhole. ☐ ☐

9. Unable to learn to tie laces one-handed when other hand is paralyzed. This may be the reason for refusing to try the method. ☐ ☐

10. Attempts to turn shirt front to back with the shirt on by pulling at the bottom of the shirt, not realizing that the shirt will not turn while arms are in the sleeves. Similarily, may try to turn pants front to back after placing one leg into leghole, by pulling at the waist opening. ☐ ☐

11. Places foot in the wrong leghole. ☐ ☐

FIG. 10-4, cont'd

Continued.

| ADL FUNCTIONS | NEUROBEHAVIORAL IMPAIRMENT SCORE | | |
| DRESSING (continued) | PRESENT | ABSENT | COMMENT |

UNILATERAL SPATIAL NEGLECT

1.   Does not pay attention to clothes placed in the visual field opposite to the lesion.   ☐   ☐

(c)   Other spatial-relations problems: ☐   ☐

PERSEVERATION

1.   Repeats movements or acts and cannot stop them once initiated. Attempts, for example, to put on shirt without any progress. May pull the front edge of a long sleeve up arm way past the wrist.   ☐   ☐

2.   Attempts to button many buttonholes onto the same button.   ☐   ☐

3.   Attempts to put the same arm into both sleeves.   ☐   ☐

4.   Persists motorically in looking for the hole of a sock on the toe side, although the hole cannot be found there.   ☐   ☐

(d)   Other perseveration problems: ☐   ☐

ORGANIZATION AND SEQUENCING

1.   Has difficulty sequencing the steps of the activity. Will, for example, dress the unaffected arm before the affected one, then run into trouble dressing the affected arm.   ☐   ☐

2.   Does not include all steps of the activity. Does not, for example, complete the fastenings (buttons, zippers, laces) as required by the nature of the activity.   ☐   ☐

3.   Will stop the activity after each step and will have to be "programmed" by the therapist to continue.   ☐   ☐

4.   Will put on the shoes before putting on the trousers.   ☐   ☐

(e)   Other organization problems: ☐   ☐

FIG. 10-4, cont'd

ADL FUNCTIONS	NEUROBEHAVIORAL IMPAIRMENT SCORE		
GROOMING AND HYGIENE	PRESENT	ABSENT	COMMENT

MOTOR APRAXIA

1. Unable to open water taps but understands the concept and has sufficient hand strength to perform. ☐ ☐

2. Unable to change the position of the comb, razor, or toothbrush to a functional one when holding it or to adjust the grasp when reaching to the other side, although the comb does not turn right. ☐ ☐

3. Unable to change an awkward grasp when holding the washcloth. Right or left side involvement? Both sides? ☐ ☐

IDEATIONAL APRAXIA

1. Does not understand what to do with the washcloth or the soap. ☐ ☐

2. Holds the washcloth and reaches for the toothpaste. ☐ ☐

3. Cannot figure out what to use to turn the water on. Pulls or attempts to turn in the wrong places. ☐ ☐

4. Places the washcloth where the water should be running to wet it, although the water is not running. ☐ ☐

5. Uses the washcloth to wash the sink instead of face. ☐ ☐

6. Uses tools inappropriately, for example, toothbrush for combing hair, shaves hair or eyebrows with razor, or smears toothpaste over face. ☐ ☐

7. Gets confused if grasping incorrect object, e.g., glass instead of toothbrush, ending up by squeezing the toothpaste into the glass or stirring the toothpaste in the glass. ☐ ☐

FIG. 10-4, cont'd

Continued.

ADL FUNCTIONS	NEUROBEHAVIORAL IMPAIRMENT SCORE		
GROOMING AND HYGIENE (continued)	PRESENT	ABSENT	COMMENT
8. Does not realize how to wet the deodorant when it is dry, that is, by turning it upside down. Tries to put it under the running water.	☐	☐	
9. Grabs the therapist's hand and puts it toward the mouth when the therapist points to his/her mouth to get him to take out the dentures.	☐	☐	
10. Patient bites on toothbrush as it is placed into patient's mouth.	☐	☐	
11. Patient automatically places the washcloth in the paralyzed hand and uses the unparalyzed hand to move the paralyzed one, in an attempt to wash.	☐	☐	
(f) Other apraxia:	☐	☐	
UNILATERAL BODY NEGLECT			
1. Washes, combs, or shaves only half of the body or face.	☐	☐	
2. May not use the affected hand for assistance when performing bilateral activities.	☐	☐	
3. Spills liquid from after-shave bottle held by the affected hand, while looking at his own face in mirror.	☐	☐	
SOMATOAGNOSIA			
1. Brushes teeth on the mirror instead of own, or washes mirror image.	☐	☐	
2. Washes only one part of the body at a time and then dries before going on to the next part; that is, washes face first, then neck, then only one arm, then the other arm, and finally chest. Divides the body into fragments.	☐	☐	
(g) Other body-scheme impairments:	☐	☐	

FIG. 10-4, cont'd

ADL FUNCTIONS	NEUROBEHAVIORAL IMPAIRMENT SCORE		
GROOMING AND HYGIENE (continued)	PRESENT	ABSENT	COMMENT

UNILATERAL SPATIAL NEGLECT

1. Does not use object located on the affected side. Is not aware that a part of the visual field in neglected. ☐ ☐

2. Does not use the instrument correctly; e.g., does not use handle of a brush if the handle is located in the neglected visual field before he/she picks it up. ☐ ☐

SPATIAL-RELATION DYSFUNCTION

1. Puts glasses on turning them upside down. Attempts to put bottom part of dentures into the roof of mouth. ☐ ☐

2. Over or underestimates distances. Example: reaches i.e. with washcloth for water above as well as below the faucet. ☐ ☐

3. Grabs the wrong object when two or more objects are placed on the sink, e.g., glass instead of toothbrush. ☐ ☐

(h) Other spatial relation impairments: ☐ ☐

PERSEVERATION

1. Repeats movements or acts and cannot stop them once initiated. May wash face, complete the activity, and then start washing face over again from the beginning (perseverates actions) or may be unable to stop washing face (perseverates movements). ☐ ☐

2. May be unable to stop movement of putting soap on washcloth. ☐ ☐

(i) Other perseveration problems: ☐ ☐

FIG. 10-4, cont'd

Continued.

ADL FUNCTIONS	NEUROBEHAVIORAL IMPAIRMENT SCORE		
GROOMING AND HYGIENE (continued)	PRESENT	ABSENT	COMMENT

ORGANIZATION AND SEQUENCING

		PRESENT	ABSENT
1.	Does not turn off water after washing or turn off electric shaver.	☐	☐
2.	Does not wring out washcloth after washing.	☐	☐
3.	Washes only one part of the body at a time; e.g., fragments activity into more than face and upper body.	☐	☐
4.	Does not complete one activity before starting the next; e.g., stops washing in the middle of the process when sees uncombed hair in the mirror.	☐	☐
5.	Does not take off glasses to wash face. Does not wet hands before putting on soap when washing hands.	☐	☐
(j)	Other organization problems:	☐	☐

ADL FUNCTIONS	NEUROBEHAVIORAL IMPAIRMENT SCORE		
TRANSFER ABILITY AND MOBILITY	PRESENT	ABSENT	COMMENT

MOTOR APRAXIA

		PRESENT	ABSENT
1.	Has trouble orienting body in terms of directions according to the intended activity.	☐	☐

IDEATIONAL APRAXIA

		PRESENT	ABSENT
1.	Does not know what to do to move. Does not know how to move. Gets trapped, for example, in the sheets without knowing why or what to do.	☐	☐
2.	Gets into bed by turning sideways. Does not realize that this is not the right position.	☐	☐
3.	Does not know how to use stool to climb into a high bed, although motoric function is intact.	☐	☐

FIG. 10-4, cont'd

TRANSFER ABILITY AND MOBILITY (continued)	PRESENT	ABSENT	COMMENT
4. Attempts to wheel wheelchair by grabbing and pushing down the arm rest.	☐	☐	
(k) Other apraxia:	☐	☐	

UNILATERAL BODY NEGLECT

	PRESENT	ABSENT	COMMENT
1. Does not account for one side of the body when moving. Walks into doorways. When transferring over to a chair patient may only move unaffected side to the chair. The affected side or a part of it may end up off the chair.	☐	☐	
2. When sitting up in bed to transfer, may place blanket over the affected hand as if it were not there.	☐	☐	
3. Lying in bed, the patient may claim that the arm beside him is not his own and that it belongs to somebody else. He may also refer to it as an object such as "an old wreck of a car."	☐	☐	
(l) Other body-scheme disorders:	☐	☐	

UNILATERAL SPATIAL NEGLECT

	PRESENT	ABSENT	COMMENT
1. Does not account for objects in the visual field on the affected side when moving. Wheels into walls.	☐	☐	

TOPOGRAPHICAL DISORIENTATION

	PRESENT	ABSENT	COMMENT
1. Does not know her way to the room or to the bathroom. Cannot locate closet and drawers in own room.	☐	☐	

SPATIAL-RELATION DISORDERS

	PRESENT	ABSENT	COMMENT
1. Has trouble orienting body in terms of directions according to the intended activity. Leans forward instead of backward when assisting with getting out of bed.	☐	☐	
2. May grab the armrest of the wheelchair instead of the wheel and push down on it.	☐	☐	
(m) Other spatial-relation symptoms:	☐	☐	

FIG. 10-4, cont'd

Continued.

ADL FUNCTIONS	NEUROBEHAVIORAL IMPAIRMENT SCORE		
TRANSFER ABILITY & MOBILITY (continued)	PRESENT	ABSENT	COMMENT

PERSEVERATION

1.   May wheel into things because of inability to stop the movement of wheeling after the desired destination has been reached. ☐ ☐

(n)   Other perseveration problems: ☐ ☐

ORGANIZATION AND SEQUENCING

1.   Does not put the brakes on the wheelchair when transferring. Sits up in bed and attempts to get out of it without taking blanket off. ☐ ☐

(o)   Other organization problems: ☐ ☐

ADL FUNCTIONS	NEUROBEHAVIORAL IMPAIRMENT SCORE		
FEEDING	PRESENT	ABSENT	COMMENT

MOTOR APRAXIA

1.   Uses clumsy, inflexible movements that lack goal-directed sequencing to hold cup, fork, or spoon. ☐ ☐

2.   Spills food because of inablity to adjust movement when getting food to mouth. ☐ ☐

IDEATIONAL APRAXIA

1.   Misuses utensils; e.g., uses knife instead of fork. ☐ ☐

2.   Takes a long time because of delay in conceptualization about what to do. ☐ ☐

3.   Does not know what to do with utensils or food. ☐ ☐

4.   Eats egg with a knife, or bread with a spoon. ☐ ☐

(p)   Other apraxia: ☐ ☐

FIG. 10-4, cont'd

UNILATERAL BODY NEGLECT

1.   Does not attend to or use affected arm when eating, so it is placed in the food or in awkward positions.   ☐ ☐

(q)   Other somatoagnostic impairments: ☐ ☐

UNILATERAL SPATIAL NEGLECT

1.   Does not attend to food or utensils located on the affected side.   ☐ ☐

2.   Does not attend to a person speaking on the affected side. Looks either straight forward or to the unaffected side when listening and answering.   ☐ ☐

3.   Person turns all the way to the unaffected side when eating, or to the visual field that is not neglected.   ☐ ☐

SPATIAL RELATIONS

1.   Over- or underestimates distances when reaching for cup or utensils or when bringing them to mouth.   ☐ ☐

(r)   Other spatial-relations impairments: ☐ ☐

PERSEVERATION

1.   Unable to stop movements or actions. May keep stuffing food into mouth without swallowing.   ☐ ☐

2.   May use a spoon to eat soup and be unable to let go of the spoon, using it for a coffee cup too instead of drinking from the cup.   ☐ ☐

(s)   Other perseveration problems: ☐ ☐

ORGANIZATION AND SEQUENCING

1.   Attempts to eat food without cutting it or asking for it to be cut. Keeps stuffing food into mouth without swallowing between.   ☐ ☐

(t)   Other organization problems: ☐ ☐

FIG. 10-4, cont'd

Continued.

ADL FUNCTIONS	NEUROBEHAVIORAL IMPAIRMENT SCORE		
COMMUNICATION	PRESENT	ABSENT	COMMENT

LANGUAGE DISORDERS

		PRESENT	ABSENT	
1.	**WERNICKE'S APHASIA:** Difficulty comprehending spoken language; does not understand one- or two-word commands (or more). Does not perform according to verbal instruction.	☐	☐	
2.	**JARGON APHASIA:** Uses unintelligible speech.	☐	☐	
3.	**ANOMIA:** Difficulty finding names of objects.	☐	☐	
4.	**PARAPHASIA:** Replaces words with incorrect similar or dissimilar words.	☐	☐	
5.	**CIRCUMLOCUTION:** Uses lengthy descriptions instead of exact words.	☐	☐	
6.	**ECHOLALIA:** Repeats words or phrases from the environment and adds to own sentences.			
7.	**PERSEVERATION:** Repeats the same words or syllables over and over. Difficulties switching to other words or syllables.	☐	☐	
8.	**BROCA'S APHASIA:** Total expressive aphasia or nonfluent speech. Unable to express oneself verbally.	☐	☐	
9.	**DYSARTHRIA:** Problems with articulation of speech musculature.	☐	☐	
10.	**ORAL APRAXIA:** Difficulties planning and sequencing oral movements necessary for smooth speech.	☐	☐	
11.	**MUTISM:** No attempt to express verbally, nor by other means.	☐	☐	
(u)	Other language disorders.	☐	☐	

FIG. 10-4, cont'd

Exhibit 10-1. Apraxias and Locations of Cortical Dysfunction

Apraxias	Locations of dysfunction
Motor apraxia (ideomotor)	Left inferior parietal lobule
	Left premotor frontal cortex
	Left supplementary motor cortex
	Anterior corpus callosum
	Right supplementary motor area
	Right premotor frontal area
Ideational apraxia	Left inferior parietal lobe
	Left premotor frontal cortex
	Left prefrontal cortex
	Corpus callosum
	Right premotor frontal cortex
	Right prefrontal cortex

EVALUATIVE CONSIDERATIONS FOR DIFFERENTIATION OF APRAXIA TYPES

Does the patient have an idea of what to do (ideation)?

Does the patient know which objects to use (ideation)?

Does the patient know how to perform or how to use the objects (ideation)?

Do the movements appear to be clumsy (motoric)?

Can the patient adjust grasp according to altered requirements during object use (motoric)?

Are there problems with sequencing and organization of activity steps (ideation)?

Are there problems with sequencing of movements (motoric)?

Ideational apraxia

Ideational apraxia refers to impaired knowledge or lack of an idea regarding what needs to be done in order to perform a particular activity. Rule out auditory comprehension problems.

0 No neurobehavioral deficits appear.

1 The patient hesitates or takes a long time to perform (that is, to wash the face or turn on water faucets) because of a delay in conceptualizing what to do to perform the activity. However, the patient is able to complete the activity without the therapist's interference.

2 The therapist must tell the patient what to do so that she will understand what to do with the washcloth when she is sitting by a sink. Note that the sequencing and organization of an activity are related to ideation, but should be scored separately on the scale.

3 The therapist must physically assist the patient (that is, wet the washcloth and guide the patient's hand toward his face) in order for the patient to understand that he is expected to wash.

4 The patient does not understand what to do, or how to wash the face despite extra verbal and physical cues. The therapist must perform the activity for the patient. Exhibit 10-1 illustrates how one can differentiate between motor and ideational apraxia. It further reviews apraxia types and the cerebral localization of possible dysfunction.

Common scoring mistakes. Make sure to differentiate between motor (ideomotor) and ideational apraxia. Also try to differentiate between ideational apraxia and its subcomponents of sequencing and organization.

Exhibit 10-2. Body-Scheme Disorders and Locations of Cortical Dysfunctions

Body-scheme disorders	Locations of dysfunction
Unilateral body neglect	Inferior parietal lobule (usually right) Dorsolateral frontal lobe Cingulate gyrus
Somatoagnosia	Right inferior parietal lobule (somatosensory and visuospatial problems) Left parieto-temporal area (language problems)

EVALUATIVE CONSIDERATIONS FOR DIFFERENTIATION OF BODY SCHEME DISORDERS

Does the patient take care of and account for the paralyzed side during performance (unilateral body neglect)?

Does the patient use the body side contralateral to the affected cerebral hemisphere in proportion to physical capabilities of those body parts, including strength (unilateral body neglect/inattention)?

Does the patient have to attend specifically, for example, to a paralyzed hand by vision during performance (sensory impairment/unilateral body neglect)?

Does the patient account for the affected body side, for example, leave the left side off the chair while transferring over to the right side (unilateral body neglect)?

Does the patient account for the extrapersonal space or objects in the environment during performance (unilateral spatial neglect)?

Does the patient understand and correctly use spatial concepts in relation to his or her own body (somatoagnosia/right-left discrimination problems/pure comprehension problems)?

Is there any evidence of fragmented organization in activities that relate to the patient's body (somatoagnosia/sequencing and organization impairment)?

Does the patient grasp the therapist's arm and attempt to dress it instead of his or her own arm (somatoagnosia)?

Is there any manifestation of visual-spatial problems (provoked, e.g., by a mirror) that interfere with the person's performance when he or she is relating tasks to his or her own body (somatoagnosia/spatial-relations problems)?

Unilateral body neglect

Unilateral body neglect is a failure to attend, respond, or orient to a unilateral stimulus presented to the body side or extremities contralateral to the cerebral lesion.

0 No neurobehavioral deficits are observed.

1 The patient does not use both hands when feeding although he or she has enough muscle power in the affected hand and arm to assist the other hand. However, the activity is completed without the therapist's interference. The patient may not attend to an arm or may not position it correctly while using the other arm when feeding.

2 The therapist gives the patient verbal cues regarding the use of the neglected hand (for example, to use the neglected hand to stabilize a sandwich while buttering it, or a cup while pouring into it). The therapist has to tell the patient to lift a neglected arm that has fallen off a table top and must ask him to place it on the table.

3 The therapist needs to show the patient how to use the neglected hand, for example, to stabilize things.

4 The therapist must do activities that require bilateral involvement for the patient, such as buttering. Notice that this would be necessary as a result of unilateral body neglect in this case, not because of motor paralysis or spasticity. Exhibit 10-2 reviews possible cerebral location of dysfunction when unilateral body neglect is manifested.

Somatoagnosia

Somatoagnosia refers to impaired structural awareness of the body, the failure to recognize one's body parts and their relation to each other in a coherent way.

0 No neurobehavioral deficits appear.

1 The patient makes a movement indicating that he intended to move the toothbrush toward a mirror instead of toward his own face.

2 Verbal interference is needed to direct the patient's hand toward her own mouth.

3 The therapist must physically point to the toothbrush and then to the patient's mouth, or take the patient's hand and guide it to his mouth in order to get him to overcome the somatoagnosia and perform.

4 The therapist must perform the activity for the patient because neither verbal nor physical cues are sufficient to assist the patient in performing (see Exhibit 10-2).

Unilateral spatial neglect

Unilateral spatial neglect refers to the failure to attend, respond, and orient to a unilateral visual stimulus presented to the visual field contralateral to the cerebral lesion. Rule out hemianopsia or loss of visual field.

0 No neurobehavioral deficits are observed.

1 The patient needs to look around and turn his head to locate things in the neglected visual field. However, the patient will complete the activity without the therapist's interference.

2 The therapist must tell the patient that, for example, the comb is located on her left side, or remind the patient to look to the affected side when she can't find the comb.

3 The therapist must point to the comb and make the patient visually follow the movement of a pointing finger from the intact visual field over to the comb in the neglected visual field or must turn the patient's head in order for him to see it.

4 The therapist must bring the object into the patient's visual field (Exhibit 10-3).

   Note: Chapter 7 provides a description of the loss of a visual field and indicates how it can be ruled out.

Spatial relation disorders

Spatial relation disorders refers to problems in the perception of spatial relationships and distances between objects or between the self and objects. Check for ideational problems.

0 No neurobehavioral deficits appear during performance.

1 The patient initially attempts to reach for a glass, but goes too far or not far enough, misjudging the distance before grasping the glass itself. However, no assistance or interference from the therapist is necessary to correct and complete the act.

2 The person needs verbal assistance to correct a mistake, for example, the attempt to open a sock at the toe end instead of at the opening; or verbal assistance may be needed for the patient to turn the heel part of the sock from the dorsum of the foot to the plantar surface because the patient does not recognize that it is turned wrong.

3 Physical assistance is needed, for example, taking the sock away from the person and handing it back so the opening is turned up, or giving physical assistance to turn the heel down from the dorsum of the foot.

4 The therapist must more or less put the sock on the patient's foot (Exhibit 10-3).

   Note: For the A-ONE, spatial-relations impairment of visual-spatial origin is synonymous with visual-spatial agnosia.

Topographical disorientation

Topographical disorientation refers to difficulty in understanding and remembering the relationships of places to one another, resulting in the difficulty of finding one's way in space.

0 No neurobehavioral deficits appear.

1 The patient shows hesitation regarding directions when going from one place to another (for example, to the dining room) but is able to get to the right place without the therapist's intervention. This could also refer to difficulties in find-

Exhibit 10-3. Spatial-Relations Impairments and Locations of Cortical Dysfunctions

Spatial-relations impairments	Locations of dysfunction
Unilateral spatial neglect	Right inferior parietal lobule (left one also possible) Dorsolateral frontal lobe Cingulate gyrus
Spatial-relation disorders	Inferior parietal region (usually right side) Parieto-occipital association cortex
Topographical disorientation	Posterior parietal area (usually right) if visual problem Temporal lobe (usually right) if memory problem

EVALUATIVE CONSIDERATIONS FOR DIFFERENTIATION OF SPATIAL-RELATIONS IMPAIRMENT TYPES

Does the patient attend visually to objects in both visual fields (unilateral spatial neglect)?

Does the patient spontaneously compensate for presence of visual defect/neglect by turning the head appropriately, and complain about it (awareness of defect points to visual-field defect; unawareness to visual-field inattention or neglect)?

Does the patient drive into things because of unilateral spatial neglect, or walk into things because of unilateral body neglect (visual-spatial or somatic disorder)? Both deficits are commonly present simultaneously.

Does the patient respond correctly to spatial concepts (comprehension/use of spatial concepts)?

Does the patient over- or underestimate distances (visual-spatial agnosia/spatial-relations impairment)?

Does the patient perform according to the direction needed for the activity, i.e., pull a shirt on instead of off the arm or lean body in the correct direction according to required activity performance (spatial-relations impairment)?

Does the patient differentiate between front and back, top and bottom of objects (spatial-relations impairment)?

Is the patient able to differentiate between foreground and background (figure-ground/spatial-relations impairment/visual-spatial agnosia)?

Is the patient able to verbally describe a plan of action (ideational apraxia)?

Is the patient able to perceive his or her own body and body parts as a whole, relate to it as such, and differentiate between its parts (somatoagnosia)?

Is the patient attending adequately to the performance and attempting to utilize available information regarding spatial relations during performance (attentional deficit)?

Is the patient able to differentiate right performance from wrong one (lack of judgment)?

Is the patient able to realize the significance of mistakes for the purpose of improving performance (concrete thought)?

Is the patient able to spatially move body in directions required by an activity or organize movements according to activity requirements (with or without objects) where comprehension of spatial information is not required (motor apraxia/ideational apraxia/spatial-relations impairment/somatoagnosia)?

Which of the following describes the patient's performance errors: lack of comprehension of spatial concepts, attention deficit, ideational apraxia, motor apraxia, somatoagnosia, spatial relation problems (visual/motoric) concrete thought, lack of judgment?

Does the patient remember the way around in the environment, or the location of specific objects (topographical disorientation, memory problems)?

Does the patient visually perceive the environment correctly (visual-spatial problems)?

ing the objects needed for ADL skill performance in the room.

2 The patient needs verbal instructions from the
therapist in order to find the right direction or
the right destination.

3 The therapist must point or physically direct the
patient to the right direction or destination.

4 The therapist must physically direct the patient
without the patient's active involvement as to
where he or she is going (Exhibit 10.3).

Note: If the patient is *physically* unable to go
by herself from one place to another, that does not
mean that she is topographically disoriented. In that
case, the therapist should ask the patient where the
dining room is or where the bathroom is to get a
feeling for the presence of topographical disorientation.

Abnormal tone

Abnormal tone refers to flaccidity, decreased
strength, rigidity, spasticity, ataxia, athetosis, and
tremor, as defined in the glossary. Make sure to
indicate which deficits are noted in the *Comments*
section. Observe how deficits affect functional performance. Note weakness or observable abnormalities in muscle patterns. Note errors in rate of
movement, range, direction, and force when objects are approached. If in doubt after observing a
patient's performance, check out the involved extremity by passive or active manipulation (muscle
strength, range of movement, spasticity, or rigidity). Also compare the two upper extremities by
grasping the patient's hands and providing resistance to movements where needed to evaluate
weakness.

0 No neurological deficits are observed in extremities during performance.

1 Flaccidity, decreased strength, rigidity, spasticity, ataxia, or tremor are observed during performance, even though these conditions, which
can affect any extremity, do not interfere with
the completion of a functional task. For example,
a person may have a flaccid left arm but still be
able to comb his hair with the right arm, or even
be able to comb it with a weak or partially spastic

arm. Make sure to indicate which deficits are
noted in the *Comments* section. If in doubt,
check out the extremity involved by passive or
active manipulation.

2 Abnormalities are observed, such as flaccidity
or spasticity, but the individual is able to perform
with verbal guidance only. For example, a person who has a flaccid left arm asks the therapist
for assistance in order to open a tube of toothpaste. The therapist verbally instructs the patient
how the tube can be held in order to open it by
a one-handed technique.

3 Physical assistance is needed in order for the
person to complete the activity. Examples would
be helping to pull a sleeve all the way up a flaccid
arm when a patient attempts to dress, or pulling
a shirt that gets stuck on the patient's shoulder,
or providing assistance in pulling a shirt down
at the patient's back or sides.

4 The therapist must dress the patient because of
a neuromuscular disability.

Common scoring mistakes. A patient with a flaccid
arm or unilateral neglect may be able to perform
an activity more or less one-handed. However, that
does not mean that the deficits are not present,
although they did not interfere with function in this
particular activity. Thus a score of 1 should be
given for abnormal tone of the particular extremity,
if manifested during these activities. One sound
arm does not mean that both arms are unimpaired.
Use the items of *Right and Left tone* to differentiate
between the two body sides. Make sure to differentiate between neuromuscular and neurobehavioral interference with ADL task performance, and
score accordingly. A person with weakness of
grasp can appear "clumsy," and this should not be
confused with motor apraxia.

Perseveration

Perseveration refers to difficulties in starting and
stopping actions and in shifting from one pattern
of response to another, whether for particular
movements or for whole tasks. Although the evaluation format does not differentiate between perseveration of a movement and perseveration of an

Exhibit 10-4. Perseverations and Locations of Cortical Dysfunctions

Perseverations	Locations of dysfunction
Premotor perseveration	Premotor frontal areas
Prefrontal perseveration	Prefrontal areas

EVALUATIVE CONSIDERATIONS FOR DIFFERENTIATION OF PERSEVERATIVE TYPES

Does the patient repeat some movements beyond the task requirements or have trouble stopping movements (premotor).

Does the patient repeat whole acts or activity steps after completing them (prefrontal).

action or task, therapists should consider which form the impairment takes and use that information if needed for localization purposes.

0 No perseverations are observed during function.

1 The patient perseverates; for example, she washes the face two or three times but is able to complete the activity without the therapist's interference.

2 The therapist needs to tell the patient that he has already finished washing the face in order to get the patient to stop the movements of washing the face, and continue to the next step in the sequence.

3 The therapist must point to another body part or take the patient's hand and direct it to washing arms and chest when the patient perseverates in washing the face.

4 The therapist must wash the patient because perseverations make the patient unable to move from one activity step to the next (Exhibit 10-4).

   Note: Field-dependent behavior is a form of perseveration. It can manifest both as motor perseveration and as perseveration of actions. Further, field dependency interferes with attention, as will be discussed later in this chapter.

Organization and sequencing problems

Organization and sequencing refer to the inability to organize one's thoughts in order to perform an activity and to perform in an organized way with the activity steps properly sequenced and timed.

0 No difficulties with organization or sequencing appear during the activity.

1 Problems with organization and/or sequencing do appear. The patient, for example, may not include all the steps of an activity, may show hesitation regarding their order (the sequencing), or may not include the steps in the usual sequence, but nevertheless succeeds in finishing the activity. An example would be a patient who takes a bar of soap and starts to use it without wetting the hands first, before realizing the mistake, or a patient who leaves for the dining room with a shirt tangled at the back.

2 The therapist must tell the patient which step is next or verbally interfere with performance if the patient skips steps. An example would be saying, "The soap is still on your body," after a patient has put the soap on body and then takes the towel to dry off. Another example would be "Dress your affected arm before the unaffected one," when a patient has a paralyzed arm. The therapist may also have to ask the patient to take off her glasses while washing the face.

3 The therapist must physically interfere with the activity sequence, that is, show the patient how to undress an unaffected arm and guide him in dressing the affected arm first when he cannot complete a dressing activity because he started

dressing the unaffected arm and then got into trouble with the affected side.

4 The therapist has to more or less dress the patient because of problems in organization and sequencing.

Note: Sequencing and organization are partially related to ideation. Thus, the signs of impaired organization and sequencing will often appear simultaneously with ideational apraxia. However, in the A-ONE they are scored separately. Ideational apraxia is a more global and severe dysfunction than sequencing or organization problems. A patient can have problems with sequencing an activity although she has a general idea of what to do. In terms of both ideation and organization, be aware of when the patient is performing automatically. If in doubt, check whether she can deal with a little alteration in the requirements of the activity. Also note that organizational and sequencing problems can be a sign of a very mild ideational problem if these are considered on a continuum. It can also be a residual effect after more severe signs of ideational apraxia have subsided, when a patient has made progress.

Common scoring mistakes. Pay attention to the organization, sequencing, and timing of activity components and steps. Manifestations of impaired organization and sequencing are easily overlooked.

• • •

When scoring neurobehavioral deficits, note that a patient can obtain a score of 4 or 3 on the Functional Independence Scale, even though an impairment may be present. A deficit that does not interfere with completion of a functional task is scored a 1. Further, if a patient needs *verbal* assistance for putting on a shirt, for example, because of motor apraxia, but needs *physical* assistance for putting on pants, because of the same deficit, the item of *Motor apraxia* under the dressing domain is scored according to the need for physical assistance (the more severe manifestation).

The language disorders are presented as a part of the Neurobehavioral Specific Impairment Subscale because they relate specifically to the category of communication. However, in many ways they have more in common with the items on the Neurobehavioral Pervasive Impairment Subscale. This is because the language deficits may be manifested throughout the evaluation, as well as in the introduction prior to the ADL task performance. Further, these items are only scored as present (1) or absent (0). The Neurobehavioral Specific Impairment Checklist in Fig. 10-4 describes these deficits and provides more possibilities of different types of impairments than does the Neurobehavioral Specific Impairment Subscale. Thus, under the item *Other,* specify the additional deficits observed. The checklist provides guidance for detecting deficits, and the conceptual definitions for these can be found in the glossary at the end of the text.

Checklists

Two checklists were developed as guidelines to aid therapists in the detection of neurobehavioral deficits. The checklists are reported to be particularly useful while therapists are familiarizing themselves with the concepts used in the evaluation procedures and in the differentiation of deficits by therapists who use the instrument. See Fig. 10-4 for the Neurobehavioral Specific Impairment Checklist and Fig. 10-5 for the Neurobehavioral Pervasive Impairment Checklist. The checklists are a part of the training material for the instrument. After having administered the evaluation several times, these checklists are used as references only. Deficits are checked as either present or absent on the checklists. The information obtained can aid therapists in scoring the neurobehavioral subscales.

Neurobehavioral Pervasive Impairment Subscale

The Neurobehavioral Pervasive Impairment Subscale includes items that can be detected during any of the ADL domains. Specific questions to elicit responses that can reveal, for example, the deficits of orientation, memory, insight, and judgment should be addressed prior to the patient's

Name_____ Date_____

Scoring criteria: Circle one
0 = Impairment is absent
1 = Impairment is present

Pervasive signs may be observed or noted in any activities of daily living (ADL) domain, according to specific instructions in the manual

NEUROBEHAVIORAL IMPAIRMENT	NB	SCORE			COMMENTS AND REASONING
MOTOR DYSFUNCTION					
1. Abnormal tone: right side	0	1			
2. Abnormal tone: left side	0	1			
SENSORY DYSFUNCTION					
1. Tactile/astereognosis	0	1			
2. Motor impersistence	0	1			
3. Visual object agnosia	0	1			
4. Associative visual agnosia	0	1			
5. Visual-spatial agnosia	0	1			
6. Anosognosia	0	1			
BODY-SCHEME DISTURBANCES					
1. Right-Left disorientation	0	1			
2. Body part identification	0	1			
EMOTIONAL/AFFECTIVE DISTURBANCES					
1. Lability	0	1			
2. Euphoria	0	1			
3. Apathy	0	1			
4. Depression	0	1			
5. Aggression	0	1			
6. Irritability	0	1			
7. Frustrations	0	1			
8. Restlessness	0	1			
COGNITIVE DISTURBANCES					
1. Concrete thinking	0	1			
2. Decreased insight	0	1			
3. Impaired judgment	0	1			
4. Confusion	0	1			
OTHER DYSFUNCTIONS					
1. Impaired alertness	0	1			
2. Impaired attention	0	1			
3. Distractibility	0	1			
4. Impaired initiative	0	1			
5. Impaired motivation	0	1			
6. Performance latency	0	1			
7. Absentmindedness	0	1			

FIG. 10-5 Neurobehavioral Pervasive Impairment Subscale. (Copyright © 1988 by Guðrún Árnadóttir.) Please see order form on page following the Index for ordering test pads.

NEUROBEHAVIORAL IMPAIRMENT	NB SCORE				COMMENTS AND REASONING
MEMORY DISTURBANCES					
1. Short-term memory loss	0	1			
2. Long-term memory loss	0	1			
3. Disorientation	0	1			
4. Confabulations	0	1			

Summary:

FIG. 10-5, cont'd

performance of the ADL tasks. The deficits are scored only in terms of presence (1) or absence (0). When appropriate, however, it is possible to use the same scoring scale as is used in the Neurobehavioral Specific Impairment Subscale in order to provide more detailed information. This is indicated by the empty boxes on the Neurobehavioral Pervasive Impairment Subscale (Fig. 10-6). An example of this is astereognosis. It can either be scored as simply present or absent or more thoroughly, as follows.

Tactile agnosia/astereognosis

Tactile agnosia, or astereognosis, is a failure of tactile recognition. For scoring, rule out pure sensory loss. It may be necessary for the therapist to check out astereognosis and motor impersistence according to the Neurobehavioral Pervasive Impairment Checklist in order to differentiate between astereognosis and other deficits.

0 No neurobehavioral deficits appear.
1 The patient needs to observe performance in order to be able, for example, to button a shirt because of decreased tactile recognition in the hand. However, the patient completes the activity without intervention from the therapist.
2 The therapist must tell the patient to observe what he is doing when he exhibits difficulties in buttoning a shirt.
3 The therapist must indicate physically to the patient what she is to observe when buttoning. This could be done by pointing to the buttons. The therapist may have to demonstrate the first two buttons or guide the patient's movements.
4 The therapist must button the shirt for the patient.

Note: If movements are clumsy, motor apraxia may also be present. Try to differentiate between the two impairments. Also check stereog-

Text continued on p. 258.

Name_____   Date_____

NEUROBEHAVIORAL IMPAIRMENT   NEUROBEHAVIORAL IMPAIRMENT SCORE

	PRESENT	ABSENT	COMMENT

MOTOR DYSFUNCTION

1. ABNORMAL TONE: RIGHT SIDE
Circle: flaccidity, weakness, spasticity, rigidity, tremor, apraxia.   ☐   ☐

2. ABNORMAL TONE: LEFT SIDE
Circle: flaccidity, weakness, spasticity, rigidity, tremor, apraxia.   ☐   ☐

3. ABNORMAL TONE; OTHER: specify:_____
Right-left-side involvement?   ☐   ☐

SENSORY DYSFUNCTION

1. TACTILE/ASTEREOGNOSIS: ☐   ☐
Tactile and proprioceptive deficit. Needs to observe performance in order to accomplish the dressing activity.
Unable to button shirt, unless observing performance. If in doubt check by having the patient recognize objects of different shape, size and texture while eyes are closed. Examples: coins, ring, pen.

2. MOTOR IMPERSISTANCE: ☐   ☐
Unable to make use of proprioceptive information. Lack of kinesthetic feedback. Check by having the patient oppose two fingers and hold for one minute.

3. VISUAL OBJECT AGNOSIA: ☐   ☐
Does not identify objects in either visual field on verbal command but can if allowed to touch them. A patient asked to shave may not be able to locate an electric razor until he reaches out with his hand and touches the objects around the sink.

4. ASSOCIATIVE VISUAL AGNOSIA: ☐   ☐
Able to perform but unable to name the objects used.

5. VISUAL-SPATIAL AGNOSIA: ☐   ☐
Misjudges direction and distances. May reach out for a cup but hand grasps several centimeters away from cup.

NOTE: All definitions are in the Evaluation Manual

FIG. 10-6 Neurobehavioral Pervasive Impairment Checklist. (Copyright © 1988 by Gudrún Árnadóttir.)
Please see order form on page following the Index for ordering test pads.

SENSORY DYSFUNCTION (continued)

	PRESENT	ABSENT	COMMENT

6. **ANOSOGNOSIA:** Does not identify a paralyzed body part as own. May deny it completely as a separate object, or recognize it and reject it. ☐ ☐

BODY-SCHEME DISTURBANCES

1. **RIGHT-LEFT DISORIENTATION:** Does not differentiate between right and left side of body on verbal command. ☐ ☐

2. **BODY-PART IDENTIFICATION:** Does not attend to instructions relating to specific body parts correctly. ☐ ☐

EMOTIONAL/AFFECTIVE DISTURBANCES

1. **LABILITY:** Shows mood swings; cries or laughs inappropriately. ☐ ☐

2. **EUPHORIA:** Inappropriate gaiety. ☐ ☐

3. **APATHY:** Shallow affect, psychomotor slowing, lack of interest in the environment, and inaction. ☐ ☐

4. **DEPRESSION:** Sad affect or expression. ☐ ☐

5. **AGGRESSION:** Shows hostility or aggression towards activity or people. May throw things at the therapist when therapist tries to motivate patient to perform. ☐ ☐

6. **IRRITABILITY:** Patient appears annoyed. May verbally express dislike or be physically agitated. This may be out of proportion to the stimulus that evoked the behavior. ☐ ☐

7. **FRUSTRATIONS:** Patient gets excited or intolerant when trying hard to perform or when unable to perform. This may be manifested emotionally, verbally, or physically. Not uncommon with aphasic people. ☐ ☐

8. **RESTLESSNESS:** Patient may be impatient, i.e.; cannot wait for therapist to start. May have trouble staying in one place during activity. ☐ ☐

FIG. 10-6, cont'd

Continued.

COGNITIVE DISTURBANCES

1. **CONCRETE THINKING:**
   Inflexible thinking. Unable to generalize from one situation to another. Patient may ask what time it is while eating breakfast. Cannot think of simple solutions that require some thought. Wets deodorant under water taps. Washes body with ice-cold water without liking cold water. Can answer concrete questions about things that he or she can see, such as, What is the weather like today? when patient can look out the window, but not regarding more abstract content.

   ☐ ☐

2. **DECREASED INSIGHT:**
   Does not have the insight into disease or disability. Does not make realistic statements regarding future plans. Makes unrealistic comments regarding disability.

   ☐ ☐

3. **IMPAIRED JUDGMENT:**
   Does not turn off water taps after washing. Does not put brakes on wheelchair while transferring or standing up. Goes to dining-room without dressing or combing hair. Does not pay attention to clothes turned inside out. Has no sense of social environment. May walk in hospital hallways without clothes, undress without closing doors, or urinate in hallways.

   ☐ ☐

4. **CONFUSION:**
   Talks about past as present. Talks out of context. Is not oriented towards time and place.

   ☐ ☐

OTHER DYSFUNCTIONS

1. **IMPAIRED ALERTNESS:**
   Patient is more or less unaware of what is going on around him.

   ☐ ☐

2. **IMPAIRED ATTENTION:**
   Does not continue an activity. Does not attend to instruction or activity. Does not attend to mistakes. May focus attention on irrelevant details and not on the global environment. These may be details such as light switches or bread crumbs. May result in perseveration of thought once details have been attended to.

   ☐ ☐

FIG. 10-6, cont'd

3. **DISTRACTIBILITY:** Talks and becomes distracted by environmental stimuli such as conversation in next room or somebody entering the room. Cannot continue the activity without being reminded to continue, although the patient understands the concept of the act.

☐   ☐

4. **IMPAIRED INITIATIVE:** Sits without initiating any activity. Has no need to perform. Can be caused by inertia of initiation if patient is mentally ready to perform. In such cases the patient may be annoyed with repeated instructions.

☐   ☐

5. **IMPAIRED MOTIVATION:**
Does not initiate or continue an activity, unless really accepting the need, although the physical ability to perform is present. For example, does not attempt to eat at mealtimes and may refuse to participate in the activity.

☐   ☐

6. **PERFORMANCE LATENCY:** Patient is slow in responding to instructions and takes an abnormally long time when performing ADL tasks.

☐   ☐

7. **ABSENTMINDEDNESS:** Exhibits brief periods of "absentmindedness"; i.e., sits for a few moments as if not aware of the environment. This may occur between activity steps or after the entire performance. This can be related to epileptic episodes.

☐   ☐

MEMORY DISTURBANCES

1. **SHORT-TERM MEMORY LOSS:**
Does not remember instructions through-out the evaluation. Shows evidence of failure of storage of new information.

☐   ☐

2. **LONG-TERM MEMORY LOSS:**
Demonstrates failure in retrieving informaiton that was processed prior to disability. This inability of retrieval also refers to information that should have been mobilized from short- to long-term memory after disability occurred.

☐   ☐

3. **DISORIENTATION:** Inability to give personal information regarding self, disability, hospital stay, or time without language problems. This disorientation can refer both to short- and long-term memory processes.

☐   ☐

4. **CONFABULATIONS:** Makes up stories or excuses. Fills in memory gaps to cover up.

☐   ☐

FIG. 10-6, cont'd

nosis of both hands and indicate in the *Comment* section which hand is involved. Score according to the side with more severe astereognosis.

Definitions for all the deficits can be obtained from the glossary at the end of the book. The Neurobehavioral Pervasive Impairment Subscale provides further examples of the ways these deficits manifest. The following items from the Pervasive Impairment Subscale, in addition to astereognosis, can be scored 0 1 2 3 4, as was outlined for tactile agnosia, and not simply as 1 or 0, as were the remainder of the items: visual-object agnosia, visual-spatial agnosia, aggression, irritability, frustration, restlessness, concrete thinking, decreased insight, and impaired judgment, as well as the deficits listed under the categories of *Other* and *Memory*. Note that verbal cuing becomes important if further breakdown of scores is considered for these deficits. Thus outcome or behavioral responses are observed, and the way in which the outcome can be modulated by sensory information is noted to provide information for scoring.

The sensory deficits of astereognosis and motor impersistence are tested specifically, according to the Neurobehavioral Pervasive Impairment Checklist (Fig. 10-5). The body-scheme disturbances of right-left disorientation and body-part identification are examined by the therapist, referring to at least one body part, and to the right or left side during instruction. If there is any indication of disturbance, follow-up instructions may be used. The results from a normative study of performance on right-left discrimination tasks that included 20 items (A.L. Benton et al., 1983), revealed that 96% of the 234 subjects examined had scores of 17 to 20. No individual in the normative group made more than one error in distinguishing the left and right sides of his or her own body, as tested by 12 items. Thus, any error on the A-ONE question relating to one's own body should be followed up by another question, as this would indicate a strong potential for dysfunction. No specific procedures are used to elicit emotional and affective disorders through the A-ONE. Examples of how cognitive dysfunction as well as other impairments and memory disturbances may be detected by use of the A-ONE are provided by the Neurobehavioral Pervasive Impairment Checklist (Fig. 10-5). For the item of *Disorientation*, it should be kept in mind that A.L. Benton et al. (1983) reported that the majority of a normative group had perfect scores on their Test of Temporal Orientation, including questions regarding date, weekday, and time; 93% had an error score of less than 3 points, each point referring to either one day removed from the correct day, or each 30-minute period removed from the correct time. An error in months exceeds the three points. Thus any mistake of more than a couple of days suggests defective temporal orientation. Questions addressing the patient's present employment, family size, home address, phone number, present location, and length of stay in hospital should be included for the evaluation of *Disorientation* in addition to the questions referring to orientation in time.

Attention refers to different sensory modalities. The type of attentional deficit should be noted. The following procedures have been used to differentiate attentional problems when in doubt. Auditory attention may be checked by digit repetition, where repetition of at least five consecutive digits is required. Visual attention can be checked by holding a visual stimulus, such as a partially pulled-out measuring tape, about 50 cm in front of the patient and requiring undivided attention for at least 20 sec, which is the minimum of time required for visual attention (Siev et al., 1986). Similarly for the item of *Distraction,* make note of what type of stimuli (visual, auditory, or tactile) cause the distraction. Remember that field-dependent behavior interferes with attention; for example, the visual stimulus of a comb may so distract a patient in the middle of putting on his shirt that he stops that task and begins combing his hair. When scoring the memory items, keep in mind that attention affects memory storage, and there are different types of sensory memory, that is, visual, auditory, and somatosensory, which all contribute to the concept of memory.

Note that if a patient has a comprehension

or speech problem, it may be impossible to make a decision regarding the presence or absence of other deficits, such as disorientation, memory, and insight. In such cases, just leave the items unscored (indicated by *not tested* [NT]), but comment on why this is done.

When scoring the evaluation the therapist should try to differentiate between things such as decreased attention or motor perseveration and stubbornness when patients ignore a verbal command, believing that their own method is better or that they are right as compared to the therapist, rather than just not attending to the instruction. An example of this would be when a patient believes that he is holding a sock correctly in terms of spatial relations (up/down) in order to find the opening and put the sock on.

Also note that some of the items could be regarded as being on a continuum. For example, aggression is a more severe impairment than irritability, and irritability is a more severe impairment than restlessness. Thus an aggressive patient could also (but not necessarily) express other impairments on the continuum. Restlessness can show up, for example, in action and perhaps verbally, but a negative verbal statement is not expressed toward an activity or the therapist, as one might observe in the irritable patient, nor does the patient indicate physical or verbal aggression. Further, striking out at the therapist, throwing equipment, or expressing verbal threats, such as one might experience with an aggressive patient, do not occur with restlessness only. On the other hand, the aggressive patient may be restless and irritable as well as aggressive.

Therapists should try to make realistic requirements and use their own judgment. A person who has little hair as a result of brain surgery should not be suspected of an organization problem, when he does not attempt to use a comb. A person who is not motivated for grooming and hygiene and refuses to comb on the basis of never having done it previously, should, on the other hand, be suspected of both lack of motivation and confabulation. Remember that asking for more information

regarding why patients perform in a specific way, or why a patient does not perform particular tasks, can add helpful facts to the information provided by the evaluation.

When attempting to differentiate between ideational apraxia and concrete thinking, keep in mind that these concepts are related. Ideation refers to whether the person has an idea of the required plan of action. In the A-ONE, *Concrete thinking* refers to whether the plan of action is confined to a narrow field of a few available stimuli or whether there is any evidence of the ability to generalize from one stimuli to another or from one situation to another. Further, a patient who experiences concrete thinking may not recognize his own mistakes and may not have the flexibility to make corrections in the action plan according to the mistakes. Thus *Concrete thinking* refers to a limited scope of ideas bound by available stimuli or a narrow field of action.

In the A-ONE, *Decreased insight* refers to the patient's disability (disease) and ideas related to planning the future. It is a subcomponent of the concept of impaired judgment. However, *Impaired judgment* in the A-ONE is scored separately from *Decreased insight*, which refers to judgment related to performance and consequences of actions. Further, *Impaired judgment* overlaps somewhat with *Impaired attention*, as attention is a necessary prerequisite for the opportunity to judge environmental, situations, actions, and their consequences.

In general, one should keep in mind that deficits may and will overlap. Further, some deficits are composed of more than one factor that may be common to other deficits too. For example, the phenomenon of right-left discrimination has, as mentioned in the previous chapters, at least three components: verbal, sensory, and visuospatial. Thus, the deficit may be a result of different factors. For nonaphasic patients with right-hemisphere lesions, visuospatial disability seems to be the underlying cause for left-right discrimination, whereas mental impairment seems to be the cause of the impairment in aphasics (Benton, 1985b).

When scoring, one should keep in mind that deficits may and will occur simultaneously, and one must attempt to isolate each of them and score them separately. The overlap, however, makes it hard to provide mutually exclusive operational definitions for some neurobehavioral impairments.

When looking at the two scales of neurobehavioral deficits and functions, one should note that they are inversely related. That is, if one receives a score of 3 or 4 on all items on the functional scale, indicating independence in a particular activity such as dressing, one would expect to see scores of 0 or 1 on the neurobehavioral scale for that particular activity. That would be an indication of no (or barely observable) impairments that do not interfere with function. If, on the other hand, a score of 3 or 4 is seen on the neurobehavioral scale, this would indicate inconsistency as a result of an error in scoring on the two scales. The therapist must then recheck the scoring. Similarly, if the person is not independent on the function scale but has no neurobehavioral nor neuromuscular deficits, this would indicate inconsistency in scoring or inappropriate use of the instrument (which is intended for patients with cortical CNS damage) for patients of incorrect diagnostic groups. Thus the therapist could quickly confirm the accuracy of the scoring by glancing at the scales (see Fig. 10-7).

INSTRUCTIONS FOR USING THE A-ONE

Fill in the patient's name, birthdate, age, gender, ethnicity, hand dominance, and the date of the evaluation on the title page of the evaluation (Fig. 10-8). Note any medication the patient is taking, because this may affect function. Also note the time of day of the evaluation and the activities performed by the patient prior to the evaluation the same day, because fatigue will affect function. As mentioned earlier, it is desirable to use more than one observation for the evaluation if that is possible. When a therapist starts scoring the evaluation, questions may arise, and going back to the patient for another observation may add to the information and give a better picture of the dysfunction. An average of three evaluations is ideal.

State the patient's vocation or profession (past vocation or profession if applicable), as well as the social situation. Include information such as housing and with whom the patient lives, as well as what his or her responsibilities are in the household. The summary sections on the title page regarding functional independence and neurobehavioral deficits are left until all the evaluation forms have been filled out. Then the summaries are based on all the information obtained by the entire evaluation. Similarly the section on treatment consideration is left until the end.

The forms for the Functional Independence Scale and the Neurobehavioral Specific Impairment Subscale are scored for independence (IP Score) and type and severity of neurobehavioral dysfunction (NB Score) during or immediately after the ADL observation. The appropriate score is circled. If necessary, the neurobehavioral checklists could also be brought along, and the presence or absence of deficits indicated by a checkmark, but it is assumed that therapists have already familiarized themselves with the different types of deficits and how they are manifested during ADL. Familiarity would eliminate turning pages during the assessment and the consequent loss of the continuous observation of the patient's performance. Less-experienced therapists should review the checklists just before the beginning of the evaluation; others, if not marking throughout the evaluation, should go through the checklist *immediately* after the observation. This should be sufficient for visualizing and remembering whether or not the deficit appeared. It is *important* to do the scoring *immediately* after the evaluation, not later during the day or the next day, as the kind of information obtained has a tendency to fade quickly and does not enter the "long-term memory stores" of the therapist in any detail. Do remember to list all the helping aids used on the form for the Functional Independence Scale. Check off whether or not deficits appeared, and score them according to the level of assistance provided. Make sure to mention results from specific sensory and motor tests and consider information on visual-field defects in the same section.

CORRECT SCORING:

DRESSING	IP SCORE					
Shirt (or dress)	4	3	2	1	0	
Pants	4	3	2	1	0	
Socks	4	3	2	1	0	
Shoes	4	3	2	1	0	
Fastenings	4	3	2	1	0	
Other						

NB IMPAIRMENT	NB SCORE					
Motor apraxia	0	1	2	3	4	
Ideational apraxia	0	1	2	3	4	
Unilateral body neglect	0	1	2	3	4	
Somatoagnosia	0	1	2	3	4	
Spatial relations	0	1	2	3	4	
Unilateral spatial neglect	0	1	2	3	4	
Abnormal tone: Right	0	1	2	3	4	
Abnormal tone: Left	0	1	2	3	4	
Perseveration	0	1	2	3	4	
Organization/Sequencing	0	1	2	3	4	
Other						

INCORRECT SCORING: Does the patient need physical assistance or supervision?

DRESSING	IP SCORE					
Shirt (or dress)	4	3	2	1	0	
Pants	4	3	2	1	0	
Socks	4	3	2	1	0	
Shoes	4	3	2	1	0	
Fastenings	4	3	2	1	0	
Other						

NB IMPAIRMENT	NB SCORE					
Motor apraxia	0	1	2	3	4	
Ideational apraxia	0	1	2	3	4	
Unilateral body neglect	0	1	2	3	4	
Somatoagnosia	0	1	2	3	4	
Spatial relations	0	1	2	3	4	
Unilateral spatial neglect	0	1	2	3	4	
Abnormal tone: Right	0	1	2	3	4	
Abnormal tone: Left	0	1	2	3	4	
Perseveration	0	1	2	3	4	
Organization/Sequencing	0	1	2	3	4	
Other						

FIG. 10-7 Inverse Relation of Functional Independence Scores and Neurobehavioral Specific Impairment Scores

Árnadóttir OT-ADL
Neurobehavioral Evaluation
(A-ONE)

Name _____ Date _____

Birthdate _____ Age _____

Gender _____ Ethnicity _____

Dominance _____ Profession _____

Medication:

Medical Diagnosis:

Social Situation:

Summary of Independence:

Summary of Neurobehavioral Impairments:

Treatment Considerations:

FIG. 10-8 Front Page of Evaluation. (Copyright © 1988 by Guðrún Árnadóttir.) Please see order form on page following the Index for ordering test pads.

Similarly, fill in the Neurobehavioral Pervasive Impairment Subscale.

As mentioned earlier, therapists have found the checklists very useful while they are familiarizing themselves with the concepts and thought process used in the A-ONE. After evaluating several patients, however, they usually feel so familiar with the concepts that they can fill out the scoring sheets and the summary sheet, using the checklists as a reference only when in doubt.

After scoring the Functional Independence Scale (IP Scores), it is possible but not necessary to fill in the total independence score for each category (dressing, grooming and hygiene, transfers and mobility, feeding, and communication) and the percentage score. This possibility was supported by a study examining item correlations within domains. Then take the neurobehavioral impairment score (NB Score) for each impairment under each ADL category of the Functional Independence Scale and enter it into the table on the Summary Sheet of the Neurobehavioral Scale. List the scores directly as they appear through the different functional categories (for example 3, 3, 3, 2 for ideomotor apraxia). Then take note of the most frequent score in order to make suggestions for processing level and treatment considerations. The scores represent the type of assistance patients need to enable them to finish an activity. A score of 2, for example, indicates that the patient can process and make use of verbal information to perform an activity. The scores are interpreted in the summary section of the title page, and the section on treatment consideration should take into account the processing type that enables a person to perform a functional activity.

The information gathered in the Functional Independence Scale, Neurobehavioral Specific Impairment Subscale and the Neurobehavioral Pervasive Impairment Subscale is sufficient for determining functional level and neurobehavioral dysfunction. If the therapist wishes to relate this information to the CNS disorder in order to set more precise treatment goals, the neurobehavioral impairments should be compared to the localization table included in Part II of the A-ONE, which is reviewed in Chapter 12. The following chapter includes results from research studies that have been performed during the development of the A-ONE (see Fig. 12-1 for the Neurobehavioral Scale Summary Sheet).

CONSIDERATIONS FOR SCORING AND COMMON SCORING MISTAKES

Make sure that scores agree with the written comments. Remember that Functional Independence scores and Neurobehavioral Impairment scores are inversely related. Be sure not to reverse them, and take a minute to check whether they are consistent.

Do consider possible cultural aspects or habits. It is, for example, possible that some people are accustomed to applying soap directly on their bodies without using a washcloth, although this may indicate a lack of sequencing, organization, and ideation. Further, some people may not dry their bodies with a towel after washing, although most people do; thus such behavior may not necessarily indicate a neurobehavioral deficit. Further, in some cultures people may comb their hair first with a comb and then brush it. Thus, this performance does not necessarily indicate a perseveration of action. However, it is usually possible to differentiate between neurobehavioral deficits and habits from general performance and patient's explanations. Further, the therapist should be able to tell how reliable the patient's information is. If still in doubt after the evaluation, it is possible to question relatives regarding specific aspects related to habits.

Look critically at behavior, and do not take it for granted that all "abnormal" behavioral reflections indicate neurobehavioral impairments. Take into account the testing situation, fatigue, and factors that may have previously upset the patient, as well as the possibility that the patient is nervous or frustrated because of the testing situation.

Sometimes there is not enough information to make a decision regarding a neurobehavioral deficit. In such cases, leave blanks rather than guess and fill in uncertain things. Go back and retest the patient at another time, or repeat parts of the evaluation. It is always better to base the judgment on more than one observation, and sometimes in very complicated cases, or in questionable cases, more than one observation is necessary.

Remember that some things, such as astereognosis and motor impersistence, must be tested separately. Always keep small items in your pocket (such as a coin, key, paperclip, ring, and pen) to be prepared for such testing. Also the therapist must be aware of the kinds of questions to ask the patient in order to gather information regarding memory and confabulations according to the patient's responses during the evaluation and the patients' history and background. It is therefore not considered desirable to standardize questions to gather such information for the purpose of the A-ONE.

The score of 3 is given on the Functional Independence scale when a person is borderline-dependent, but the therapist does not trust the person 100% to perform without supervision at all times. A patient may for example be able to transfer over to a wheelchair without assistance, but therapist may note balance problems indicating that supervision would be desirable for safety reasons. Similarly, a patient who has recently started walking may be able to walk without physical assistance, although somebody will need to walk beside or close to her for safety reasons.

A score of 0 on the Functional Independence Scale indicates that no active performance is provided by the patient. A score of 1 indicates that the patient does provide some work and actively assists the therapist. Be sure to give the patient an opportunity to reveal the dysfunction. Do not jump in too fast with assistance. Try to stand back, but be ready to intervene when needed. For example, if a therapist immediately provides physical assistance to correct a patient who starts dressing the wrong arm and guides the patient toward correct action, she will not learn whether the patient will be able to correct the mistake, and the patient may be given lower marks than he deserves.

Do not add up scores for the different ADL domains. A person can have total expressive aphasia and yet be independent in domains other than communication. Thus if these groups were added up, information would get lost, and the patient would not get full credit for independence. Language problems only enter scoring in other functional domains than communication if the patient needs assistance with performance. In such cases the type of assistance becomes important, and if the patient does not have sufficient auditory processing and therefore does not understand verbal instructions, scoring drops to the level of physical assistance. Note however, that a patient may have comprehension deficits, and yet be able to perform independently because he understands how to perform the tasks he is faced with.

Note that when using the A-ONE to report progress, the therapist may find that a patient seems to regress temporarily when helping aids are changed. For example, a patient who is independent in a wheelchair may need supervision or physical assistance when starting to walk. However, this change should be temporary, and it is important to use the *Comment* section to explain the scores.

The above mentioned "mistakes" are things that have become apparent with use of the A-ONE. Mistakes provide a basis for corrections, a learning experience, and it is hoped that these examples will provide clarification and answers for therapists who have similar doubts.

GENERAL CONSIDERATIONS

When deciding which scales to use for patient evaluation, there are several points that should be considered. Two of the most important are (1) for what patient population is the scale intended, and how sensitive is it for the specific characteristics of that population? and (2) what is the purpose of the scale? Is it to be used clinically or for research purposes. Is it intended to identify factors that can be used to contribute to decisions about treatment and the planning of goals, to evaluate clinical change, or to evaluate outcome status, future placement, or level of assistance. The purpose of the

A-ONE spans many of these factors. It is primarily intended to provide information that is necessary to form effective treatment goals and aid in decisions about pertinent treatment. It has also been used to record clinical change. In that respect, it is no different from other ADL evaluations and rehabilitation instruments in sampling the training program where ADL training is a part of the treatment. This should be kept in mind as a possible practice or training effect when considering progress. Thus an extension of the A-ONE that evaluates secondary activities of daily living would be a natural one. Such an instrument could, for example, be used to check out whether neurobehavioral improvement on the A-ONE carries over to other activities when patients have reached a ceiling on the A-ONE.

The A-ONE is a behavioral instrument, not neuropsychological in nature. It can identify problems that interfere with functional independence and differentiate between gross deficits, but it should not be taken for a complete test of specific deficits, such as memory.

When choosing instruments for research purposes, the goals of the research have to be considered. If the intention is to compare different patient groups with respect to functional independence, measures such as the Klein-Bell ADL scale might be appropriate, but such measures as the ADL scales are not very informative regarding the specifics of each patient group. Further, many scales are intended for quick information gathering, based on questioning patients regarding ADL performance. Such measures are not very reliable information regarding actual performance, and actual

problems, especially not when gathering information on brain damaged individuals. In such cases it is necessary to *observe* the performance.

It should be mentioned, that I have not experienced a negative attitude toward the A-ONE from the total of over 200 patients who have been evaluated so far. However, such attitudes have been noticed toward some of the "traditional" cognitive perceptual tests by some of these patients. Complete refusal to participate in such testing has also been observed.

As was stressed throughout Part I, the subject matter is a complicated one. For various reasons, there is considerable overlap, both in the types of neurobehavioral deficits that can be observed during behavior and in the locations of dysfunctions within the CNS. Thus, for all interpretation, it should be kept in mind that there need not be only one correct answer, as there is in many multiple choice assignments. Rather, there may be multiple "correct" answers regarding the same question. This fact, of course reduces reliability, but it is essential for the clinical flexibility required by the nature of the subject matter.

As stated by Diller and Ben-Yishay (1987), "Because the major thrust of rehabilitation is decreased dependency in activities of daily living, the amount of dependence required to perform an act successfully becomes a matter of practical, as well as scientific interest" (pp. 150–151). I agree with these authors, and I also believe that the factors that interfere with the successful performance of daily activities are of further practical and scientific interest, as well as is the relation between these factors and ADL performance.

CHAPTER
11

A-ONE, Part I: Research

Several studies have been performed in order to establish the validity and reliability of the Árnadóttir OT-ADL Neurobehavioral Evaluation (A-ONE) instrument. These include content validity, interrater reliability, normative study, discriminant validity, test-retest reliability and interitem correlations. The presently available results from the different studies are reviewed in this chapter.

CONTENT VALIDITY

As mentioned in Chapter 9, the literature on the test construct for the A-ONE (which is primary ADL performance and how it relates to brain structure and function) was reviewed. Open-ended questions provided by the author's previous experience with patients who had CNS dysfunctions due to various causes were modified in order to form the instrument's objectives. These were then developed into the neurobehavioral evaluation. Content validation was provided by a literature review and expert opinion in 1986.

Literature review

The literature review of functional neuroanatomy, neurophysiology, and neurobehavioral dysfunction provided a foundation for the neurobehavioral concepts used in the instrument to detect neurobehavioral deficits that interfere with ADL performance. It also provided a foundation for the methodology used to convert these neurobehavioral deficits to an ADL hypothesis of CNS dysfunction, as will be reviewed in Chapter 12. The literature review is presented in Part I of this book.

Expert opinion

Three experts in occupational therapy and neurology examined the content of Part I of the A-ONE. All three experts agreed that the evaluation was valid to detect neurobehavioral deficits on the basis of the ADL observations. The validation included all items of the entire evaluation. Several suggestions for future consideration were made. (See Table 11-1 for an overview of research studies for A-ONE, Part I.)

INTERRATER RELIABILITY

The kappa coefficient was used to determine the degree of agreement between the ratings of two raters using the A-ONE instrument simultaneously to observe and score the performance of the same patients. In a study of 20 subjects, the criteria for all the subscales were surpassed, and the instrument was determined to have interrater reliability. The average kappa coefficients for the degree of agreement between raters for all items of all scales was .84. See Table 11-2 for the exact subscale values. All but five items on the multiscore scales showed a statistically significant degree of agreement between raters at $P < .01$. Three of these items reached statistical significance at $P < .05$, and the remaining two did not reach statistical significance. This and subsequent reliability studies and analysis of therapists' scoring have provided information for refinements of the instrument. These include suggestions for item improvement and the training of therapists. As mentioned earlier, reliability depends on several factors. One factor is the items themselves, but reliability also depends on the training of therapists who are using the test. This is in agreement with Berk (1979) who states that "the reliability index, in general, reflects the effectiveness of observer training and the degree of objectivity with which the target behavior can be measured" (p. 460).

NORMATIVE STUDY

A normative control study was performed in order to investigate how individuals who do not have CNS disorders perform on the evaluation. The study was performed by therapists at four different hospitals in Iceland. A sample of convenience composed of 79 individuals was used. This included patients admitted for a short time to the acute and rehabilitation wards of the four hospitals who had nonneurologic disorders, and staff volunteers. Iceland has a population of 240,000 people. Reykjavík, which is the capital city, houses half of the population. Patients at the Reykjavík City Hospital, the National Hospital of Iceland, and Reykjalundur Rehabilitation Center, were included in the study, thus providing the possibility of a cross section of subjects from all socio-economic groups, both rural and urban. The results of the study indicate that a score of 4 can be expected during "normal" performance on all items of the Functional Independence Scale, which indicates complete independence, and a score of 0 can be expected on all items of the neurobehavioral subscales, which indicates the absence of neurobehavioral deficits. A few of the patients used helping aids, including reachers, clothes pins, stocking aids, crutches, walkers, a cane, and a raised toilet seat. However, their disabilities did not interfere with independence when they were allowed to use aids, which is acceptable without affecting the scores on the A-ONE. Tables 11-3 through 11-5 present the distributions of the psychometric characteristics of the normative sample including age distribution, sex distribution, occupation and diagnosis of subjects.

Lezak (1983) describes norms that he believes can be considered "species-wide performance expectations for adults" (p. 88). These norms develop long before adulthood, and refer to functions that are "taken for granted" as components of the "normal adult behavioral repertory" (p. 88). Further, according to Lezak, establishment of a premorbid functional performance level can be done easily for such "species-wide" norms. Although the ADL items were considered to be "species-wide," and neurobehavioral deficits were not expected to manifest during performance, it was considered necessary to examine the assumptions by samples from the population. The results certainly supported the notion that the functions tested are "species-wide" for Icelandic individuals, and maximum performance with no indication of neurobehavioral deficits is to be expected from the normal population. The sample used was biased because it was composed of hospitalized individuals, although they were getting ready for discharge. Thus, one would expect this sample to be less independent than the normal population, if anything. The variables of age were thought to have a potential for affecting performance, or the manifestation of neurobehavioral dysfunctions, whereas educational level, vocational training, and occupation were not thought to affect development of the functions. Neither age nor occupation were found to affect the scoring. The sample was also culturally and ethically biased, since it included only Icelanders, all of whom are Caucasian.

FURTHER VALIDATION

A concurrent validity study was performed in order to determine whether the A-ONE could differentiate between the average performance of normals and the performance of individuals with neurobehavioral dysfunction. The average performance of a sample including 50 patients with the diagnosis of CVA was examined and compared to the average performance of a normative control group. See Table 11-6 for the distribution of scores in the samples and Table 11-7 for results from the group comparison. The results obtained by a Mann-Whitney U-test indicated a high significance of group differentiation for most of the items on all three scales. However, there were a few variables that were not

TABLE 11-1 A-ONE, Part I: Research Studies

Study	Purpose	Research questions	Design
Content validation Literature review (1986)	Provide content validation for A-ONE, Part I.		
Content validation Expert opinion California (1986)	Provide content validation for A-ONE, Part I.	Does Part I of the A-ONE possess content validity according to the experts?	Three experts from occupational therapy and neurology evaluated the instrument.
Interrater reliability Reykjavík (1987)	Provide interrater reliability for A-ONE, Part I.	Does Part I of the A-ONE have interrater reliability?	Four occupational therapists rated 20 patients (two therapists at the time). Sample of convenience.
Normative study Iceland (1988)	Provide normative standards.	How do normal individuals perform on the different scales of the evaluation?	Seven therapists rated 79 individuals.
Concurrent validation Iceland/USA (1987-1989)	To determine whether the average test scores of CNS-damaged patients differ from the test scores of a normative sample.	Are the average test scores of CVA patients different from the average test scores of a normative sample?	Average performance from a group of CVA patients was compared to average performance of normative control subjects.
Pilot study of stability and test-retest reliability. Reykjavík (1988)	Explore stability of the instrument during two independent observations performed within one week.	How stable is the evaluation over two independent observations performed within the same week?	Subjects were evaluated twice within the same week and r_s calculated.
	Explore test-retest reliability over time and subsequent sensitivity of the instrument to detect progress.	Can the instrument reveal change in performance over time?	Improvement of subjects evaluated twice within the same week was compared with improvement of subjects evaluated twice with more than 3 weeks elapsing between evaluations with a Mann-Whitney U-test.

Subjects	Results	Contribution to instrument development
	References providing content validation for A-ONE, Part I.	Establishment of content validity.
	Part I of the A-ONE does have content validity.	Establishment of content validity.
Twenty CNS-damaged patients.	Part I of A-ONE does have interrater reliability (kappa = .84).	Establishment of interrater reliability.
Seventy-nine volunteers of both sexes with age range from 19 to 90. No neurological diagnosis.	Mean score on Functional Independence Scale = 4. Mean score on Neurobehavioral Scales = 0.	Normative standards.
Fifty CVA patients and 79 normal control subjects.	Mann-Whitney U-test indicated high significance of group discrimination for all items of the Functional Independence Scale and all but six items of each of the neurobehavioral subscales.	Establishment of concurrent validity for a CVA population.
Two independent groups of 10 subjects with CNS disorders.	r_s for test stability within 1 week were .85 or higher for all items ($P < .05$).	Indication of test stqability for two independent observations performed close in time.
	The A-ONE instrument is also able to detect change in patients' performance over time with significance level of .05 or more for 14 out of 22 items on the Functional Independence Scale. Ceiling effects of some items contributed to the nonsignificant statistics.	Indication of the instrument's ability to detect change in performance over time manifesting patient's progress.

Continued.

TABLE 11-1 A-ONE, Part I: Research Studies—cont'd

Study	Purpose	Research questions	Design
Item correlations Iceland/USA (1986-89)	Examine interitem correlations.	What are interitem correlations within ADL domains? What are interitem correlations across domains? What are item correlations across scales?	Scores from 89 subjects were correlated.
Exploratory factor analysis Iceland/USA (1986-1989)	Explore factors. Contribute to construct validity.	Which factors emerge from the different scales of the A-ONE?	Factor analysis: Varimax rotation.

TABLE 11-2 A-ONE, Part I: Interrater Reliability (Average Kappa Coefficients for Each Subscale): Reykjavík Study (1987)

Study	Scale	n	Kappa
Reyk-javík (1987)	Functional Independence	20	.83
	Neurobehavioral Specific Impairment Subscale	20	.86
	Neurobehavioral Pervasive Impairment Subscale	20	.84

Average kappa coefficient for A-ONE: .84

TABLE 11-3 Age Distribution of the Normative Sample

Age group	Number of cases	Mean	Standard deviation
19–29	6	23.3	4.2
30–39	16	34.6	2.6
40–49	12	42.4	3.3
50–59	10	54.2	3.2
60–69	17	63.1	2.4
70–79	12	74.8	2.9
80–89	6	83.7	2.8
TOTAL	79 individuals		

Subjects	Results	Contribution to instrument development
Eighty-nine subjects with cortical neurological diagnosis.	Item correlations within domains ranged from .3 to .9. Item correlations across domains ranged from .1 to .8. Item correlations across scales (independence/neurobehavior) were significant three times as often as nonsignificant.	Support for the theoretical statement of neurobehavioral dysfunction affecting performance in self-care activities, resulting in diminished independence.
Eighty-nine subjects with CNS diagnosis.	Three factors emerged from Functional Independence Scale. Two factors emerged from the Neurobehavioral Specific Impairment Subscale.	Contribution to construct validity.

TABLE 11-4 Sex Distribution of the Normative Sample

Age group	Number of cases	Females	Males
19–29	6	3	3
30–39	16	15	1
40–49	12	11	1
50–59	10	5	5
60–69	17	11	6
70–79	12	9	3
80–89	6	5	1
TOTAL	79	59	20
Percent	100	74.7	25.3

TABLE 11-5 Occupations and Diagnoses of the Normative Sample

OCCUPATIONS	Number of cases	DIAGNOSES	Number of cases
Homemakers	24	Lumbago, discus prolapse, myosis	29
Health-care workers	11	Hip prosthesis/fractures	13
Hard-labor workers	10	Other orthopedic disabilities	12
Clerical workers	9	Cardiopulmonary diseases	12
Retired	7	No diagnosis	6
Industrial workers	4	Arthritis	5
Sailors/fishermen	2	Systemic infections	2
Business/commerce	2	TOTAL	79
Students	2		
Disabled	2		
Civil-service workers	1		
Waitresses	1		
Educational workers	1		
Drivers	1		
Social-service employees	1		
Unknown	1		
TOTAL	79		

significantly sensitive to differences between the two samples. Some of these have been removed from the evaluation. Others are known to be more sensitive when evaluating patients with other neurological diagnoses, such as head-injured individuals. The results from the study thus support the ability of the A-ONE instrument to differentiate between the performance of patients with CVA and normal individuals both in terms of functional independence and the presence of neurobehavioral dysfunction.

FURTHER RELIABILITY

Two pilot studies were conducted in order to examine how stable the test was for two independent observations and to determine its potential for detecting change in ADL performance and neurobehavioral deficits over time. Two samples of ten subjects each were used for the comparison. In the first sample (see Table 11-1) therapists evaluated each patient twice within 1 week. A coefficient of stability obtained by the Spearman rank-order correlation coefficient (r_S) statistic correlating the scores on the two observations indicated stability of all items on all three scales of the test. Test-retest reliability over time, indicating the instrument's ability to detect change in performance, revealed significant results when two groups were compared, one that obtained the two observations within the same week and one that obtained the two observations with more than a 3-week interval between tests. For this comparison significant results were obtained by a Mann-Whitney U-test for those items on the Functional Independence Scale that did not reach the ceiling of the scale (highest possible score) on the initial evaluation. Test-retest reliability over time for the neurobehavioral scales requires a larger sample size.

TABLE 11-6 Performance of CVA Patients Compared to Normal Individuals

	Normal sample			CVA		
	Mean	**Standard deviation**	**Number of cases**	**Mean**	**Standard deviation**	**Number of cases**
AGE	53.4	18.1	79	68.0	8.72	48
FUNCTIONAL INDEPENDENCE SCALE						
Shirt	4.0	0.0	79	2.2	1.4	50
Pants	4.0	0.0	79	1.7	1.6	47
Socks	4.0	0.0	79	1.8	1.7	45
Shoes	4.0	0.0	79	1.9	1.8	46
Fastenings	4.0	0.0	79	1.9	1.6	34
Wash	4.0	0.0	79	2.5	1.3	48
Comb hair	4.0	0.0	79	2.9	1.3	46
Brush teeth	4.0	0.0	79	2.6	1.5	42
Shave	4.0	0.0	79	2.6	1.2	36
Bath	4.0	0.0	79	1.2	1.5	15
Continence	4.0	0.0	79	3.3	1.5	19
Sit up in bed	4.0	0.0	79	2.2	1.5	47
Get out of bed	4.0	0.0	79	2.3	1.5	47
Maneuver	4.0	0.0	79	2	1.6	50
Toilet	4.0	0.0	79	2.2	1.5	26
Tub transfers	4.0	0.0	79	1.7	1.5	16
Drink	4.0	0.0	79	3.8	0.5	46
Finger feeding	4.0	0.0	79	3.9	0.4	46
Fork	4.0	0.0	79	3.7	0.6	47
Knife	4.0	0.0	79	1.6	1.6	43
Comprehension	4.0	0.0	79	3.4	1.1	50
Speech	4.0	0.0	79	3.1	1.3	50
NEUROBEHAVIORAL SPECIFIC IMPAIRMENT SUBSCALE						
Dressing						
Motor apraxia	0.0	0.0	79	0.7	1.1	48
Ideation	0.0	0.0	79	1.0	1.4	49
Astereognosis	0.0	0.0	79	0.9	1.3	33
Unilateral body neglect	0.0	0.0	79	0.7	1.2	49
Somatoagnosia	0.0	0.0	79	0.1	0.6	48
Spatial relations	0.0	0.0	79	1.1	1.3	48
Unilateral spatial neglect	0.0	0.0	79	0.4	1.0	46
Tone	0.0	0.0	79	1.7	1.5	48
Perseveration	0.0	0.0	79	0.2	0.7	34
Organization	0.0	0.0	79	1.7	1.3	49
Grooming						
Motor apraxia	0.0	0.0	79	0.7	1.0	50
Ideation	0.0	0.0	79	1.0	1.4	50
Visual-object agnosia	0.0	0.0	79	0.1	0.6	38
Unilateral body neglect	0.0	0.0	79	0.4	0.9	48

Continued.

TABLE 11-6 Performance of CVA Patients Compared to Normal Individuals—cont'd

	Normal sample			CVA		
	Mean	Standard deviation	Number of cases	Mean	Standard deviation	Number of cases
NEUROBEHAVIORAL SPECIFIC IMPAIRMENT SUBSCALE—CONT'D						
Grooming—cont'd						
Somatoagnosia	0.0	0.0	79	0.1	0.5	48
Spatial relations	0.0	0.0	79	0.4	1.0	47
Unilateral spatial neglect	0.0	0.0	79	0.5	1.0	48
Tone	0.0	0.0	79	1.6	1.0	48
Perseveration	0.0	0.0	79	0.5	1.0	34
Organization	0.0	0.0	79	1.6	1.1	56
Transfers						
Motor apraxia	0.0	0.0	79	0.3	0.9	44
Ideation	0.0	0.0	79	0.6	1.1	43
Unilateral body neglect	0.0	0.0	79	0.2	0.6	41
Spatial relations	0.0	0.0	79	0.2	0.7	41
Unilateral spatial neglect	0.0	0.0	79	0.4	0.8	43
Topographical disorientation	0.0	0.0	79	0.1	0.7	37
Tone	0.0	0.0	79	2.0	1.4	48
Perseveration	0.0	0.0	79	0.2	0.5	30
Organization	0.0	0.0	79	1.5	1.3	42
Feeding						
Motor apraxia	0.0	0.0	79	0.5	0.8	47
Ideation	0.0	0.0	79	0.3	0.8	47
Visual-object agnosia	0.0	0.0	79	0.0	0.0	37
Visual association	0.0	0.0	79	0.0	0.0	35
Unilateral body neglect	0.0	0.0	79	0.3	0.7	45
Spatial relations	0.0	0.0	79	0.0	0.0	42
Unilateral spatial neglect	0.0	0.0	79	0.4	1.0	45
Tone	0.0	0.0	79	1.8	1.5	46
Perseveration	0.0	0.0	79	0.2	0.6	32
Organization	0.0	0.0	79	0.5	1.0	46
NEUROBEHAVIORAL PERVASIVE IMPAIRMENT SUBSCALE						
Perseveration	0.0	0.0	79	0.3	0.5	50
Bradykinesia	0.0	0.0	79	0.2	0.4	50
Tone	0.0	0.0	79	0.8	0.4	48
Lability	0.0	0.0	79	0.1	0.2	50
Euphoria	0.0	0.0	79	0.0	0.0	34
Apathy	0.0	0.0	79	0.1	0.3	49
Depression	0.0	0.1	79	0.0	0.2	47
Aggression	0.0	0.0	79	0.0	0.1	50
Irritability	0.0	0.0	79	0.1	0.2	50
Frustration	0.0	0.0	79	0.1	0.2	49
Restlessness	0.0	0.0	79	0.1	0.2	49

TABLE 11-6 Performance of CVA Patients Compared to Normal Individuals—cont'd

	Normal sample			CVA		
	Mean	Standard deviation	Number of cases	Mean	Standard deviation	Number of cases
NEUROBEHAVIORAL PERVASIVE IMPAIRMENT SUBSCALE—CONT'D						
Concrete thought	0.0	0.0	79	0.4	0.5	39
Insight	0.0	0.0	79	0.4	0.5	36
Judgment	0.0	0.0	79	0.8	0.4	44
Confusion	0.0	0.0	79	0.1	0.3	29
Alertness	0.0	0.0	79	0.0	0.1	49
Attention	0.0	0.0	79	0.3	0.4	49
Distraction	0.0	0.0	79	0.2	0.4	47
Initiative	0.0	0.0	79	0.1	0.4	49
Motivation	0.0	0.0	79	0.0	0.0	49
Right/left discrimination	0.0	0.0	79	0.0	0.2	44
Performance latency	0.0	0.0	79	0.2	0.4	32
Absent mindedness	0.0	0.0	79	0.2	0.4	34
Wernicke's aphasia	0.0	0.0	79	0.2	0.4	50
Jargon aphasia	0.0	0.0	79	0.0	0.2	46
Anomia	0.0	0.0	79	0.2	0.4	46
Paraphasia	0.0	0.0	79	0.1	0.2	41
Circumlocution	0.0	0.0	79	0.0	0.0	30
Expressive aphasia	0.0	0.0	79	0.2	0.4	50
Disarticulation	0.0	0.0	79	0.3	0.4	30
Short-term memory	0.0	0.0	79	0.4	0.5	41
Long-term memory	0.0	0.0	79	0.3	0.5	38
Disorientation	0.0	0.0	79	0.3	0.5	29
Confabulation	0.0	0.0	79	0.1	0.3	46

TABLE 11-7 Significance Levels Indicating Ability of All Items on the A-ONE, Part I, Discriminate between Normal Control Groups and Individuals with CVA

	Discriminant validity: Normal/CVA							
Scale	Significance level							
	.0000	.0001	.0005	.001	.005	.01	.05	NS
ADL (22)	20		2					
NBS (39)	21	4	1	4		1	2	6
NBP (34)	14	3	2	2		4	3	6

$n_1 = 50$; $n_2 = 79$ Mann-Whitney U-test
Frequencies refer to items

ITEM CORRELATIONS

Item analysis was performed on scores from 89 subjects with a cortical CNS diagnosis. Item correlations were highly significant for most of the computations on the functional scale. Correlations for items within domains were higher than correlations across domains, indicating the possibility of adding up item scores within domains for specific purposes. Variability within the *Feeding* domain was higher than within other domains. This is because some of the feeding items, such as finger feeding, drinking, and eating from a spoon could be performed independently by most patients in the sample, providing support for the view that these items are components of early development, whereas cutting was an item with which many patients had trouble. The items that could be performed by many individuals (including most feeding items and the communication items) often reached a ceiling effect on an initial evaluation, and thus they are not as sensitive to changes due to progress as are many of the other items.

Correlations for items across domains had a greater range than correlations within domains. Feeding had lower correlations with the other self-care domains—that is, dressing, grooming and hygiene, and transfer and mobility—and so did communication; the correlation of communication items to items of other domains was often insignificant. These findings support the view that adding up items across domains cannot be justified, and thus it is discouraged for the A-ONE.

The correlation of items from the functional scale to items of the specific neurobehavioral scale revealed significant results about three times as often as nonsignificant results: correlation coefficients ranged from .18 to .78. These results support the theoretical statement that neurobehavioral dysfunctions affect performance in self-care activities, resulting in diminished independence.

An exploratory factor analysis was performed on the different scales of the A-ONE on scores from the 89 subjects mentioned previously (Table 11-2). Three factors emerged for the Functional Independence Scale. Factor 1 was represented by dressing, grooming, hygiene, and transfer behavior items; Factor 2 included most of the feeding items, as well as continence; and Factor 3 included the communication items. Two factors emerged for the Neurobehavioral Specific Impairment Subscale. Factor 1 had high loadings of the apraxia items, *Tone* and *Organization*. Factor 2 included spatial-relations and body scheme items, in addition to *Perseveration* and *Organization*. For the version of the instrument used for this study, items classified as *Aphasia* were included in the Neurobehavioral Pervasive Impairment Subscale.

CHAPTER
12

A-ONE, Part II

Part II of the Árnadóttir OT-ADL Neurobehavioral Evaluation (A-ONE) instrument is needed to relate the results from Part I of the evaluation to the location of lesions and processing dysfunctions within the CNS. This part is optional for those therapists who are interested in such information. The relationship between functional performance, neurobehavioral deficits, and localization allows the therapist to understand the underlying CNS dysfunction and to be better able to speculate about and subsequently select the most appropriate treatment methods. Here impairments identified on the neurobehavioral subscales can be transferred to the Neurobehavioral Scale Summary Sheet of the evaluation (Fig. 12-1), and its results can subsequently be compared to the localization table at the end of this chapter to relate the neurobehavioral impairment to CNS dysfunction. The table was constructed to aid therapists in relating the neurobehavioral impairments to the locations of lesions and processing dysfunctions of the CNS. Possible sites of processing abnormalities are checked off on the summary sheet according to the table. The table shows possible lesion sites or sites of processing dysfunctions. This information is based on expert opinion and a literature review. The numbers refer to references in the reference list accompanying the table. The shades indicate the level of agreement among the experts who provided the content validation for the instrument. The darker the shade, the stronger the agreement. However, *all* indications, regardless of level of agreement, should be

considered as possible lesion sites; therefore, all the information has been retained in the table.

It is important that therapists be familiar with the literature review in Part I of this book, including the relationship between the localization of dysfunctions and the processing pathways, in order to use the information in the localization table effectively. Further, all the processing models provided throughout Chapters 4 and 8 should be used as references to pull together patterns from the localization table. Fig. 12-2, a flowchart of the procedures used in the A-ONE, includes the detection of impairments, as well as the use of the localization table and illustrations of processing models.

Turning back to the localization table, although many lobes may be indicated as possible lesion sites for a particular deficit, the patient does not necessarily have a lesion of all the lobes. Rather, there is a possibility of a lesion or dysfunction in one or more of them. In such cases, therapists should look at the complete picture when hypothesizing, including all the impairments observed. A man with left hemiplegia is, for example, more likely to have ideational apraxia due to involvement of the right frontal lobe than the left one, although ideational apraxia can occur in both cases. Therapists should look for a deficit that gives clues with regard to a specific hemisphere, or lobe, such as hemiplegia or motor apraxia, and go from there. If a specific hemisphere or lobe(s) is obvious as a potential lesion site (determined by identifi-

Name_____ Date _____

Fill in scores from neurobehavioral scales for present impairments or check off in score column.
Use localization table to fill in possible lesion site by (✔).

IMPAIRMENT	SCORE												POSSIBLE LESION SITE*
	D	G	F	T	RP	LP	RF	LF	RO	LO	RT	LT	OTHER
APRAXIA													
Ideomotor													
Ideational													
Oral													
AGNOSIA													
Astereognosis													
Visual-object agnosia													
Visual-spatial agnosia													
Associative visual agnosia													
Anosognosia													
BODY-SCHEME DISORDERS													
Unilateral body neglect													
Somatoagnosia													
R/L discrimination													
SPATIAL RELATIONS													
Unilateral spatial neglect													
Spatial relations													
Topographical disorientation													
MOTOR													
Perseveration													
Abnormal tone: Left/Right?													
Other:													
APHASIA													
Wernicke's aphasia													
Jargon aphasia													
Anomia													
Paraphasia													
Perseveration													
Broca's aphasia													
Other:													
MEMORY													
Short-term													
Long-term													
Disorientation													
Confabulation													

FIG. 12-1 A-ONE, Part II: Neurobehavioral Scale Summary Sheet. (Copyright© 1988 by Guðrún Árnadóttir.) Please see order form on page following the Index for ordering test pads.

IMPAIRMENT	SCORE												POSSIBLE LESION SITE
	D	G	F	T	RP	LP	RF	LF	RO	LO	RT	LT	OTHER
EMOTION													
Lability													
Apathy													
Depression													
Aggressiveness													
Irritability													
Frustration													
Restlessness													

COGNITION													
Concrete thinking													
Decreased insight													
Impaired judgment													
Confusion													

OTHER													
Impaired alertness													
Impaired attention													
Distractibility													
Impaired initiative													
Impaired motivation													
Performance latency													
Absentmindedness													
Impaired organization													

Comments and reasoning:

Types of Neuroimaging performed and results:

KEY: D = dressing domain, G = grooming domain, F = feeding domain, T = transfer domain, R = right, L = left, P = parietal lobe, F = frontal lobe, O = occipital lobe, T = temporal lobe.

FIG. 12-1, cont'd.

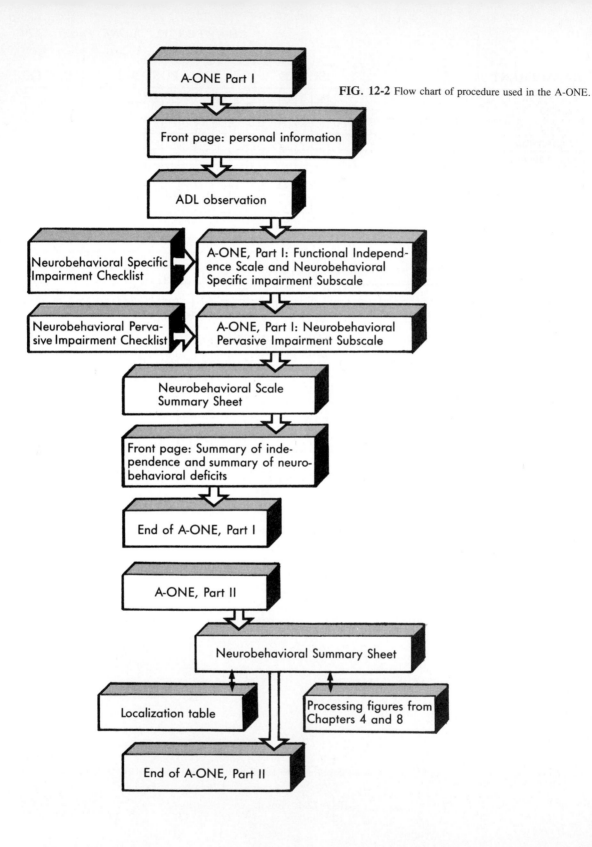

FIG. 12-2 Flow chart of procedure used in the A-ONE.

cation of an impairment that strongly suggests specific laterality for origin of cerebral dysfunction), other deficits are more likely to belong to similar locations, even though the table indicates more common lesion sites in the other lobes or hemispheres. The relative severity of impairments may also be useful in differential localization. A patient with severe bilateral motor apraxia (score of 3) and weak signs of spatial-relation dysfunction (score of 1) is more likely to have dysfunction of the left hemisphere than the right one, although spatial-relation disorders are commonly manifested in dysfunction of the right hemisphere.

Therapists should check all possible lesion sites in the column for possible lesion sites on the Neurobehavioral Scale Summary Sheet and then rule out some of them according to the entire picture. In cases where neurobehavioral deficits and possible lesion sites do not seem to fit, therapists should keep in mind the indicated handedness of

---

Exhibit 12.1 *Cerebral Vascular Dysfunctions*

Types

Ischemia
  Thrombosis
  Embolism

Hemorrhage
  Subarachnoid
  Intracerebral

Artery	Common impairment
Middle cerebral artery	Contralateral hemiplegia especially in upper extremity
	Hemisensory loss
	Impaired visual field
	Apraxia
	Unilateral neglect
	Spatial relations disorders
	Aphasia
	Attentional disorders
	Impaired judgment
Anterior cerebral artery	Contralateral paralysis especially in foot
	Apraxia
	Inertia of speech
	Behavioral disturbances
Posterior cerebral artery	Homonymous hemianopsia
	Associative visual agnosia
	Prosopagnosia
	Color agnosia
	Right/left discrimination
	Finger agnosia
	Alexia
	Anomia
	Acalculia
	Memory impairment

the person, which could complicate the picture, as well as the medical diagnosis or possible cause for the dysfunction, which might give a further clue to an explanation of the pattern of the dysfunction. This would include for example, CVA affecting (most frequently) one hemisphere at the time; head injury having a possibility of bilateral presentation, or contrecoup effect; or dementia, which could affect many lobes bilaterally. Further, two vascular lesions from different origins are possible, and may clarify an unexpected pattern of the location of a CNS dysfunction. Demographic data could also be useful; for example, a patient's age could be an indication of cerebral deterioration, although the patient does not have the primary diagnosis of dementia. The information provided in Chapter 5 in Part I of the book will be useful for localization purposes (see also Exhibits 12-1 to 12-4).

If things do not seem to fit, remember that other diseases, such as Parkinsonism or dementia, may be present, and these can affect subcortical as well as cortical structures such as white matter connections, basal ganglia, thalamus, cerebellum, and the brain stem. These should be specified in the column labeled *Other* on the Summary Sheet. It should be kept in mind that neurobehavior is a result of neuronal processing, which can take place at different levels of the CNS, both cortical and subcortical. Subcortical dysfunction can lead to neurobehavioral deficits such as impaired attention or memory as well as emotional disturbances, which resemble signs of cortical dysfunction because of common neuronal pathways involved in processing for these functions. The A-ONE may be able to detect the effects of an interrupted pro-

---

Exhibit 12-2 Anoxia Effects

Diffuse cerebral dysfunction
Affects watershed areas in particular

Exhibit 12-3. Head Injury*

PRIMARY EFFECTS
Gray matter	Coup: located at cortical point of impact
	Contrecoup: located at cortical sites opposite to point of impact especially at frontal and temporal tips
White matter	Tearing of connecting fibers

SECONDARY EFFECTS
Hemorrhage	Subdural
	Subarachnoid
	Intracerebral
Increased intracranial pressure	Parahippocampal gyri
	Cingulate gyri
	Medial occipital cortex
	Structures surrounding the ventricular system
Hypoxia	Bilateral damage to hippocampus, calcarine area, watershed areas

*Cortical dysfunction and the resulting neurobehavioral impairments depend on the site of the primary effects and the results of the accompanying secondary effects. The frontal lobes are particularly vulnerable in any type of head injury, including closed head injuries.

Exhibit 12-4. Cortical Dementia

Type	Impairment	Sites
ALZHEIMER DISEASE		
Stage 1	Memory deficit Impaired judgment Spatial and temporal disorientation Anomia Emotional changes (apathy, sadness, depression)	Mainly posterior association areas of parietal, temporal, and occipital lobes, as well as temporo-limbic association cortex and posterior cingulate gyrus. Later involvement of frontal association cortex. See also Fig. 5-3
Stage 2	Short- and long-term memory deficits Ideational apraxia Ideomotor apraxia Aphasia (paraphasia, anomia, decreased comprehension) Agnosia Restlessness Visual-spatial deficits	
Stage 3	Severe intellectual deficits Motor impairment (rigidity, spasticity) Language impairment (echolalia, perseveration, disarthria, mutism) Impaired concentration, reasoning, abstraction and judgment Possible personality changes Possible incontinence	
PICK DISEASE		
Stage 1	Personality changes Emotional alterations (loss of fear, decreased affective responses) Impaired judgment Socially inappropriate behavior Impaired language (anomia, circumlocution)	Frontal and temporal association areas. Left-sided involvement predominant
Stage 2	Aphasia (comprehension deficits)	
Stage 3	Substantial intellectual impairment Memory deficits Impaired visual-spatial skills Language impairment (mutism) Extrapyramidal symptoms Incontinence	

cessing pathway in these instances, but often it will not be able to differentiate a subcortical origin of a dysfunction from a cortical one. For example, it may be impossible to differentiate between cortical or subcortical origin of some impairments that have been related to the prefrontal lobes in Chapters 7 and 8.

On the basis of information from Part II of the A-ONE, therapists could speculate regarding treatment choices, depending on their beliefs. Some references were made to treatment in Chapter 8 of Part I, although treatment is beyond the spectrum of this book. Treatment could, for example, be geared toward facilitating the mechanisms affected by the lesioned area and/or facilitating areas that can compensate for the missing function, rather than focusing only on environmental compensation. Further, therapists could analyze environmental stimuli, according to information provided by Chapter 4 and results of the A-ONE, and present specific stimuli combined with functional activities. This could be done based on principles from the Sensory Integration Theory, or the Affholter methods. See Exhibit 12-5 for an example of how the results of the A-ONE could be used to form a treatment plan. By combining functional evaluations and knowledge of the cerebral localization of dysfunctions, we can start to study the mechanisms of recovery. Combining such studies with high technology is a promising future direction. Remember that the A-ONE is intended to provide *questions* that facilitate clinical decision making—for example, regarding treatment methods, prognosis, and independence level—not to provide specific *answers* regarding treatment.

Use the *Comments and Reasoning* section to write the conclusions from the A-ONE, Part II, along with the section on treatment considerations on the title page, regarding specific treatment principles, if applicable.

RESEARCH STUDIES

Content validity was provided for the A-ONE, Part II, by a literature review and by expert opinion. An interrater reliability study was also conducted to establish reliability among raters. Further validation was provided by a comparative study of results from A-ONE, Part II, and results from neuroimaging.

Content validation

As just mentioned, content validation was provided for the A-ONE, Part II (as well as for Part I) by a literature review and expert opinion.

Literature review

The literature review in Part I of this book provided a foundation for the neurobehavioral concepts used in the instrument, as mentioned earlier. It further provided a foundation for the methodology used to relate these neurobehavioral deficits to CNS dysfunctions. A table in which deficits were related to dysfunctions of cortical location, whether caused by structural lesions or processing abnormalities, was constructed according to the literature. This table provided the form for the expert reviewers mentioned in the next section. Further, models of likely processing pathways for some behavior and possible sites of dysfunction were also synthesized on the basis of the literature review (see processing models in Chapters 4 and 8).

Expert opinion

Four experts from the fields of neurology and occupational therapy assigned neurobehavioral deficits to specific CNS locations. A percentage of agreement was calculated for a possible lesion site for each item in each lobe. A 75% agreement (three of four experts) for at least one lobe per item was considered sufficient for validation. All impairments, except for confabulation, reached this predetermined level and can be considered localizable. The localization table at the end of this chapter summarizes the results from the content validation. The numbers in the table are references that have identified a particular lesion site.

The experts were encouraged to note all possible cortical sites of the neurobehavioral deficits. High agreement thus indicates a lesion site that is considered a probability by the expert group. Per-

---

Exhibit 12-5. *Example of How the Results of* A-ONE *Can Be Used to Form a Treatment Program*

CASE
The case involves a young man who sustained a head injury.

SUMMARY OF INDEPENDENCE
Patient needs verbal or physical assistance for some items of dressing and grooming and hygiene, as well as
   with transfers and mobility. Is able to eat independently.

SUMMARY OF NEUROBEHAVIORAL IMPAIRMENTS
The following impairments manifested themselves through the patient's performance, many of which interfered
   with independent functional performance:
   Impaired initiative
   Impaired motivation
   Impaired organization and sequencing
   Impaired attention
   Distractibility and field-dependent behavior
   Impaired judgment
   Concrete thinking
   Lack of insight into disability
   Perserveration and reluctance to change
   Irritability
   Aggressiveness
   Low frustration tolerance
   Impaired short-term memory
   Confabulations
Patient is able to make use of a few clear step-by-step verbal instructions within levels of frustration tolerance,
   and within limits of concrete thinking.

TREATMENT CONSIDERATIONS
Make use of knowledge of impairments and normal cerebral function to structure treatment program. Lack of
   executive control frontal lobe functions interfere with performance (initiative, motivation, organization, and
   sequencing). Providing such control externally by a rigid program (including desirable tasks from a rehabilitation point of view, in an organized way) presented by an authoritative person should help the patient
   to structure a plan of action. By making use of the perseverations and lack of flexibility it may be possible
   to implement the program as a routine to gain certain desirable behavior. Because of tendencies to perseverate,
   the patient will be expected to adhere to the program, which simultaneously fulfills the need of an external
   control figure. Such a program will address lack of initiative and lack of motivation. It will also diminish
   possibility of socially unacceptable behaviors (frustrations, irritability, and aggression) as the structure
   provides safety and thus protects the patient from being threatened by unexpected requests (which could be
   a result of a memory problem) for which he can neither organize nor control a plan of desired action.

---

fect agreement (100%), indicating a lobe that is considered to be a lesion site by all four experts, is reported in the darkest shade. The acceptable level of validation, 75% agreement, is indicated by a slightly lighter shade. Note that more than one lobe may have been identified at 100% or 75% agreement as possible sites for a lesion that results in a particular deficit. Lobes indicated by 50% or 25% of the experts were retained for the table, assuming that they might offer suggestions for alternative sites or areas of processing dysfunctions that could also result in the deficit. Thus on the basis of the content validation studies, Part II of the A-ONE was considered to have content validity.

Interrater Reliability

For the interrater reliability study of Part II of the A-ONE, 20 case studies were summarized from patients who had been evaluated by the A-ONE, Part I. The total average kappa of .76 for all raters indicated that Part II of the A-ONE can be considered reliable. Six lobes surpassed the predetermined level of .70, as indicated in Table 12-1. The temporal lobes, however, did not surpass this level, indicating that further refinement of the instrument was desirable and that additional information regarding the relation of a patients' behavior to the CNS localization of a lesion, in the form of a textbook (which was not available at the time) and training seminar, were needed for therapists.

Further Validation

Further validation of the A-ONE was provided by a comparative study of the results of Part II of the evaluation and neuroimaging. The study explored the brain-behavior linkage assumed as the basis of the A-ONE and the extent to which the localization from the A-ONE agrees with other evaluation methods that are used to detect and localize dysfunction. It was questioned that viewing the individual from all possible aspects—including behavior as well as CNS structure and processing patterns—would provide a more complete evaluation than any of these alone.

The imaging methods of computerized tomography (CT scans) and computerized mapping of EEG (CMEEG), both of which were described in Chapter 6, were chosen for the initial comparison. These are computerized techniques used to evaluate structural changes and dysfunctions in neuronal activity, respectively. Results from these evaluations were employed in the study as they offer both static and dynamic information on the brain and its function. Further, they are considered

TABLE 12-1 The Average Kappa Coefficients for Lobes for All Pairs of Raters in Part II of the A-ONE

Lobe	Number of cases	Value
Right frontal	20	1.000
Left frontal	20	.949
Right parietal	20	.900
Left parietal	20	.800
Right temporal	19	.565
Left temporal	20	.389
Right occipital	20	.759
Left occipital	20	.717

Total average weighted kappa for all lobes = .76

to be of minimal risk to the patient, and they were routine procedures at the hospitals where the data was gathered. Data from these procedures, which were interpreted by a neurologist and an x-ray specialist, were compared to the therapist-generated hypotheses about the localization of cerebral dysfunction based on the dynamics of the observed neurological impairments as they affected function during administration of the A-ONE. The results of the evaluations were in the form of localization in eight major cortical lobes of the brain.

A pilot study was performed at two locations: 17 patients were evaluated at the UCLA Medical Center in Los Angeles, California, and 10 patients were evaluated at the Reykjavík City Hospital in Iceland. Thus 27 patients provided the total sample: 20 of the patients had diagnoses of CVA (74.1%), 6 of TIA (22.2%), and 1 of head injury (3.7%). The kappa coefficient statistic was used to detect the degree of agreement for the localization in each lobe as determined by the different evaluation methods. Table 12-2 summarizes the average kappa coefficients from this study. A subsequent study with 10 additional subjects confirmed these results.

TABLE 12-2 Comparison of the Degree of Agreement between the A-ONE, CMEEG, and CT Scans

Comparison	Number of cases	Average kappa
A-ONE/CT	21	.55
A-ONE/CMEEG	17	.36
CT/CMEEG	12	− .02

The results from the study suggest that CT scans measuring structure and the OT-ADL hypothesis based on the A-ONE agree moderately as to the localization of a particular CNS dysfunction. The association is not very strong, which suggests that the tests are also measuring different things, and thus would seem to provide supplementary information, all of which is necessary to obtain a complete picture of the dysfunction. The CMEEG, however, which measures neuronal activity, does not seem to be as accurate for localizing a particular CNS dysfunction. This is not surprising, as the CMEEG is more sensitive to laterality than to the precise site of dysfunction. However, there is a mild association between the CMEEG and the A-ONE, although it is lower than the one between the A-ONE and CT. This association would support the ability of the A-ONE to detect some processing abnormalities as detected by CMEEG in addition to structural ones. The reader is referred to Chapter 6 for information on the CT and CMEEG.

A follow-up study of agreement on cerebral laterality as compared to the previous lobe localization revealed that the CMEEG is a stronger predictor of the laterality of a dysfunction than of exact lobe localization. By retrospective examination of the data, several explanations of the disagreement became apparent, among them that changes on CT scans may not become evident until 2 days after the onset of impairments, and that CMEEG detects abnormalities in patients with transient ischemic attack (TIA) after clinical neurological impairments

have subsided. It should be emphasized that a considerable proportion of the CVA sample, which was a sample of convenience, was composed of TIA patients who did not present with neurological signs on the day the A-ONE was administered. Further, the CMEEG misclassified parietal and frontal lobes as temporal at times, thus detecting laterality correctly but not the specific lesion site.

As the strength of the association was not high, it suggests that the different methods may provide complementary information, and no one of them can be used to replace another. That is, a CT scan may detect the structural location of a lesion but not the resulting processing abnormalities that may be caused by disrupted connections with other lobes. The A-ONE is, to a degree, also sensitive to the localization of such dysfunctions. The CMEEG and the A-ONE detect some of the processing abnormalities that result from CNS lesions. In addition, the A-ONE detects the behavioral deficits that result from both the structural and processing abnormalities, and it measures their interference with functional independence.

Thus the results support the importance of analyzing all available information to enhance knowledge regarding the CNS—knowledge upon which therapists will eventually base their treatment models. One should keep in mind that the process of validation and establishment of reliability is never-ending, and that there is no absolute goal or standard that one can use for comparison, neither for the CMEEG nor the ADL evaluation.

CONCLUSION FROM RESEARCH STUDIES

The development of the A-ONE has been reported in the previous chapters. The A-ONE is considered to meet its aims of providing an assessment of both the functional and neurobehavioral status of patients. It is further considered helpful in aiding therapists to understand the mechanisms that underlie patient dysfunction and in providing them with a basis for speculation regarding suitable treatment methods. It was pointed out that test reliability is dependent on the training of therapists for test administration and scoring. This view was supported by the therapists who have used the evaluation and their indication of the need for further training. Lack of therapist training would thus be one of the major limitations for using an instrument such as the A-ONE.

It is felt that the A-ONE has potential for use by therapists who are specifically interested in shifting their approach to the evaluation of patients with neurobehavioral deficits. It is further felt that the instrument has a considerable potential to initiate rethinking in terms of treatment strategies. This is because it identifies neurobehavioral deficits and the extent of their interference with functional independence, and it relates the neurobehavioral impairments to CNS dysfunctions. Such analysis may stimulate ideas regarding how, for example, sensory stimuli may be used to affect CNS processes.

In conclusion, a process of instrument development within the field of occupational therapy for neurobehavioral evaluation of ADL has been initiated. Little research has been published regarding suitable treatment methods for neurobehavioral impairments. The basis for such studies is, of course, the existence of instruments suitable for evaluating the dysfunctions as well as measuring progress.

Those who have written most about neurobehavioral deficits are neurologists and neuropsychologists. However, occupational therapists are focused on the neurobehavioral rehabilitation of these patients. Thus it is their responsibility to evaluate the treatment methods they use and to contribute to the development of new methods. Nobody is in a better position than the occupational therapist to evaluate the occupational performance skills of these patients, to see how they are affected by neurobehavioral deficits, and in turn to develop and evaluate suitable treatment methods for occupational therapy.

However, viewing the individual from all possible aspects, by using a combination of evaluation methods to explore behavior, as well as CNS structure and processing patterns, would provide a more complete evaluation of patients than any method alone. This could be done with combinative studies that examine the findings of both behavioral and technological evaluations. Such combinative studies will provide more effective evaluation, and this might lead to the development of more effective treatment strategies based on enhanced CNS knowledge. Studies to explore and experiment with treatment strategies in order to obtain information regarding the mechanisms that underlie neurobehavior and functional progress are therefore needed. Thus, despite the advent of technological diagnostic tools, a viable place remains for behavioral assessment.

The next chapter presents the practical implications of the research studies as well as need for additional studies. Further, the possibilities for using the instrument will be outlined.

A-ONE Part II: LOCALIZATION TABLE
Localization of Dysfunction within the Cerebral Cortex

DYSFUNCTION	PARIETAL LOBE Left	Right	FRONTAL LOBE Left	Right	OCCIPITAL LOBE Left	Right	TEMPORAL LOBE Left	Right	CORP. CALL.*	THALAMUS*	RETICUL. F.*	BASAL GANG.*	CEREBELLUM*
MOTORIC													
Perseveration			3	4			7	8					
Hyper/hypotonia			11	12						a			b
Bradykinesia			19	20									
Motor impersistence*		26		28									
Tremor/rigidity*												c	d
Dysarthria *			35	36									
APRAXIA													
Ideomotor	1		3	4					a			b	
Ideational	9		11	12					c				
Constructional	17	18	19	20	21	22							
AGNOSIA													
Sensory Disorders*	1	2			5	6	7	8					
Astereognosis	9	10											
Visual object*	17	18			21	22	23	24	a				
Visual spatial*	25	26											
Associative visual					37	38	39		b				
Anosognosia		42		44									
Prosopagnosia					53	54	55	56					
Color agnosia					61	62	63	64					
Auditory agnosia							71	72					
BODY SCHEME													
Unilateral body neglect		2		4				8		a	b		
Somatoagnosia		10											
L/R discrimination	17	18	19	20	21	22	23						
Finger agnosia	25	26	27	28	29	30	31						
SPATIAL RELATION													
Unilateral spatial neglect	1	2	3	4				8		a		c	
Spatial relations	9	10	11	12	21	22	16						
Topographical disorientation		18			21	22	24						

Continued.

A-ONE PART II: LOCALIZATION TABLE (continued)
Localization of Dysfunction within the Cerebral Cortex

DYSFUNCTION	PARIETAL LOBE		FRONTAL LOBE		OCCIPITAL LOBE		TEMPORAL LOBE		CORP. CALL.*	THALAMUS*	RETICUL. F.*	BASAL GANG.*	CEREBELLUM*
	Left	Right	Left	Right	Left	Right	Left	Right					
APHASIA													
Wernicke's	1						7						
Jargon							15			a			
Anomia	17		19		21		23						
Paraphasia	25		27				31						
Perseveration*			35	36			39						
Broca's(*)			43										
Circumlocution*	49												
Echolalia*			59	60									
Oral apraxia*			67	68									
Mutism*			75	76					b	c		d	
MEMORY													
Short term	1		3	4			7	8					
Long term							15	16	a	b			
Orientation problems*			19	20									
Confabulation			27	28									
EMOTION													
Lability			3	4									
Apathy			11	12			15	16		a			
Depression			19	20			23						
Aggressiveness			27	28			31	32		b			
Irritability			35	36			39	40		c			
Frustration*			43	44			47	48		d			
Restlessness			51	52									
Euphoria*			59	60									
COGNITION													
Concrete thinking			3	4									
Decreased insight			11	12									
Impaired judgment			19	20									
Confusion*	25	26	27	28	29	30	31	32		a	b		

A-ONE PART II: LOCALIZATION TABLE (continued)
Localization of Dysfunction within the Cerebral Cortex

DYSFUNCTION	PARIETAL LOBE Left	PARIETAL LOBE Right	FRONTAL LOBE Left	FRONTAL LOBE Right	OCCIPITAL LOBE Left	OCCIPITAL LOBE Right	TEMPORAL LOBE Left	TEMPORAL LOBE Right	CORP. CALL.*	THALAMUS*	RETICUL. F.*	BASAL GANG.*	CEREBELLUM*
OTHER													
Impaired alertness			3	4					a				
Impaired attention		10	11	12				16		b	c		
Distractibility*			19	20									
Impaired initiative			27	28									
Impaired motivation			35	36			39	40		d			
Performance latency*			43	44									
Absent–mindedness*			51	52									
Impaired organization			59	60									
Lack of social awareness			67	68									
Altered personality*			75	76									
Lack of inhibition*			83	84									
AGRAPHIA		90	91	92	93		95	96	f				
ALEXIA	97	98			101	102	103		e				
ACALCULIA	105	106	107	108	109	110	111						

Key to expert opinion:
- ▧ Most frequent lesion site
- ▨ Possible lesion site
- ▢ Possible lesion site
- ☐ Possible lesion site
- # Reference number from literature review
- * Not included at time of expert opinion
- (*) Altered terminolgy from time of expert opinion

© 1988, Guðrún Árnadóttir

NOTE: The table is primarily concerned with cortical location of dysfunction, although an occasional reference is given for subcortical structures. The information for the expert opinion study only included the four cerebral lobes. The limbic lobe was considered to be a part of frontal and temporal lobes. Several dysfunctions have been added to the table since the time of content validation by the experts. The table is to be used in combination with the A-ONE processing models in Chapter 4 and Chapter 8.

REFERENCES FOR CELLS IN LOCALIZATION TABLE[*]

MOTOR

3. Damasio, 1985; Luria, 1980; Strub and Black, 1985; Walsh, 1987.
4. Damasio, 1985; Luria, 1980; Strub and Black, 1985; Walsh, 1987.
7. Luria and Thomas Hutton, 1977.
8. Luria and Thomas Hutton, 1977.
11. Barr and Kiernan, 1983; Daube and Sandok, 1978; Geschwind, 1979; Ingvar and Philipson, 1977; Olesen, 1971; Roland et al., 1980.
12. Barr and Kiernan, 1983; Daube and Sandok, 1978; Geschwind, 1979; Ingvar and Philipson, 1977; Olesen, 1971; Roland et al., 1980.
19. Damasio, 1979; Luria, 1980.
20. Damasio, 1979; Luria, 1980.
26. Carmon, 1970.
28. Carmon, 1970; Stuss and Benson, 1986.
35. Geschwind, 1979.
36. Geschwind, 1979.
a. Barr and Kiernan, 1983.
b. Barr and Kiernan, 1983; Daube and Sandok, 1978.
c. Daube and Sandok, 1978.
d. Barr and Kiernan, 1983; Daube and Sandok, 1978.

APRAXIA

1. Ayres, 1985; Basso et al., 1980; Geschwind, 1975; Heilman et al., 1982; Heilman and Rothi, 1985; Ingvar and Philipson, 1977; Kimura and Archibald, 1974; Roy, 1983; Siev et al., 1986.
3. Ayres, 1985; Basso et al., 1980; Damasio, 1985; Daube and Sandok, 1978; Geschwind, 1975; Heilman et al., 1982; Heilman and Rothi, 1985; Ingvar and Philipson, 1977; Kimura and Archibald, 1974; Luria, 1980; Roland et al., 1980; Roy, 1983; Stuss and Benson, 1986.
4. Ayres, 1985; Basso et al., 1980; Damasio, 1985; Daube and Sandok, 1978; Geschwind, 1975; Heilman et al., 1982; Heilman and Rothi, 1985; Ingvar and Philipson, 1977; Kimura and Archibald, 1974; Luria, 1980; Roland et al., 1980; Roy, 1983; Stuss and Benson, 1986.
9. Ayres, 1985; Heilman and Rothi, 1985; Ingvar and Philipson, 1977; Walsh, 1987.

---

[*]For full bibliographic information, see the references at the end of this book.

11. Ayres, 1985; Ingvar and Philipson, 1977; Luria, 1980; Roland et al., 1980; Roy, 1983; Stuss and Benson, 1986.
12. Ayres, 1985; Ingvar and Philipson, 1977; Luria, 1980; Roland et al., 1980; Roy, 1983; Stuss and Benson, 1986.
17. Ayres, 1985; Benton, 1985a; Black and Bernard, 1984; Black and Strub, 1976; Dee and Benton, 1970; Siev et al., 1986; Walsh, 1987.
18. Ayres, 1985; Benton, 1985a; Black and Bernard, 1984; Black and Strub, 1976; Dee and Benton, 1970; Piercy et al., 1960; Siev et al., 1986; Walsh, 1987.
19. Ayres, 1985; Benton, 1985a; Black and Bernard, 1984; Black and Strub, 1976; Luria, 1980; Walsh, 1987.
20. Ayres, 1985; Benton, 1985a; Black and Bernard, 1984; Black and Strub, 1976; Luria, 1980; Piercy et al., 1960; Walsh, 1987.
21. Bauer and Rubens, 1985; Geshwind, 1979a,b; Siev et al., 1986; Walsh, 1987.
22. Bauer and Rubens, 1985; Geschwind, 1979; Siev et al., 1986; Walsh, 1987.
a. Geschwind, 1975; Heilman and Rothi, 1985.
b. Ayres, 1985.
c. Heilman and Rothi, 1985.

AGNOSIA

1. Ayres, 1985; Barr and Kiernan, 1983; Daube and Sandok, 1978; Werner, 1980.
2. Ayres, 1985; Barr and Kiernan, 1983; Daube and Sandok, 1978; Werner, 1980.
5. Daube and Sandok, 1978.
6. Daube and Sandok, 1978.
7. Barr and Kiernan, 1983.
8. Barr and Kiernan, 1983.
9. Barr and Kiernan, 1983; Daube and Sandok, 1978; Geschwind, 1979; Roland et al., 1980; Williams and Warwick, 1980.
10. Barr and Kiernan, 1983; Daube and Sandok, 1978; Geschwind, 1979; Roland et al., 1980; Williams and Warwick, 1980.
17. Siev et al., 1986.
18. Siev et al., 1986.
21. Bauer and Rubens, 1985; Siev et al., 1986; Strub and Black, 1985; Walsh, 1987.

22. Bauer and Rubens, 1985; Strub and Black, 1985; Walsh, 1987.
23. Bauer and Rubens, 1985; Walsh, 1987.
24. Walsh, 1987.
25. Siev et al., 1986.
26. Siev et al., 1986.
37. Bauer and Rubens, 1985; Strub and Black, 1985.
38. Bauer and Rubens, 1985; Strub and Black, 1985.
39. Bauer and Rubens, 1985; Strub and Black, 1985.
42. Siev et al., 1986.
44. Stuss and Benson, 1986.
53. Bauer and Rubens, 1985; Geschwind, 1979.
54. Bauer and Rubens, 1985; Geschwind, 1979.
55. Bauer and Rubens, 1985; Geschwind, 1979.
56. Bauer and Rubens, 1985; Geschwind, 1979.
61. Strub and Black, 1986.
62. Strub and Black, 1986.
63. Strub and Black, 1986.
64. Strub and Black, 1986.
71. Bauer and Rubens, 1985; Siev et al., 1986.
72. Bauer and Rubens, 1985; Siev et al., 1986.
  a. Barr and Kiernan, 1983; Walsh, 1987.
  b. Bauer and Rubens, 1985; Stuss and Benson, 1985.

BODY-SCHEME DISORDERS

2. Siev et al., 1986; Heilman et al., 1985.
4. Heilman et al., 1985.
8. Heilman et al., 1985.
10. Siev et al., 1986.
17. Benton, 1985b; Heilman, 1979; Siev et al., 1986; Walsh, 1987.
18. Benton, 1985b; Heilman, 1979; Siev et al., 1986; Walsh, 1987.
19. Benton, 1985b; Heilman, 1979; Walsh, 1987.
20. Benton, 1985b; Heilman, 1979; Walsh, 1987.
21. Benton, 1985b; Heilman, 1979; Walsh, 1987.
22. Benton, 1985b; Heilman, 1979; Walsh, 1987.
23. Benton, 1985b; Heilman, 1979; Walsh, 1987.
25. Benton, 1985b; Siev et al, 1986; Walsh, 1987.
26. Benton, 1985b; Walsh, 1987.
27. Benton, 1985b; Walsh, 1987.
28. Benton, 1985b; Walsh, 1987.
29. Benton, 1985b; Walsh, 1987.
30. Benton, 1985b; Walsh, 1987.
31. Benton, 1985b; Walsh, 1987.
  a. Heilman et al., 1985.
  b. Heilman et al., 1985.

SPATIAL-RELATIONS DISORDERS

1. Walsh, 1987.
2. Benton, 1985a; Heilman et al., 1985; Siev et al., 1986; Walsh, 1987.
4. Heilman et al., 1985.
8. Heilman et al., 1985.
9. Luria, 1973; Luria, 1980.
10. Benton, 1985a Kinsbourne, 1978; Luria, 1973; Semmes, et al., 1963.
11. Luria, 1973; Luria, 1980.
12. Kinsbourne, 1978; Luria, 1973; Semmes et al., 1963.
16. Kinsbourne, 1978; Luria, 1973; Semmes et al., 1963.
18. Walsh, 1987.
21. Siev et al., 1986.
22. Siev et al., 1986; Walsh, 1987.
24. Walsh, 1987.
  a. Heilman et al., 1985; Walsh, 1987.
  b. Heilman et al., 1985.
  c. Walsh, 1987.

APHASIA

1. Benson, 1985; Geschwind, 1979; Luria, 1980; Williams and Warwick, 1980.
7. Benson, 1985; Brown and Perecman, 1986; Daube and Sandok, 1978; Geschwind, 1979; Liebman, 1979; Luria and Thomas Hutton, 1977; Luria, 1980; Strub and Black, 1985; Werner, 1980.
15. Walsh, 1987.
17. Benson, 1985; Luria and Thomas Hutton, 1977.
19. Benson, 1985.
21. Luria and Thomas Hutton, 1977; Mayeux and Kandel, 1985.
23. Benson, 1985; Luria and Thomas Hutton, 1977; Mayeux and Kandel, 1985.
25. Benson, 1985; Luria and Thomas Hutton, 1977.
27. Luria and Thomas Hutton, 1977.
31. Benson, 1985; Luria and Thomas Hutton, 1977.
35. Luria, 1980; Luria and Thomas Hutton, 1977.
36. Luria, 1980.
39. Luria and Thomas Hutton, 1977.
43. Barr and Kiernan, 1983; Brown and Perecman, 1986; Daube and Sandok, 1978; Geschwind, 1979; Netter, 1983; Strub and Black, 1985.
49. Benson, 1985.

59. Luria, 1980.
60. Luria, 1980.
67. Ayres, 1985.
68. Ayres, 1985.
75. Damasio, 1985.
76. Damasio, 1985.
 a. Brown and Perecman, 1986.
 b. Bogen, 1985.
 c. Benson, 1985; Brown and Perecman, 1986.
 d. Benson, 1985.

MEMORY

 1. Kolb and Wishaw, 1980.
 3. Damasio and Van Hoesen, 1983; Damasio, 1985; Kolb and Wishaw, 1980; Luria, 1973.
 4. Damasio and Van Hoesen, 1983; Damasio, 1985; Kolb and Wishaw, 1980; Luria, 1973.
 7. Butters, 1979.
 8. Butters, 1979.
15. Butters, 1979; Geschwind, 1979; Kolb and Wishaw, 1980; Srebro, 1985; Walsh, 1987.
16. Butters, 1979; Geschwind, 1979; Kolb and Wishaw, 1980; Walsh, 1987.
19. Luria, 1980.
20. Luria, 1980.
27. Baddeley et al., 1987; Walsh, 1987.
28. Baddeley et al., 1987; Walsh, 1987.
 a. Sperry, 1964.
 b. Goldberg et al., 1981.

EMOTION

 3. Damasio and Van Hoesen, 1983; Damasio, 1985; Gainotti, 1972; Luria, 1980.
 4. Geschwind, 1979; Kaupfermann, 1985a.
11. Damasio, 1985; Stuss and Benson, 1985.
12. Damasio, 1985; Stuss and Benson, 1985.
15. Kaupfermann, 1985b.
16. Kaupfermann, 1985b.
19. Damasio and Van Hoesen, 1983; Damasio, 1985; Geschwind, 1979; Gainotti, 1972; Kaupfermann, 1985a.
20. Damasio and Van Hoesen, 1983; Damasio, 1985.
23. Kaupfermann, 1985a.
27. Damasio and Van Hoesen, 1983; Damasio, 1985; Stuss and Benson, 1985.
28. Damasio and Van Hoesen, 1983; Damasio, 1985; Stuss and Benson, 1985.
31. Kaupfermann, 1985b.
32. Kaupfermann, 1985b.

35. Damasio and Van Hoesen, 1983; Damasio, 1985; Stuss and Benson, 1985.
36. Damasio and Van Hoesen, 1983; Damasio, 1985; Stuss and Benson, 1985.
39. Kaupfermann, 1985b.
40. Kaupfermann, 1985b.
43. Damasio and Van Hoesen, 1983; Damasio, 1985; Kaupfermann, 1985b.
44. Damasio and Van Hoesen, 1983; Damasio, 1985; Kaupfermann, 1985b.
47. Kaupfermann, 1985b.
48. Kaupfermann, 1985b.
51. Damasio, 1985.
52. Damasio, 1985.
59. Damasio and Van Hoesen, 1983; Damasio, 1985; Stuss and Benson, 1985.
60. Damasio and Van Hoesen, 1983; Damasio, 1985; Kaupfermann, 1985a; Stuss and Benson, 1985.
 a. Kaupfermann, 1985b.
 b. Kaupfermann, 1985b.
 c. Kaupfermann, 1985b.
 d. Kaupfermann, 1985b.

COGNITION

 3. Damasio, 1985; Luria, 1980; Walsh, 1987.
 4. Damasio, 1985; Luria, 1980; Walsh, 1987.
11. Luria, 1980.
12. Luria, 1980.
19. Barr and Kiernan, 1983; Damasio and Van Hoesen, 1983; Damasio 1985; Luria, 1980; Walsh, 1987.
20. Barr and Kiernan, 1983; Damasio and Van Hoesen, 1983; Damasio, 1985; Luria, 1980; Walsh, 1987.
25. Strub and Black, 1985.
26. Strub and Black, 1985.
27. Strub and Black, 1985.
28. Strub and Black, 1985.
29. Strub and Black, 1985.
30. Strub and Black, 1985.
31. Strub and Black, 1985.
32. Strub and Black, 1985.
 a. Strub and Black, 1985.
 b. Strub and Black, 1985.

OTHER

 3. Luria, 1980.
 4. Luria, 1980.
10. Heilman and Van Den Abell, 1980; Heilman et al., 1985.
11. Luria, 1980.

12. Heilman and Van Den Abell, 1980; Heilman et al., 1985; Luria, 1980.
16. Heilman et al., 1985.
19. Luria, 1980.
20. Luria, 1980.
27. Luria, 1980; Damasio and Van Hoesen, 1983; Stuss and Benson, 1986.
28. Damasio and Van Hoesen, 1983; Luria, 1980; Stuss and Benson, 1986.
35. Kaupfermann, 1985c.
36. Kaupfermann, 1985c.
39. Lezak, 1987.
40. Lezak, 1987.
43. Damasio, 1979; Luria, 1980.
44. Damasio, 1979; Luria, 1980.
51. Damasio, 1985; Luria, 1980.
52. Damasio, 1985; Luria, 1980.
59. Damasio, 1985; Luria, 1980; Walsh, 1987.
60. Damasio, 1985; Luria, 1980; Walsh, 1987.
67. Luria, 1980; Stuss and Benson, 1985.
68. Luria, 1980; Stuss and Benson, 1985.
75. Damasio, 1985; Kaupfermann, 1985b; Luria, 1980; Strub and Black, 1985; Stuss and Benson, 1986.
76. Damasio, 1985; Kaupfermann, 1985b; Luria, 1980.
83. Damasio, 1985; Kaupfermann, 1985b; Luria, 1980.

84. Damasio, 1985; Kaupfermann, 1985b; Luria, 1980.
89. Roeltgen, 1985.
90. Roeltgen, 1985.
91. Luria and Thomas Hutton, 1977.
93. Roeltgen, 1985; Siev et al., 1986.
95. Roeltgen, 1985; Walsh, 1987.
96. Roeltgen, 1985; Walsh, 1987.
97. Friedman and Albert, 1985; Geschwind, 1979.
98. Friedman and Albert, 1985.
101. Friedman and Albert, 1985; Siev et al., 1986.
102. Friedman and Albert, 1985; Geschwind, 1979; Siev et al., 1986.
103. Friedman and Albert, 1985.
105. Levin and Spiers, 1985.
106. Levin and Spiers, 1985.
107. Luria, 1980.
108. Luria, 1980.
109. Levin and Spiers, 1985; Siev et al., 1986.
110. Levin and Spiers, 1985; Siev et al., 1986.
111. Levin and Spiers, 1985.
  a. Lezak, 1987.
  b. Gronwall, 1987; Heilman and Van Den Abell, 1980.
  c. Lezak, 1987.
  d. Kaupfermann, 1985c.
  e. Friedman and Albert, 1985.
  f. Roeltgen, 1985.

CHAPTER
13

Utilization and Future Development

The background and development of the Árnadóttir OT-ADL Neurobehavioral Evaluation (A-ONE) has been outlined in the preceding chapters. From the review it is evident that the instrument is only starting its developmental course. This chapter outlines its potential use as a clinical instrument as well as a research tool. In addition, some suggestions for future research are made.

CLINICAL USE

The instrument is intended to be used to gather clinical information regarding patients' performance and the types of neurobehavioral impairments that interfere with task performance. It is informative in terms of the origin of the disorder within the CNS, so that therapists can speculate regarding the most effective treatment for the underlying problem. It is further intended to be used to measure progress. Fig. 13-1 illustrates how progress can be recorded for different variables of importance in a particular clinical case. It would be desirable if at least three observations supported the information provided for each point.

Thus, as stated earlier, the A-ONE has potential for use by occupational therapists who are specifically interested in shifting their approach to the evaluation of patients with neurobehavioral deficits. The instrument also has a considerable potential to initiate rethinking in terms of treatment strategies. This is because it identifies neurobe-havioral deficits (performance component dysfunctions), their interference with functional independence (performance skills dysfunctions), and the possible relation of performance impairments to the original CNS dysfunctions. Such analysis may stimulate ideas regarding how treatment may be used to affect CNS processes. When a single-subject recording format is used, and treatment methods based on neurological rationales are monitored, it may be possible to review the cases later and look at which independence items and neurobehavioral deficits improved. Further, this can be related to the treatment methods used as well as medical diagnoses and different demographic data. Such studies of multiple cases may generate important information regarding the effectiveness of treatment strategies and the importance of specific clinical information for prognosis.

It should be noted that the A-ONE is an evaluation of skill performance. It can be used to examine how neurobehavioral dysfunctions interfere with task performance. It can also identify problem areas that could be tested in a more focused way if necessary. Thus, it is not intended to replace other forms of evaluation, such as neuropsychological tests or neuroimaging.

RESEARCH USE

The test can be used for research purposes to reveal changes in patients' progress over time (as already

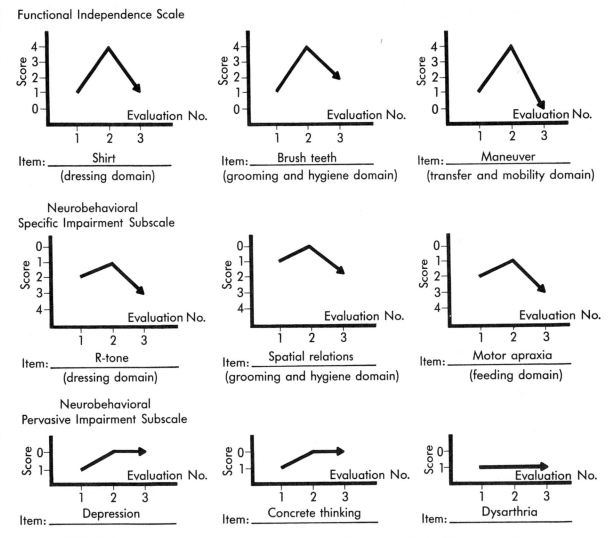

FIG. 13-1 An Example of a Graphic Progress Report (the performance of a single subject on several variables [items] from the different scales of the A-ONE, Part I). The subject had sustained a left cerebral vascular accident. The initial evaluation was performed upon admission to the rehabilitation center. The second evaluation was performed after 6 weeks of rehabilitation preparing for discharge. The third evaluation was performed several days after the second one, after the subject had sustained a second stroke. Note that these are only samples of a few items. All the items should be recorded in order to explore interrelations.

mentioned), the relationship between different variables, and potentially the effectiveness of different treatment approaches. When using the A-ONE to examine treatment effectiveness, several things should be kept in mind. When ADL treat-

ment is examined, the A-ONE may sample the treatment program as do many other evaluation tools used in rehabilitation medicine. A single-subject recording format with multiple baseline design, where ADL treatment is withheld for different lengths of time, could be used to minimize this sampling effect. Patient performance on all items or variables of all scales should, of course, be matched on the initial evaluation, not just for the variable under study. When considering the sampling effect, one should keep in mind that ADL training varies with different hospital settings. Many therapists train patients in performing all the self-care tasks within the daily routine. However, some therapists provide ADL training that isolates some ADL aspect, such as putting on a shirt, and the patient is made to repeat that isolated performance numerous times during the same session. The A-ONE would sample such treatment programs to various degrees. Further comparison of different ADL training approaches could be studied. If the effectiveness of other treatment methods, such as block construction and sensory integration and how they affect improvement in self-care skills is being studied, the ADL program should be kept constant for the patients receiving different experimental treatments. The A-ONE provides a long-needed opportunity to match patients on many different variables. The previous gaps in matching patients for other variables than those under study as well as for severity of dysfunction has contributed to nonsignificant results in some studies that examine the efficacy of different treatment methods.

Studies of treatment effectiveness or prognostic factors would be more powerful if behavioral measures were combined with brain-imaging methods such as CT scans, MRI, mappings of evoked potentials, and EEGs, as well as blood-flow measurements, such as PET. Thus, the CNS mechanisms can be studied from a holistic view, looking at neurobehavior as well as CNS structure and information processing. Complimentary results from such comparisons might contribute valuable information in terms of understanding the nervous system and its processing functions and dysfunctions. When such a relationship has been established, subsequent studies with repeated measures over time may reveal information with regard to the mechanisms that underlie neurobehavioral deficits and the improvement of performance components

in dysfunctions affecting skill performance. This may lead in turn to theories from which more effective treatment can evolve.

Note that when the instrument is used for research purposes, criteria with less flexibility than those for pure clinical use should be used to maintain standardized procedures.

FURTHER RESEARCH

The A-ONE instrument is only starting its course. Refinements have been made according to the findings of the available research studies. However, much work is still ahead in terms of establishing further reliability and validity. Studies to further establish reliability and to determine interitem correlations have already been initiated. Here items relating to neurobehavioral deficits can be correlated to look for clusters. In addition, neurobehavioral items can be correlated directly with items of functional independence to study the effects of neurobehavioral impairments on independence in skill performance. Fig. 13-2 presents graphic displays of some case examples, illustrating the kind of information that can be obtained by studying the information provided by the different variables. Such information is much more direct than that arising from correlating items from different tests, such as block building and ADL. Further, the performance on the A-ONE of different diagnostic groups could be examined and compared. This could subsequently be related to progress, as could any examination of performance or of the type and severity of deficits.

Most of the studies that have been conducted include samples involving Icelandic subjects and Icelandic occupational therapists. This population is composed of an all-white ethnic group. It would be interesting to repeat the studies in mixed or different ethnic groups and examine the differences. In the meantime, therapists should keep in mind that most of the samples are biased toward one nationality and one ethnic group, contributing to limitations on the extent to which results can be generalized.

In addition to the previously mentioned need

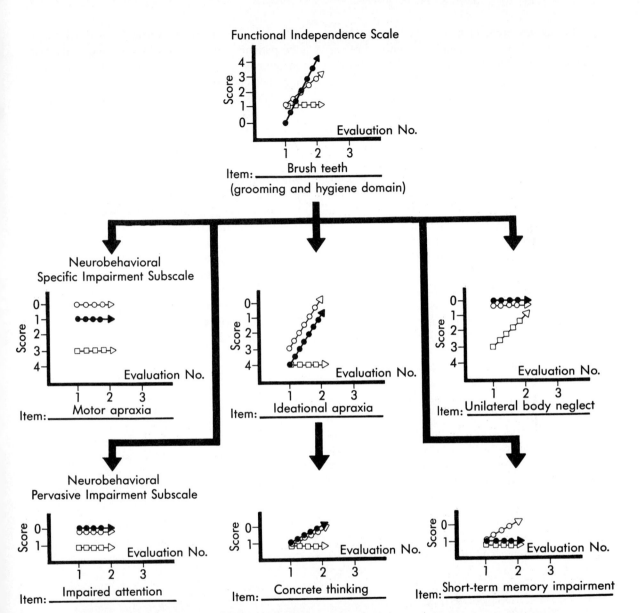

FIG. 13-2 General Comparison of Scores (three aphasic patients who had sustained a left CVA at the same time). All had complete expressive aphasia and severe impressive aphasia. The initial evaluation was performed upon admission to rehabilitation services. The second evaluation was performed after two months of treatment. When examining improvement in the different subjects on one of the performance skill variables (brushing teeth), two patients had improved; one had not. Can the explanation for the differences be found in the neurobehavioral ratings (indicating performance component dysfunction)? A few items from each neurobehavioral subscale are provided. These are only a few examples. All the variables need to be studied along with their interrelations in order to explore the differences. A wealth of such studies may eventually provide answers to questions regarding which neurobehavioral components are important factors for prognosis.

for further research, there is a need for the development of a parallel evaluation composed of secondary activities of daily living. Such an evaluation should be based on the same methodology as that used in the A-ONE and is necessary for patients who have less severe dysfunctions. It would also be a natural continuation of the A-ONE. As patients improve in primary ADL activities, secondary ADL activities could be used to determine whether some neurobehavioral deficits are still present and how they affect new environmental requirements.

The A-ONE does make it possible to associate a patient's neurobehavioral deficits to performance of self-care. This information could be associated with probable lesion sites as identified by other disciplines, either by using technological methods or neuropsychological assessments. The possibility of comparative studies was mentioned previously in relation to research. The relation of occupational therapy behavioral observations to neuroimaging must be further examined; the comparative study in Chapter 12 only served to initiate that process. Combinative studies to explore and experiment with treatment strategies in order to obtain information regarding the mechanisms that underlie neurobehavioral or functional progress are needed. However, such measures of change are quite feasible when technological methods such as the ones described in the study reviewed in Chapter 12 are used, as these are repeatable without risk to the patients. Such studies may subsequently lead to theories from which more effective treatment methods can evolve.

Presently, the evaluation of the electrophysiological CNS events during functional activity has a long way to go in terms of validity and repeatability. These studies are at present very hard to control in order to obtain acceptable results. Later, when these techniques have evolved, it may be possible to use electrophysiological or chemical measurements while patients are engaged in daily activties and thus obtain more clearly related measures of neuroanatomical, neurophysiological, and neurobehavioral analyses of ADL.

To conclude the review of the background and development of the A-ONE instrument, it is appropriate to remember the words of the leader of neurobehavioral theory development and instrumentation in occupational therapy, Dr. Ayres, who said,

> "Truth, like infinity, is to be forever approached and never met."*

---

*From a poster created by Charlotte DePenne (OTR) and Nav Jiwan Khalsa (OTR) of GRD Graphics. Reprinted by permission of Charlotte DuPenne and GRD Graphics.

References

Adams, K. M. (1980). In search of Luria's battery: A false start. *Journal of Consulting and Clinical Psychology, 48*(4), 511–516.

American Occupational Therapy Association. (1974). *A curriculum guide for occupational therapy educators.* The Association.

Avlund, K. (1988). Funktionnsevnemåling inden for Gerontologisk forskning: 1. Physical activities of daily living. *Ergoterapeuten, 8,* 340–349.

Ayres, A. J. (1972). *Sensory integration and learning disorders.* Los Angeles, Western Psychological Services.

Ayres, A. J. (1979). Sensory integration and the child. Los Angeles: Western Psychological Services.

Aryes, A. J. (1985). *Developmental dyspraxia and adult onset apraxia.* Torrance, CA: Sensory Integration International.

Ayres, A. J. (1989). *Sensory integration and praxis tests*: SIPT. Los Angeles: Western Psychological Services.

Bach, R. (1973). *Jonathan Livingston Seagull: a story.* London: Pan Books Ltd.

Baddeley, A., Harris, J., Sunderland, A., Watts, K. P., & Wilson, B. A. (1987). Closed head injury and memory. In H.S. Levin, J. Grafman, & H. M. Eisenberg (Eds.), *Neurobehavioral recovery from head injury* (pp. 295–317). New York: Oxford University Press.

Barr, M. L., & Kiernan, J. A. (1983). *The human nervous system: An anatomical viewpoint.* Philadelphia: Harper & Row.

Basso, A., Luzzatti, C., & Spinnler, H. (1980). Is ideomotor apraxia the outcome of damage to well-defined regions of the left hemisphere? *Journal of Neurology, Neurosurgery and Psychiatry, 43,* 118–126.

Bauer, R. M. and Rubens, A. B. (1985). Agnosia. In K. M. Heilman & E. Valenstein (Eds.), *Clinical neuropsychology* (2nd ed., pp. 187–242). New York: Oxford University Press.

Baum, B., & Hall, K. M. (1981). Relationship between constructional praxis and dressing in the head-injured adult. *American Journal of Occupational Therapy, 35*(7), 438–442.

Benson, F. D. (1985) Aphasia. In K. M. Heilman & E. Valenstein (Eds.), *Clinical neuropsychology.* (2nd ed., pp. 17–48). New York: Oxford University Press.

Benson, J., & Clark, F. (1982). A guide for instrument development and validation. *American Journal of Occupational Therapy, 36*(12), 789–800.

Benton, A. (1985a). Visuoperceptual, visuospatial, and visuoconstructive disorders. In K. M. Heilman & E. Valenstein (Eds.), *Clinical Neuropsychology* (2nd ed., pp. 151–186). New York: Oxford University Press.

Benton, A. (1985b). Body-schema disturbances: Finger agnosia and right-left disorientation. In K. M. Heilman & E. Valenstein (Eds.), *Clinical neuropsychology* (2nd ed., pp. 115–130). New York: Oxford University Press.

Benton, A. L. (1987). Thoughts on the application of neuropsychological tests. In H. S. Levin, J. Grafman & H. M. Eisenberg (Eds.), *Neurobehavioral recovery from head injury* (pp. 111–115). New York: Oxford University Press.

Benton, A. L., Hamsher, K. deS., Varney, N. R., &

Spreen, O. (1983). *Contributions to neuropsychological assessment*. New York: Oxford University Press.

Bergland, R. (1985). *The fabric of mind*. Victoria: Penguin Books of Australia, Ltd.

Berk, R. A. (1979). Generalizability of behavioral observations: A clarification of interobserver agreement and interobserver reliability. *American Journal of Mental Deficiency, 83*(5), 460–472.

Black, F. W., & Bernard, B. A. (1984). Constructional apraxia as a function of lesion locus and size in patients with focal brain damage. *Cortex, 20*, 111–120.

Black, F. W., & Strub, R. L. (1976). Constructional apraxia in patients with discrete missile wounds of the brain. *Cortex, 12*. 212–220.

Bogen, J. E. (1985). The callosal syndromes. In K. M. Heilman & E. Valenstein (Eds.), *Clinical neurology* (2nd ed., pp. 295–338). New York: Oxford University Press.

Boller, F., Vrtunski, P. B., Kim, Y., & Mack, J. L. (1978). Delayed auditory feedback and aphasia. *Cortex, 14*, 212–226.

Boys, M., Fisher, P., Holzberg, C., & Reid, D. W. (1988). The OSOT Perceptual Evaluation: A research perspective. *The American Journal of Occupational Therapy, 42*(2), 92–98.

Bradshaw, J. (1985). *Brain CT: An introduction*. Bristol: John Wright and Sons, Ltd.

Brown, J. W., & Perecman, E. (1986). Neurological basis of language processing. In R. Chapey (Ed.), *Language intervention strategies in adult aphasia* (2nd ed., pp. 12–27). Baltimore: Williams & Wilkins.

Brun, A., & Gustafson, L. (1978). Limbic lobe involvement in presenile dementia. *Archives of Psychiatry and Neurological Sciences, 226*, 79–93.

Brust, J. C. M. (1985). Stroke: Diagnostic, anatomical and physiological considerations. In E. R. Kandel & J. H. Schwartz (Eds.), *Principles of neural science* (2nd ed., pp. 853–862). New York: Elsevier.

Bryden, M. P., & Ley, R. G. (1983). Right-hemispheric involvement in the perception and expression of emotion in normal humans. In K. M. Heilman & P. Satz (Eds.), *Neuropsychology of human emotion* (pp. 6–44). New York: The Guilford Press.

Buchtel, H. A. (1987). Attention and vigilance after head trauma. In H. S. Levin, J. Grafman, & H. M. Eisenberg (Eds.), *Neurobehavioral recovery from head injury* (pp. 372–378). New York: Oxford University Press.

Busk, J., & Galibraith, G. C. (1975). EEG correlates of visual-motor practice in man. *Electroencephalography and Clinical Neurophysiology, 38*, 415–422.

Butters, N. (1979). Amnesic disorders. In K. M. Heilman & E. Valenstein (Eds.), *Clinical neuropsychology* (pp. 439–475). New York: Oxford University Press.

Butters, N., & Miliotis, P. (1985). Amnesic disorders. In K. M. Heilman & E. Valenstein (Eds.), *Clinical neuropsychology* (2nd ed., pp. 403–452). New York: Oxford University Press.

Caplan, L. R., & Stein, R. W. (1986). *Stroke: A clinical approach*. Boston: Butterworth Publishers.

Carmon, A. (1970). Impaired utilization of kinesthetic feedback in right hemisphere lesions. *Neurology, 20*, 1033–1038.

Carter, L. T., Oliveira, D. O., Duponte, J., & Lynch, S. V. (1988). The relationship of cognitive skills performance to activities of daily living in stroke patients. *The American Journal of Occupational Therapy 42*(7), 449–455.

Chiappa, K. H. (1983). *Evoked potentials in clinical medicine*. New York: Raven Press Books.

Clark, F., Mailloux, Z., & Parham, D. (1985). Sensory integration and children with learning disabilities. In P. N. Clark & A. S. Allen (Eds.) *Occupational therapy for children* (pp. 359–405). St. Louis: The C. V. Mosby Company.

Côté, L. (1985). Aging of the brain and dementia. In E. R. Kandel & J. H. Schwartz (Eds.), *Principles of neural science* (2nd ed., pp. 784–792). New York: Elsevier.

Cummings, J. L., & Benson, D. F. (1983). *Dementia: A clinical approach*. Boston: Butterworth Publishers.

Damasio, A. R. (1979). The frontal lobes. In K. M. Heilman and E. Valenstein (Eds.), *Clinical neuropsychology* (pp. 360–412). New York: Oxford University Press.

Damasio, A. R. (1985). The frontal lobes. In K. M. Heilman and E. Valenstein (Eds.), *Clinical neuropsychology* (2nd ed., pp. 339–376). New York: Oxford University Press.

Damasio, A. R., & Van Hoesen, G. W. (1983). Emotional disturbances associated with focal lesions of the limbic frontal lobe. In K. M. Heilman & P. Satz (Eds.), *Neuropsychology of human emotion* (pp. 80–110). New York: The Guilford Press.

Daube, J. R., & Sandok, B. A. (1978). *Medical neurosciences: An approach to anatomy, pathology and physiology by systems and levels*. Boston: Little Brown.

Dee, H. L., & Benton, A. L. (1970). A cross-modal investigation of spatial performances in patients with unilateral cerebral disease. *Cortex, 6*, 261–272.

De Renzi, E., Fabrizia, M., & Nichelli, P. (1980). Imitating gestures: A quantitative approach to ideomotor apraxia. *Archives of Neurology, 37*, 6–10.

De Renzi, E., Faglioni, P., & Sorgato, P. (1982). Modality-specific and supramodal mechanisms of apraxia. *Brain, 105*, 301–312.

Devor, M. (1982). Plasticity in the adult nervous system. In L. S. Illis, E. M. Sedgwick, & H. J. Glanville (Eds.), *Rehabilitation of the neurological patient* (pp. 44–84). Oxford: Blackwell Scientific Publications.

Dickoff, J., James, P., & Wiedenbach, E. (1968). Theory in a practice discipline. Part I: Practice oriented theory. *Nursing Research, 17*(5), 415–435.

Diller, L., & Ben-Yishay, Y. (1987). Outcomes and evidence in neuropsychological rehabilitation in closed head injury. In H. V. Levin, J. Grafman, & H. M. Eisenberg (Eds.), *Neurobehavioral recovery from head injury* (pp. 146–165). New York: Oxford University Press.

Duara, R. (1985). Brain regional localization in positron emission tomography images. *Journal of Cerebral Blood Flow and Metabolism, 5*, 343–344.

Duffy, F. H. (1981). Brain electrical activity mapping (BEAM): Computerized access to complex brain function. *International Journal of Neuroscience, 13*, 55–65.

Duffy, F. H. (1982). Topographical display of evoked potentials: Clinical application of brain electrical activity mapping (BEAM). *Annals of the New York Academy of Sciences, 388*, 183–196.

Duffy, F. H. (1985). The BEAM method for neurophysiological diagnosis. *Annals of the New York Academy of Sciences, 457*, 19–34.

Duffy, F. H., Albert, M. S., & McAnulty, G. (1984). Brain electrical activity in patients with presenile and senile dementia of the Alzheimer's type. *Annals of Neurology, 16*, 439–448.

Duffy, F. H., Albert, M. S., McAnulty, G., & Garvey, A. J. (1984). Age-related differences in brain electrical activity of healthy subjects. *Annals of Neurology, 16*, 430–438.

Duffy, F. H. Bartels, P. H., & Burchfiel, J. L. (1981). Significance probability mapping: An aid in the topographic analysis of brain electrical activity. *Electroencephalography and Clinical Neuropsychology, 51*, 455–462.

Duffy, F. H., Burchfiel, J. L., Cesare T., & Lombroso, C. T. (1979). Brain electrical activity mapping (BEAM). A new method for extending the clinical utility of EEG and evoked potential data. *Annals of Neurology, 5*(4), 309–321.

Duffy, F. H., Denckla, M. B., Bartels, P. H., Sandini, G., & Kiessling, L. S. (1980). Dyslexia: Regional differences in brain electrical activity by topographical mapping. *Annals of Neurology, 7*, 412–420.

Eisenberg, H. M., & Weiner, R. L. (1987). Input variables: How information from the acute injury can be used to characterize groups of patients for studies of outcome. In H. S. Levin, J. G. Grafman, & H. M. Eisenberg (Eds.), *Neurobehavioral recovery from head injury* (pp. 13–29). New York: Oxford University Press.

Eyzaguirre, C., & Fidone, S. J. (1975). *Physiology of the nervous system: An introductory text* (2nd ed.). Chicago: Year Book Medical Publishers.

Farver, P. F., & Farver, T. B. (1982). Performance of normal older adults on tests designed to measure parietal lobe functions. *American Journal of Occupational Therapy, 36*(7), 444–449.

Felten, D. L., and Felten, S. Y. (1982). A regional and systemic overview of functional neuroanatomy. In S. D. Farber (Ed.), *Neurorehabilitation: A multisensory approach*. Philadelphia: W. B. Saunders.

Foit, A., Larsen, B., Hattori, S., Skinhøj, E., & Lassen, N. A. (1980). Cortical activation during somatosensory stimulation and voluntary movement in man: A regional cerebral blood-flow study. *Electrophysiological and Clinical Neuropsychology, 50*, 426–436.

Friedman, R. B. & Albert, M. L. (1985). Alexia. In K. M. Heilman and E. Valenstein (Eds.), *Clinical neuropsychology* (2nd ed., pp. 49–74). New York: Oxford University Press.

Gainotti, G. (1972). Emotional behavior and hemispheric side of the lesion. *Cortex, 8*, 41–55.

Galaburda, A. M., LeMay, M., Kemper, T. L., & Geschwind, N. (1978). Right-left asymmetries in the brain: Structural differences between the hemispheres may underlie cerebral dominance. *Science, 199*, 852–856.

Geschwind, N. (1975). The apraxias: Neural mechanisms of disorders of learned movement. *American Scientist, 63*, 188–195.

Geschwind, N. (1979a). Specialization of the human brain. *Scientific American, 241*(3), 180–199.

Geschwind, N. (1979b). Specialization of the human

brain. *Scientific American* offprints #1444 (pp. 1–12).

Geschwind, N. (1985). Foreword. In R. L. Strub & F. W. Black (Eds.), *The mental status examination in neurology* (2nd ed.). Philadelphia: F. A. Davis.

Geschwind, N., & Galaburda, A. M. (1984). *Cerebral dominance: The biological foundations.* Cambridge: Harvard University Press.

Geschwind, N., & Galaburda, A. M. (1985). Cerebral lateralization: Biological mechanisms, associations, and pathology. I: A hypothesis and a program for research. *Archives of Neurology, 42,*(5), 428–459.

Geschwind, N., Galaburda, A. M. (1987). *Cerebral lateralization: Biological mechanisms, associations, and pathology.* Cambridge: The MIT Press.

Geschwind, N., & Levitsky, W. (1986). Human brain: Left-right asymmetries in temporal speech region. *Science, 161,* 186–187.

Ghez, C. (1985). Voluntary movement. In E. R. Kandel and J. H. Schwartz (Eds.), *Principles of neural science* (2nd ed., pp. 487–501). New York: Elsevier.

Goldberg, E., Antin, S. P., Bilder, R. M., Jr., Gerstman, L. J., Hughes, J. E. O., & Mattis, S. (1981). Retrograde amnesia: Possible role of mesencephalic reticular activation in long-term memory. *Science* 213: 1392–1394.

Goldberg, E., & Costa, L. D. (1981). Hemisphere differences in the acquisition and use of descriptive systems. *Brain and language, 14,* 144–173.

Golden C. J. (1980). In reply to Adam's "In search of Luria's battery: A false start." *Journal of Consulting and Clinical Psychology, 48*(4), 517–521.

Gowers, W. R. (1974). Carotid artery syndrome. In J. F. Toole & A. N. Patel (Eds.), *Cerebrovascular disorders* (2nd ed., pp. 122–140). New York: McGraw-Hill.

Grafman, J., & Salazar, A. (1987). Methodological considerations relevant to the comparison of recovery from penetrating and closed head injuries. In H. S. Levin, J. G. Grafman, & H. M. Eisenberg (Eds.), *Neurobehavioral recovery from head injury* (pp. 43–54). New York: Oxford University Press.

Gresham, G. E., Phillips, T. F., & Labi, M. L. C. (1980). ADL status in stroke: Relative merits of three standard indexes. *Archives of Physical Medicine and Rehabilitation, 61*(8), 335–358.

Gronwall, D. (1987). Advances in the assessment of attention and information processing after head injury. In H. S. Levin, J. Grafman, & H. M. Eisenberg

(Eds.), *Neurobehavioral recovery from head injury* (pp. 355–371). New York: Oxford University Press.

Harlowe, D., & Van Deusen, J. (1984). Construct validation of the St. Mary's CVA Evaluation: Perceptual measures. *American Journal of Occupational Therapy, 38*(3), 184–186.

Hécaen, H., De Agostini, M., & Monzon-Montes, A. (1981). Cerebral organization of left-handers. *Brain and Language, 12,* 261–284.

Heilman K. M. (1979). Neglect and related disorders. In K. M. Heilman and E. Valenstein (Eds.), *Clinical neuropsychology* (2nd ed., pp. 268–307). New York: Oxford University Press.

Heilman, K. M. (1983). Introduction. In K. M. Heilman & P. Satz (Eds.), *Neuropsychology of human emotion.* New York: The Guilford Press.

Heilman, K. M., & Rothi, L. J. G. (1985). Apraxia. In K. M. Heilman and E. Valenstein (Eds.), *Clinical neuropsychology* (2nd ed., pp. 131–150). New York: Oxford University Press.

Heilman, K. M., Rothi, L. J., & Valenstein, E. (1982). Two forms of ideomotor apraxia. *Neurology, 32,* 342–346.

Heilman, K. M., & Valenstein, E. (1985). *Clinical neuropsychology* (2nd ed.). New York: Oxford University Press.

Heilman, K. M., & Van Den Abell, T. (1980). Right hemisphere dominance for attention: The mechanism underlying hemispheric asymmetries of inattention (neglect). *Neurology, 30,* 327–330.

Heilman, K. M., & Watson, R. T. (1978). Changes in the symptoms of neglect induced by changing task strategy. *Archives of Neurology, 35,* 47–49.

Heilman, K. M., Watson, R. T., & Bowers, D. (1983). Affective disorders associated with hemispheric disease. In K. M. Heilman & P. Satz (Eds.), *Neuropsychology of human emotion* (pp. 45–64). New York: The Guilford Press.

Heilman, K. M., Watson, R. T., & Valenstein, E. (1985). Neglect and related disorders. In K. M. Heilman and E. Valenstein (Eds.), *Clinical neuropsychology* (2nd ed., pp. 243–294). New York: Oxford University Press.

Hughes, J. R. (1982). *EEG in clinical practice.* Woburn, MA: Butterworth Publishers.

Ingvar, D. H., & Philipson, L. (1977). Distribution of cerebral blood flow in the dominant hemisphere during motor ideation and motor performance. *Annals of Neurology, 2,* 230–237.

Jennett, B., & Teasdale, G. (1981). *Management of head injuries.* Philadelphia: F. A. Davis.

Kandel, E. R. (1979). Small systems of neurons. *The brain: A Scientific American book.* (pp. 29–38). New York: W. H. Freeman.

Kandel, E. R. (1985a). Nerve cells and behavior. In E. R. Kandel and J. H. Schwartz (Eds.), *Principles of neural science* (2nd ed., pp. 13–24). New York: Elsevier.

Kandel, E. R. (1985b). Synapse formation, trophic interactions between neurons, and the development of behavior. In E. R. Kandel & J. H. Schwartz (Eds.), *Principles of neural science* (2nd ed., pp. 743–756). New York: Elsevier.

Kandel, E. R. (1985c). Brain and behavior. In E. R. Kandel & J. H. Schwartz (Eds.), *Principles of neural science* (2nd ed., pp. 3–12). New York: Elsevier.

Kandel, E. R. (1985d). Processing of form and movement in the visual system. In E. R. Kandel & J. H. Schwartz (Eds.), *Principles of neural science* (2nd ed., pp. 366–383). New York: Elsevier.

Kandel, E. R. (1985e). Early experience, critical periods, and developmental fine tuning of brain architecture. In E. R. Kandel & J. H. Schwartz (Eds.), *Principles of neural science* (2nd ed., pp. 757–770). New York: Elsevier.

Kandel, E. R., & Schwartz, J. H. (1985). *Principles of neural science* (2nd ed.). New York: Elsevier.

Kandel, E. R. & Siegelbaum, S. (1985). Principles underlying electrical and chemical synaptic transmission. In E. R. Kandel & J. H. Schwartz (Eds.), *Principles of neural science* (2nd ed., pp. 89–107). New York: Elsevier.

Kaupfermann, I. (1985a). Hemispheric asymmetries and the cortical localization of higher cognitive and affective functions. In E. R. Kandel & J. H. Schwartz (Eds.), *Principles of neural science* (2nd ed., pp. 673–687). New York: Elsevier.

Kaupfermann, I. (1985b). Hypothalamus and limbic system. I: Peptideric neurons, homeostasis, and emotional behavior. In E. R. Kandel & J. H. Schwartz (Eds.), *Principles of neural science* (2nd ed., pp. 611–625). New York: Elsevier.

Kaupfermann, I. (1985c). Hypothalamus and limbic system. II: Motivation. In E. R. Kandel & J. H. Schwartz (Eds.), *Principles of neural science* (2nd ed., pp. 626–635). New York: Elsevier.

Kelly, D. D. (1985a). Sexual differentiation of the nervous system. In E. R. Kandel & J. H. Schwartz (Eds.), *Principles of neural science* (2nd ed., pp. 771–783). New York: Elsevier.

Kelly, J. P. (1985b). Anatomy of the central visual pathways. In E. R. Kandel & J. H. Schwartz (Eds.), *Principles of neural science* (2nd ed., pp. 356–365). New York: Elsevier.

Kelly, J. P. (1985c). Auditory system. In E. R. Kandel & J. H. Schwartz (Eds.), *Principles of neural science* (2nd ed., pp. 396–408). New York: Elsevier.

Kertesz, A. (1985). Recovery and treatment. In K. M. Heilman & E. Valenstein (Eds.), *Clinical neuropsychology* (2nd ed., pp. 481–505). New York: Oxford University Press.

Kertesz, A., Ferro, J. M., & Shewan, C. M. (1984). Apraxia and aphasia: The functional-anatomical basis for their dissociation. *Neurology, 34,* 40–47.

Kety, S. S. (1979). Disorders of the human brain. *Scientific American, 241,* 202–214.

Kimura, D. (1966). Dual functional asymmetry of the brain in visual perception. *Neuropsychologia, 4,* 275–385.

Kimura, D. (1973). The asymmetry of the human brain. *Scientific American, 228,* 70–78.

Kimura, D. (1977). Acquisition of a motor skill after left-hemisphere damage. *Brain, 100,* 527–542.

Kimura, D., & Archibald, Y. (1974). Motor functions of the left hemisphere. *Brain, 97,* 337–350.

Kinsbourne, M. (1978). *Asymmetrical function of the brain.* Cambridge: Cambridge University Press.

Klein, R.M., & Bell, B. J. (1979). *Klein-Bell activities of daily living scale: Manual.* Seattle: University of Washington, Division of Occupational Therapy.

Kolb, B., & Whishaw, I. Q. (1980). *Fundamentals of human neuropsychology.* San Francisco: W. H. Freeman.

Kuffler, S. W., Nicholis, J. G., & Martin, A. R. (1984). *From neuron to brain* (2nd ed.). Sunderland, Mass.: Sinauer Associates.

Kuhn, T. S. (1970). *The structure of scientific revolutions* (2nd ed.). Chicago: The University of Chicago Press.

Larsen, B., Skinhøj, E., & Lassen, N. A. (1978). Variations in regional cortical blood flow in the right and left hemispheres during automatic speech. *Brain, 101,* 193–209.

Lassen, N. A. (1985). Measurement of regional cerebral blood flow in humans with single-proton-emitting radioisotopes. In L. Sokoloff (Ed.), *Brain imaging and brain function,* (pp. 9–20). New York: Raven Press.

Lassen, N. A., Ingvar, D. H., & Skinhøj, E. (1978). Brain function and blood flow. *Scientific American, 239,* 62–71.

Lauder, J. N., & Krebs, H. (1986). Do neurotransmitters, neurohumors, and hormones specify critical periods? In W. T. Greenough & J. M. Juraska (Eds.), *Developmental neuropsychology* (pp. 120–174). Orlando, FL: Academic Press.

Leenders, K. L., Gibbs, J. M. Frackowiak, R. S. J., Lammertsma, A. A., & Jones, T. (1984). Positron emission tomography of the brain: New possibilities for the investigation of human cerebral pathophysiology. *Progress in Neurobiology, 23,* 1–38.

Lenzi, G. L., & Pantano, P. (1984). Neurologic applications of positron emission tomography. *Neurologic Clinics, 2*(4), 853–871.

Levin, H. S., & Spiers, P. A. (1985). Acalculia. In K. M. Heilman & E. Valenstein (Eds.), *Clinical neuropsychology* (2nd ed., pp. 97–114). New York: Oxford University Press.

Lewis, G. P., Golden, C. J., Moses, J. A., Osmon, D. C., Purisch, A. D., & Hammeke, T. A. (1979). Localization of cerebral dysfunction with a standardized version of Luria's neuropsychological battery. *Journal of Consulting Clinical Psychology, 47*(6), 1003–1019.

Lezak, M. D. (1983). *Neuropsychological assessment* (2nd ed.). New York: Oxford University Press.

Lezak, M. D. (1987). Making neuropsychological assessment relevant to head injury. In H. S. Levin, J. Grafman, & H. M. Eisenberg (Eds.). *Neurobehavioral recovery from head injury* (pp. 116–128). New York: Oxford University Press.

Liebman, M. (1979). *Neuroanatomy made easy and understandable.* Baltimore: University Park Press.

Little, M. M. (1987). The Remediation of everyday memory deficits. In J. M. Williams & C. J. Long (Eds.), *The rehabilitation of cognitive disabilities* (pp. 123–138). New York: Plenum Press.

Llorens, L. A. (1986). Activity analysis: Agreement among factors in a sensory processing model. *American Journal of Occupational Therapy, 40*(2), 103–110.

Lombroso, C. T., & Duffy, F. H. (1980). Brain electrical activity mapping as an adjunct to CT scanning. *Advances in epileptology: XIth Epilepsy International Symposium.* New York: Raven Press.

Luria, A. R. (1973). *The working brain: An introduction to neuropsychology.* New York: Basic Books.

Luria, A. R. (1980). *Higher cortical functions in man* (2nd ed.). New York: Basic Books.

Luria, A. R., & Thomas Hutton, J. (1977). A modern assessment of the basic forms of aphasia. *Brain and Language, 4,* 129–151.

Mahoney, F. I., & Barthel, D. W. (1965). Functional evaluation: The Barthel Index. *Maryland State Medical Journal, 44,* 61–65.

Martin, J. H. (1985). Cortical neurons, the EEG, and the mechanisms of epilepsy. In E. R. Kandel & J. H. Schwartz (Eds.), *Principles of neural science* (2nd ed., pp. 636–647). New York: Elsevier.

Martin, J. H., & Brust, J. C. M. (1985). Imaging the living brain. In E. R. Kandel & J. H. Schwartz (Eds.), *Principles of neural science* (2nd ed., pp. 259–283). New York: Elsevier.

Matthews, W. B., & Miller, H. (1975). *Diseases of the nervous system.* Oxford: Blackwell Scientific Publications.

Mayeux, R., & Kandel, E. R. (1985). Natural language, disorders of language, and other localizable disorders of cognitive functioning. In E. R. Kandel & J. H. Schwartz (Eds.), *Principles of neural science* (2nd ed., pp. 688–703). New York: Elsevier.

Mazziotta, J. C., & Phelps, M. E. (1985). Human neuropsychological imaging studies of local brain metabolism: Strategies and results. In L. Sokoloff (Ed.), *Brain imaging and brain function* (pp. 121–138). New York: Raven Press.

Mazziotta, J. C., Huang, S. C., Phelps, M. E., Carson, R. E., MacDonald, N. S., & Mahoney, K. (1985). A noninvasive positron computed tomography technique using oxygen-15-labeled water for the evaluation of neurobehavioral task batteries. *Journal of Cerebral Blood Flow and Metabolism, 5,* 70–78.

McGlone, L. (1978). Sex differences in functional brain asymmetry. *Cortex, 14,* 122–128.

Metter, E. J. (1986). Medical aspects of stroke rehabilitation. In R. Chapey (Ed.), *Language intervention strategies in adult aphasia* (2nd ed. pp. 141–173). Baltimore: Williams & Wilkins.

Moehle, K. A., Rasmussen, J. L., & Fitzhugh-Bell, K. B. (1987). Neuropsychological theories and cognitive rehabilitation. In J. M. Williams & C. J. Long (Eds.), *The rehabilitation of cognitive disabilities* (pp. 57–76). New York: Plenum Press.

Moore, J. C. (1986). Recovery potentials following CNS lesions: A brief historical perspective in relation to modern research data on neuroplasticity. *American*

Journal of Occupational Therapy, 40(7), 459–463.

Neistadt, M. E. (1988). Occupational therapy for adults with perceptual deficits. *American Journal of Occupational Therapy, 42*(7), 434–440.

Netter, F. H. (1983). *The Ciba collection of medical illustrations.* Vol. 1. *Nervous system.* West Caldwell, N. J.: Ciba Pharmaceutical Products.

Nishizawa, Y., Olsen, T. S., Larsen, B., & Lassen, N. A. (1982). Left-right cortical asymmetries of regional cerebral blood flow during listening to words. *Journal of Neurophysiology, 48*(2), 458–466.

Norman, D., & Brant-Zawadski, M. (1985). Magnetic resonance imaging of the central nervous system. In L. Sokoloff (Ed.), *Brain imaging and brain function* (pp. 259–269). New York: Raven Press.

Novelline, R. A. & Squire, L. F. (1987). *Living anatomy: A working atlas using computed tomography, magnetic resonance and angiography images.* St. Louis: C. V. Mosby.

Nuwer, M. R. (1988a). Quantitative EEG. I: Techniques and problems of frequency analysis and topographic mapping. *Journal of Clinical Neurophysiology, 5*(1), 1–43.

Nuwer, M. R. (1988b). Quantitative EEG. II: Frequency analysis and topographic mapping in clinical settings. *Journal of Clinical Neurophysiology, 5*(1), 45–85.

Nuwer, M. R., Jordan, S. E., & Ahn, S. S. (1987). Evaluation of stroke using EEG frequency analysis and topographic mapping. *Neurology, 37,* 1153–1159.

Oldendorf, W. H. (1985). Principles of imaging structure by NMR. In L. Sokoloff (Ed.), *Brain imaging and brain function,* (pp. 245–257). New York: Raven Press.

Ottenbacher, K. J. (1980). Cerebral vascular accident: Some characteristics of occupational therapy evaluation forms. *American Journal of Occupational Therapy, 39*(4), 368–371.

Ottenbacher, K. J. (1986). *Evaluating clinical change: Strategies for occupational and physical therapists.* Baltimore: Williams & Wilkins.

Ottenbacher, K. J., Johnson, M. B., & Hojem, M. (1988). The significance of clinical change and clinical change of significance: Issues and methods. *American Journal of Occupational Therapy, 42*(3), 156–163.

Ottenbacher, K. J., & York, J. (1984). Strategies for evaluating clinical change: Implications for practice and research. *The American Journal of Occupational Therapy, 38*(10), 647–659.

Pedretti, L. W., & Pasquinelli-Estrada, S. (1985). Foundations for treatment of physical dysfunction. In L. W. Pedretti (Ed.), *Occupational therapy practice skills for physical dysfunction* (2nd. ed., pp. 1–10). St. Louis: C. V. Mosby.

Penfield, W., and Rasmussen, T. (1949). Vocalization and arrest of speech. *Archives of Neurology and Psychiatry, 61,* 21–27.

Phelps, M. E., Kuhl, D. E., & Mazziotta, J. C., (1981a). Metabolic mapping of the brain's response to visual stimulation: Studies in humans. *Science, 211,* 1445–1448.

Phelps, M. E., & Mazziotta, J. C. (1985). Positron emission tomography: Human brain function and biochemistry. *Science, 228*(4701), 799–809.

Phelps, M. E., Mazziotta, J. C., Kuhl, D. E., Nuwer, M., Packwood, J., Metter, J., & Engel, J. (1981b). Tomographic mapping of human cerebral metabolism: Visual stimulation and deprivation. *Neurology (NY), 31,* 517–529.

Piazza, D. M. (1980). The influence of sex and handedness in the hemispheric specialization of verbal and nonverbal tasks. *Neuropsychologia, 18,* 163–176.

Piercy, M., Hècaen, H., & DeAjuriaguerra, J. (1960). Constructional apraxia associated with unilateral cerebral lesions: Left- and right-sided cases compared. *Brain, 83,* 225–241.

Ragot, R., Derouesne, C., Renault, B., & Leserve, N. (1982). Ideomotor apraxia and P300: A preliminary study. In J. Courjon, S. Mauguiere, & M. Revol (Eds.), *Clinical applications of evoked potentials in neurology* (pp. 263–269). New York: Raven Press.

Regan, D. (1979). Electrical responses evoked from the human brain. *Scientific American, 241,* 139–149.

Reivich, M., Alavi, A., Gur, R. C., & Greenberg, J. (1985). Determination of local cerebral glucose metabolism in humans: Methodology and applications to the study of sensory and cognitive stimuli. In L. Sokoloff (Ed.), *Brain imaging and brain function* (pp. 105–120). New York: Raven Press.

Restak, R. (1984). *The brain.* New York: Bantam Books.

Reynolds, P. D. (1971). *A primer in theory construction.* Indianapolis: Bobbs-Merrill Educational Publishing.

Roeltgen, D. (1985). Agraphia. In K. M. Heilman and E. Valenstein (Eds.), *Clinical neuropsychology* (2nd ed., pp. 75–96). New York: Oxford University Press.

Roland, P. E. (1985). Applications of brain blood-flow imaging in behavioral neurophysiology: Cortical field activation hypothesis. In L. Sokoloff (Ed.), *Brain im-*

aging and brain function, (pp. 87–104). New York: Raven Press.

Roland, P. E., Larsen, B., Lassen, N. A., & Skinhøj, E. (1980). Supplementary motor area and other cortical areas in organization of voluntary movements in man. *Journal of Neurophysiology, 43*, 118–136.

Roland, P. E. and Skinhøj, E. (1981). Extrastriate cortical areas activated during visual discrimination in man. *Brain Research, 222*, 166–171.

Rothi, L. J. G., & Heilman, K. M. (1985). *Ideomotor apraxia: Gestural discrimination, compensation and memory*. Amsterdam, Netherlands: Elsevier (North Holland).

Rowland, L. P. (1985). Blood-brain barrier, cerebrospinal fluid, brain edema, and hydrocephalus. In E. R. Kandel & J. H. Schwartz (Eds.), *Principles of neural science* (2nd ed., pp. 835–844). New York: Elsevier.

Roy, E. A. (1983). Current perspectives on disruptions to limb praxis. *Physical Therapy, 63*(12), 1998–2003.

Sauget, J., Benton, A. L., & Hècaen, H. (1971). Disturbances of the body scheme in relation to language impairment and hemispheric locus of lesion. *Journal of Neurology, Neurosurgery and Psychiatry, 34*, 496–501.

Sbordone, R. J. (1987). A conceptual model of neuropsychologically-based cognitive rehabilitation. In J. M. Williams & C. J. Long (Eds.), *The rehabilitation of cognitive disabilities* (pp. 3–28). New York: Plenum Press.

Scott, A. D. (1983). Evaluation and treatment of sensation. In C. A. Trombly (Ed.), *Occupational Therapy for Physical Dysfunction* (2nd ed., pp. 38–45). Baltimore: Williams & Wilkins.

Semmes, J. (1968). Hemispheric specialization: A possible clue to mechanism. *Neuropsychologia, 6*, 11–26.

Semmes, J., Weinstein, S., Ghent, L., & Teuber, H. L. (1963). Correlation of impaired orientation in personal and extrapersonal space. *Brain, 86*, 747–769.

Siev, E., Freishtat, B., & Zoltan, B. (1986). *Perceptual and cognitive dysfunction in the adult stroke patient: A manual for evaluation and treatment*. New Jersey: SLACK Incorporated.

Smith, R. O., Morrow, M. E., Heitman, J. K., Rardin, W. J., Powelson, J. L., & Von, T. (1986). The effects of introducing the Klein-Bell ADL scale in a rehabilitation service. *American Journal of Occupational Therapy, 40*(6), 420–424.

Sokoloff, L. (1985). Basic principles of imaging of regional cerebral metabolic rates. In L. Sokoloff (Ed.), *Brain imaging and brain function*. New York: Raven Press.

Sørensen, L. (1978a). *Cognitive Test*. Gentofte, Denmark: Tranehaven.

Sørensen, L. (1978b). Cognitiv test: et vigtigt hjaelpemiddel for ergoterapeuten. *Ergoterapeuten, 39*(9), 318–322.

Sørensen, L. (1983). *Practiske cognitive og ADL undersøgelser*. Gentofte, Denmark: Tranehaven.

Sørensen, L. (1984). Focus på Barthel and Cognitiv test resultater ved udskrivning. *Ergoterapeuten, 43*(20), 713–716.

Spehlman, R. (1985). *Evoked potential primer: Visual, auditory and somatosensory evoked potentials in clinical diagnosis*. Boston: Butterworth Publishers.

Sperry, R. W. (1964). The great cerebral commissure. *Scientific American, 210*, 42–52.

Springer, S. P., & Deutsch, G. (1981). *Left brain, right brain*. San Francisco: W. H. Freeman.

Srebro, R. (1985). Localization of cortical activity associated with visual recognition in humans. *Journal of Physiology, 360*, 247–259.

Stone, J., & Dreher, B. (1982). Parallel processing of information in the visual pathways: A general principle of sensory coding? *Trends in Neurosciences 5*(12), 441–446.

Strub, R. L., & Black, F. W. (1985). *The mental status examination in neurology* (2nd ed.). Philadelphia: F. A. Davis.

Stuss, D. T., & Benson, F. (1983). Emotional concomitants of psychosurgery. In K. M. Heilman & P. Satz (Eds.), *Neuropsychology of human emotion* (pp. 111–140). New York: The Guilford Press.

Stuss, D. T., & Benson, D. F. (1986). *The frontal lobes*. New York: Raven Press.

Trombly, C. A. (1983). *Occupational therapy for physical dysfunction* (2nd ed.). Baltimore: Williams & Wilkins.

Tucker, D. M. (1976). Sex differences in hemispheric specialization for synthetic visuospatial functions. *Neuropsychologia, 14*, 447–454.

Tyner, F. S., Knott, J. R., & Mayer, W. B. (1983). *Fundamentals of EEG technology*. Vol. 1. *Basic concepts and methods*. New York: Raven Press.

Van Deusen, J. (1988). Unilateral neglect: Suggestions for research by occupational therapists. *American Journal of Occupational Therapy, 42*(7), 441–448.

Van Deusen Fox, J., & Harlowe, D. (1984). Construct validation of occupational therapy measures used in CVA evaluation: A beginning. *American Journal of Occupational Therapy, 38*(2), 101–106.

Walsh, K. (1987). *Neuropsychology: A clinical approach*. Edinburgh: Churchill Livingstone.

Warren, M. (1981). Relationship of constructional apraxia and body-scheme disorders to dressing performance in adult CVA. *American Journal of Occupational Therapy, 35*(7), 431–437.

Werner, J. K. (1980). *Neuroscience: A clinical perspective*. Philadelphia: W. B. Saunders.

Williams, P. L., & Warwick, R. (Eds.) (1980). *Gray's anatomy* (33rd ed.). Edinburgh: Churchill Livingstone.

Willis, W. D., & Grossman, R. G. (1981). *Medical neurobiology: Neuroanatomical and neurophysiological principles basic to clinical neuroscience* (3rd ed.). St. Louis: The C.V. Mosby Co.

Yerxa, E. J. (1983). The occupational therapist as a researcher. In H. L. Hopkins & H. D. Smith (Eds.), *Willard and Spackman's occupational therapy* (6th ed., pp. 869–875). Philadelphia: J. B. Lippincott.

Ziporyn, T. (1985). PET scans "relate clinical picture to more specific nerve function." *Journal of the American Medical Association, 253*(7), 943–949.

Zoltan, B., Jabri, J., Meeder Ryckman, D. L., & Panikoff, L. B. (1983). *Perceptual motor evaluation for head injured and other neurologically impaired adults*. California: Santa Clara Valley Medical Center.

Glossary

abnormal tone Flaccidity, decreased strength, rigidity, spasticity, ataxia, athetosis and tremor. In the A-ONE, these deficits are observed through a performance evaluation indicating effects of such dysfunction on functional performance, not the exact strength of a particular muscle or group of muscles.

absent-mindedness Defined for the purpose of this book as brief periods of lack of awareness of the external environment or activities in which a person is engaged.

abstract thinking A mental state in which internal speech is used by an individual who has detached him- or herself from the internal and external environment. It includes use of symbolics, analysis of components, classification of concepts, and synthesis necessary for generalizing similarities between situations, grasping a general idea as a whole, planning ahead, and making predictions regarding consequences of actions. (Walsh, 1987; Zoltan et al., 1983).

acalculia Acquired disorders in solving mathematical problems. It can be produced by spatial-relation disorders, alexia or agraphia for numbers, or impaired calculation (Levin and Spiers, 1985).

activities of daily living Self-care activities of primary ADL skills, as well as occupations, including employment, household, and leisure activities that are classified here as secondary (instrumental) ADL skills. ADL skills were operationalized by the development of the A-ONE instrument. The evaluation includes the primary ADL skills of dressing, grooming and hygiene, feeding, transfers and mobility, and communication.

activity analysis The process of closely examining activities by breaking them down into their components in order to understand and evaluate them. For the purposes of this theory, activity analysis was used to develop the neurobehavioral subscales and checklists of

the A-ONE, which include guidelines to assist therapists in detecting and classifying neurobehavioral deficits. To construct the checklists, the performance skills of feeding, grooming and hygiene, transfers and mobility, and communication, were analyzed in terms of performance components necessary for task completion as well as neurobehavioral deficits that may be manifested during the performance. The neurobehavioral performance components and deficits that can be observed during ADL skill performance were further analyzed in terms of neurophysiological processing and functional localization within the cerebral cortex in order to provide a better understanding of the nature of the dysfunction. A neurobehavioral framework was used to classify the deficits.

affect According to Heilman et al. (1983), affect is characterized by the outward appearance of the inward feeling of an individual with comparatively little association to reason or ideation and a relatively stable and enduring status.

aggression Angry and destructive ideas or behaviors that are intended to be injurious physically or emotionally. Such behaviors are aimed at domination of one person by another. Aggression may be manifested by hostility as well as attacking and destructive behavior.

agnosia Impaired ability to recognize the significance of and differentiate between sensory stimuli.

agraphia Defined by Strub and Black (1985) as an acquired writing disturbance. According to them, it refers specifically to language errors, not to motoric errors in letter formation or poor handwriting.

akinesia Used as a synonym for *hypokinesia*, referring to abnormal reduction of mobility.

alertness Defined by Strub and Black (1985) as a basic arousal process "in which the awake patient is able to respond to any stimulus in the environment" (p. 41).

alexia Acquired inability to read or comprehend written language as a result of brain damage. It can be related to dysfunction of language, as well as visual processes (Friedman and Albert, 1985; Strub and Black, 1985).

anomia Loss of the ability to name objects or retrieve names of people.

anosognosia A patient's denial of a paretic extremity as his or hers, accompanied by lack of insight with regard to the paralysis. The patient may refer to paralyzed extremities as objects or may perceive the extremities out of proportion to other body parts.

apathy Shallow affect, psychomotor slowing, blunted emotional responses, lack of interest in the environment, and inaction.

aphasia Defined by Strub and Black (1985) as a defect in higher integrative language processing. It refers to disturbed comprehension or speech expression, including grammatical errors and errors in word choice, or to both. Although aphasia refers to language processing, it may be accompanied by articulation and praxis errors.

apraxia A disorder of skilled purposeful movement that is neither caused by deficits in primary motor skills nor comprehension problems. It can affect the praxic components of ideation and concept formation, as well as programming and planning of movement. Disturbances in motor execution, on the contrary, are usually related to primary motor skills (Ayres, 1985; Daube and Sandok, 1978; Heilman and Rothi, 1985; Liebman 1979; Matthews and Miller, 1975; Siev et al., 1986).

assessment Used in this book as a synonym for *evaluation*. It is the process of obtaining and interpreting data necessary for patient evaluation and treatment.

associative visual agnosia An impairment that occurs when the visual cortex has been disconnected from the language or visual memory areas in cases where there is adequate visual perception. Clinically, the object can be recognized and its use demonstrated, but it cannot be named (Strub and Black, 1985).

astereognosis Sometimes referred to as *tactile agnosia;* a failure to recognize objects, forms, sizes and shapes of objects by touch alone. It includes a failure of shape discrimination, texture, size, and weight. It refers to a failure of tactile recognition, although touch sensation is still intact.

ataxia The lack of muscular coordination or unsteadiness of movement manifested in the absence of paresis or apraxia as a result of cerebellar dysfunction. It can affect the movements of the limbs, trunk, and eyes depending on the exact lesion site.

attention disorders The inability to attend to or focus on a specific stimulus. Presence of other irrelevant environmental stimuli may thus result in distraction. According to Strub and Black (1985), an alert patient with attention disorder "will be attracted to any novel sound, movement, or event occurring in the vicinity" (p. 41). The attentive patient is able to screen out irrelevant stimuli.

auditory agnosia A defective recognition of sound differences (Siev et al., 1986). It includes both auditory verbal agnosia, or recognition problems with words, and auditory sound agnosia, referring to nonspeech sounds (Bauer & Rubens, 1985).

body-scheme disorders Perceptual deficits regarding one's own postural model. It refers to defective perception of body position, including and involving the relation of body parts to each other, according to Siev et al. (1986).

bradykinesia Slow task performance, slowness in responding to therapist's instructions, and taking an abnormally long time when performing an ADL task. It is used as a synonym for *long performance latency* in the A-ONE.

Broca's aphasia A dysfunction of Broca's motor speech area, resulting in expressive aphasia indicated by a loss of speech production. It is used in this book as a synonym for *expressive aphasia.*

concentration Defined by Strub and Black (1985) as "the ability to sustain attention over an extended period of time" (p. 41).

cognition A conscious thought process that refers to awareness and knowledge of objects, perceptions, thoughts, and memories. In addition to knowledge, it includes the abilities to understand, reason, make decisions, and apply judgment (Zoltan et al., 1983).

cognitive perceptual tests Defined for the purpose of this book as structured tests for assessment of thought processes and perception of sensory information. There are different subtests used by occupational therapists, neuropsychologists, and neurologists, including paper-and-pencil tasks, block designs, and verbal questions.

color agnosia A defective color recognition as a result of brain lesion. It can be manifested as a disability to name colors, which is a disability associated with alexia and agraphia, or as a disturbance in recognition of color (Strub and Black, 1985).

concrete thinking Inflexible thinking. The individual is unable to apply internal speech in order to generalize from similarities among situations. This style of thinking is opposite to abstract thinking on a linear continuum of thinking.

confabulations The use of imaginary experiences to fill in memory gaps in order to cover up.

confusion Lack of ability to think clearly, which results in disturbed awareness and orientation in regard to time, place, and person. Interpretation of the external environment is impaired, and responses as replies to verbal stimuli are slowed (Daube and Sandok, 1978).

constructional apraxia A failure to produce a single design or object from parts in two or three dimensions, be they drawings or block designs. The failure may manifest spontaneously, upon command, or by copying (Benton, 1985a; Siev et al., 1986).

depression An affective disorder that manifests in sadness, hopelessness, and/or loss of general interest in usual performance. It may be accompanied by loss of appetite, loss of energy, sleeping disorders, and feelings of worthlessness (Strub and Black, 1985).

disorientation The inability to give personal information regarding self, disability, or hospital stay and time, without language problems. This disorientation can refer both to short- and long-term memory after the disability occurred.

distraction Diversion of attention.

dysarthria An impairment of the muscles responsible for speech production.

dysfunction Impairment of performance skills and performance components as well as impaired cortical function.

dressing apraxia An inability to dress, caused by different types of neurobehavioral deficits. In the A-ONE, the use of subcomponents is preferred to the collective term of *dressing apraxia,* as these give a clearer picture of the specific problem.

echolalia A disorder affecting speech in which words or syllables are repeated from the environment and added to the patient's expressive content.

emotion Objective behavioral responses that combine somatic and mental activities with consciously perceived feelings. It differs from *affect,* as it does not include drive and energies that contribute to unconscious feelings (Heilman et al., 1983).

euphoria Inappropriate gaiety or a feeling of subjective well-being accompanied by self-confidence.

evaluation Used in this book as a synonym for *assessment,* which was defined earlier in this section.

expressive aphasia An impairment of verbal expression, which can result in complete inability to speak, although comprehension may be intact. It is used in this book as a synonym for *Broca's aphasia.*

field-dependent behavior Impulsiveness related to the elementary orienting reflex.

finger agnosia An uncertainty about the fingers as a result of a language disorder, not being able to name the fingers, tactile recognition, or discrimination of touch applied to the fingers (Benton, 1985b; Siev et al., 1986; Walsh, 1987; Strub and Black, 1985).

flaccidity Paralysis and loss of normal tone as a result of neurologic damage leading to disruption of the reflex arch (Daube and Sandok, 1978).

frustrations An appearance of agitation and intolerance in behavior that may manifest emotionally, verbally, or physically.

functional performance The task performance of an individual who is engaged in purposeful activity. For the purpose of this book, functional performance refers to primary ADL skills.

gnosis The ability to recognize the significance of sensory information and differentiate among sensory stimuli.

hyperkinesia Abnormal involuntary movements as a result of neurologic damage (Daube and Sandok, 1978).

hypertonia Increased muscle tone, or spasticity.

hypokinesia Abnormal reduction of mobility, which is usually accompanied by increased muscle tone, resulting in rigidity (Daube and Sandok, 1978). It is used interchangeably with *akinesia* and *dyskinesia* in this text.

hypotonia Decreased muscle tone.

ideational apraxia According to Ayres (1985), "a breakdown in knowing what is to be done in order to perform" (p. 9) due to a loss of a neuronal model or mental representation about the concept required for performance. It can occur automatically or when performing on command (Siev et al., 1986).

ideomotor apraxia Defined by Ayres (1985) as a breakdown of planning and programming of action, which is one of the three praxic components. It further presents as a defective selection and sequencing of movement, as well as difficulties with spatial orientation when gesturing, pantomiming, or performing purposeful motor tasks (Heilman and Rothi, 1985; Siev et al., 1986). Ideomotor apraxia is used as a synonym for *motor apraxia* in this book.

initiativity The ability to initiate performance of an activity when the need to perform is present.

insight A discovery stage, with increasing awareness of a person's whole self. In the A-ONE, it refers to insight into one's own condition and disability.

internal speech Conceptual interpretation and use of language.

interrater reliability The reliability between two raters evaluating the same person at the same time by use of the same procedure or instrument.

irritability Hypersensitivity to stimulation. It includes quick excitability manifested in annoyance, impatience, or anger.

jargon aphasia A language disorder that manifests in speech output that cannot be understood by others, as the sequences necessary for intelligible speech phonemes are not available. It results from a failure of comprehension, since the patient receives no feedback about his speech performance.

judgment The ability to make realistic decisions based on environmental information. When judgment is impaired, individuals are unable to make use of feedback from their own errors.

lability Pathological emotional instability. Alternating states of gaiety and sadness, including inappropriate crying.

language Communicative behavior that involves speech and comprehension as well as other forms of communication to form, express, and share thoughts and feelings.

long-performance latency Defined for the purpose of this book as a slowness in responding to instructions and taking an abnormally long time to perform ADL tasks.

long-term memory Storing, consolidation, and retention of information that has passed through short-term memory in a permanent form, as well as the ability to retrieve this information.

memory Retention and recall of previous experiences, including concepts and tasks (Hopkins and Smith, 1983). It can be divided into short- and long-term memory, as well as recent and remote memory.

motor apraxia Refers to the loss of access to kinesthetic memory patterns so that purposeful movement cannot be achieved because of defective planning and sequencing of movements, even though the idea and purpose of the task is understood. It is used as a synonym for *ideomotor apraxia* in the A-ONE instrument.

motor impersistence Impaired precision and movement, manifested in diminished ability to sustain simple motor activities, such as opposing the fingers on command, due to an inability to utilize kinesthetic feedback.

motivation A person's willingness to perform, with or without a perceived need.

mutism Dysfunction affecting speech in which a patient makes no effort to communicate.

neurobehavior Behavioral and motor responses based on CNS processing and integration of sensory stimuli from the individual and the surrounding environment with previous experiences. These responses are the basis for task performance in ADL.

neurobehavioral assessment methods Evaluation methods that measure functional task performance of individuals. These include neuropsychological testing and occupational therapy evaluations of patients with neurobehavioral dysfunctions.

neurobehavioral dysfunction Defined here as a functional impairment of an individual manifested in defective skill performance due to a neurological processing deficit that affects any of the following performance components; affect, body scheme, cognition, emotion, gnosis, language, memory, personality, praxis, or spatial relations, and visuospatial skills.

neuromuscular impairment (deficit) Muscular dysfunction as a result of neuronal disorder.

occupational performance components A concept used in the occupational performance frame of reference. It refers to behavioral patterns that are learned and based on development. These include sensory-integrative functioning, motor functioning, social functioning, psychological functioning, and cognitive functioning, all of which can be subdivided.

occupational performance skills A concept used in the occupational performance frame of reference. It refers to self-care activities, work, leisure-time activities, and play.

occupational therapy evaluations Evaluations performed by occupational therapists, using the skills and methods that are traditionally applied in that profession.

oral apraxia Difficulties with planning movements of the tongue, the cheeks, the lips, and the jaws on command.

organization The ability to organize one's thoughts in order to perform an activity, and to perform in an organized way, with activity steps properly sequenced and timed.

organization of an ADL assessment Defined for the purpose of this book as the analysis of ADL assessment components and the synthesis of these components into a coherent assessment that is sensitive to specific neurobehavioral deficits if specific guidelines or instruction are used.

orientation Defined here as awareness of personal information regarding self, disability, or hospital stay and time.

paraphasia Is an expressive speech defect characterized by misuse or replacement of words or phonemes during active speech.

paralysis (muscle weakness) Loss or impairment of the ability to move body parts voluntarily as a result of a central or peripheral neurologic lesion. Involuntary movement is also absent, and muscle tone is decreased or absent.

perception The ability to meaningfully interpret sensory information.

perseverations Repeated movements or acts during functional performance as a result of difficulty in shifting from one response pattern to another. It refers to both inertia on initiation and termination of performance. Prefrontal perseveration refers to repetition of whole actions or action components, whereas premotor perseveration refers to compulsive repetition of the same movement.

praxis Ideation, as well as the programming and planning necessary for the execution of skilled, purposeful movement.

processing A series of operations or events leading to achievement of a specific result. Processing is differentiated into serial or sequential processing, in which one event takes place after another and as a result of it, as well as parallel or simultaneous processing, in which more than one event takes place simultaneously at different cerebral locations, to achieve one function.

prosopagnosia An inability to recognize familiar faces because of impaired visual processing.

reliability Consistency, stability, and precision of a test or a method used for measurement.

restlessness Uneasiness, impatience, and the inability to relax.

right-left discrimination An ability to discriminate between right and left body sides or to apply these concepts to the external environment. The disability includes an inability to understand and use the concepts of left and right; it is composed of several factors, including a verbal component, nonverbal component of tactile sensory discrimination and stimuli location, as well as spatial-relations and visuospatial components (Siev et al., 1986; Walsh, 1987).

rigidity Difficulties initiating movements and slow performance of active movements as well as increased resistance to passive movements due to increased muscle tone. There are different types of rigidity, including cogwheel and clasp-knife rigidity (Daube and Sandok, 1978).

sensitivity of an evaluation The capacity of an evaluation to respond to certain characteristics and discriminate them from other characteristics.

sequencing The ability to sequence activity steps effectively. It refers to order and timing of events.

short-term memory The registration and short-time storing of information received by the different sensory modalities, be it somatosensory, auditory, or visual. If information is to be stored for any length of time, it is processed from short-term over to long-term memory.

somatoagnosia A disorder of body scheme. Defined by Siev et al. (1986) as diminished "awareness of body structure and the failure to recognize one's [body] parts and their relationship to each other" (p. 53).

spasticity Abnormal muscle tone. It manifests in hypertonia of muscles, resulting in increased resistance to passive movement (Daube and Sandok, 1978).

spatial-relation dysfunction Difficulties in relating objects to each other, or to the self. When such difficulties are due to visual-spatial impairment, this term becomes synonymous with spatial-relations dysfunction.

spatial-relations syndrome Defects common to apraxias and agnosias, according to Siev et al., (1986). The following deficits have been related to this dysfunction: constructional apraxia; trouble differentiating foreground from background; difficulties with form constancy; inability to interpret and deal with concepts related to spatial positioning of objects; difficulties with spatial relations; impaired spatial memory; perceptual deficits related to depth and distance, and topographical disorientation.

strength Muscle power. Muscle weakness, or diminished muscle power, may manifest itself in abnormal or compensatory movement patterns, muscle imbalance, and poor endurance during performance of physical tasks. Manual muscle testing refers to evaluation of maximal contraction of isolated muscles or muscle groups.

topographical disorientation Difficulty finding one's way in space as a result of amnestic and/or agnostic problems. It manifests in problems with finding one's way in familiar surroundings or in learning new routes.

tremor Involuntary trembling of limbs, occurring either at rest or during activity, depending on the origin of the lesion.

unilateral body neglect (unilateral body inattention) Failure to report, respond, or orient to a unilateral stimulus presented to the body side contralateral to a cerebral lesion (Heilman et al., 1985). It can be a result of either defective sensory processing or an attention deficit, resulting in ignorance or impaired use of the extremities.

unilateral spatial neglect Inattention to or neglect of visual stimuli presented in the extrapersonal space on the side contralateral to a cerebral lesion, as a result of visual perceptual deficits or impaired attention (Heilman et al., 1985). According to Siev et al. (1986), it may occur independently of visual deficits or with hemianopsia.

validity The degree to which a procedure, such as an instrument, measures what it purports to measure.

visual-object agnosia An inability to recognize objects seen, resulting from distorted visual perception regardless of visual acuity (Siev et al., 1986; Strub and Black, 1985).

visual-spatial agnosia Visual-space perception disorders resulting in distortion of relationships between objects, or objects and the self. Thus it is a subcomponent of spatial relations in the A-ONE.

Wernicke's aphasia A deficit in auditory comprehension that affects semantic speech performance, manifested in paraphasia or nonsensical syllables (Benson, 1985; Geschwind, 1979a). Repetitions are also impaired.

Index

A-ONE ORDER FORM

Each set of the **A-ONE** includes the following test forms:

- **-A-ONE** Part I   Summary Sheet
- **-A-ONE** Part I   Functional Independence Scale and Neurobehavioral Specific Impairment Subscale
- **-A-ONE** Part I   Neurobehavioral Pervasive Impairment Subscale
- **-A-ONE** Part II   Neurobehavioral Scale Summary Sheet

Please send me the following test forms:

Test forms	Cost per set	Quantity	Total
A pad with 20 sets of test forms	US $ 20.00		
Overseas shipment and handling (per pad)	US $ 10.00		
		TOTAL	

*Prices effective Dec.1989. Prices subject to change.

- ❑ Payment enclosed (US$ money orders only)
- ❑ Please charge my **VISA**
- ❑ Please charge my **MasterCard**
- ❑ Please charge my **American Express**

Card number   Expiration date

Signature

Name (please print)

Address

City   State   Zip Code

Country   Telephone

A-ONE Certificate #

Academic Degree

Mail all orders to:

A. Arnason
P.O. Box 3171
123 Reykjavík
ICELAND